Essentials of Ortho

Fourth Edition

Sam W. Wiesel · John N. Delahay
Editors

Essentials of Orthopedic Surgery

Fourth Edition

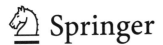 Springer

Editors
Sam W. Wiesel, MD
Department of Orthopaedic Surgery
Georgetown University Medical Center
3800 Reservoir Road, NW
Washington, DC 20007, USA
wiesels@gunet.georgetown.edu

John N. Delahay
Department of Orthopaedic Surgery
Georgetown University Medical Center
3800 Reservoir Road, NW
Washington, DC 20007, USA
delahayj@gunet.georgetown.edu

ISBN 978-1-4419-1388-3   e-ISBN 978-1-4419-1389-0
DOI 10.1007/978-1-4419-1389-0
Springer New York Dordrecht Heidelberg London

Library of Congress Control Number: 2010932335

First edition, Essentials of Orthopaedic Surgery © 1993 W.B. Saunders Company.
Second edition, Essentials of Orthopaedic Surgery © 1997 W.B. Saunders Company.
Third edition, Essentials of Orthopedic Surgery © Springer Science+Business Media, LLC 2007

Printed on acid-free paper

Springer is part of Springer Science+Business Media (www.springer.com)

Preface

The fourth edition of the *Essentials of Orthopedic Surgery* is directed to students who are beginning their study of the musculoskeletal system. This would include medical students and residents interested in orthopedic surgery, physiatry, rheumatology, emergency medicine, family medicine, and general internal medicine. Each chapter has been updated to reflect current material and we have tried to keep to a standardized format as much as possible. Every topic is presented from a practical point of view.

Decision making for each topic is highlighted. Algorithms are the key for each chapter and each decision point is based on either a standard or a guideline in the literature. We hope that when students are confronted with a specific clinical problem these algorithms will allow them to formulate both a diagnostic and a treatment plan.

We have enjoyed working with our publisher, Springer, and especially with Katharine Cacace and Flora Kim who have guided this text to publication.

Finally, it has been a wonderful and stimulating experience to work with all the members of the Department of Orthopedic Surgery at Georgetown University Hospital. The department has added several new members since the last edition, and their contributions bring a new perspective to our work. We are proud of the contributions which everyone has made to this effort.

Washington, DC
Sam W. Wiesel
John N. Delahay

Contents

Contributors

Raymond M. Carroll Cary Orthopedic Sports Medicine Specialists, 1120 S.E. Cary Parkway, Suite 100, Cary, NC 27518, USA

Paul S. Cooper Department of Orthopedic Surgery, Georgetown University Medical Center, 3800 Reservoir Road NW, Pasquerilla Healthcare Center (PHC), Ground Floor, Washington, DC 20007, USA

John N. Delahay Department of Orthopedic Surgery, Georgetown University Medical Center, 3800 Reservoir Road NW, Pasquerilla Healthcare Center (PHC), Ground Floor, Washington, DC 20007, USA

Scott G. Edwards Department of Orthopedic Surgery, Division of Hand and Elbow Surgery, Center for Hand and Elbow Specialists, Georgetown University Medical Center, 3800 Reservoir Road NW, Pasquerilla Healthcare Center (PHC), Ground Floor, Washington, DC 20007, USA

Brian G. Evans Department of Orthopedic Surgery, Georgetown University Medical Center, 3800 Reservoir Road NW, Pasquerilla Healthcare Center (PHC), Ground Floor, Washington, DC 20007, USA

Kristen L. Kellar-Graney Department of Orthopedic Oncology, Washington Cancer Institute, 430 Charles Street Avenue, Washington, DC 20010, USA

John J. Klimkiewicz Department of Orthopedic Surgery, Division of Sports Medicine, Georgetown University Medical Center, 3800 Reservoir Road NW, Pasquerilla Healthcare Center (PHC), Ground Floor, Washington, DC 20007, USA

William C. Lauerman Department of Orthopedic Surgery, Division of Spine Surgery, Georgetown University Medical Center, 3800 Reservoir Road NW, Pasquerilla Healthcare Center (PHC), Ground Floor, Washington, DC 20007, USA

Martin M. Malawer Departments of Orthopedic Surgery and Orthopedic Oncology, Georgetown University School of Medicine, 913 Frome Lane, Washington, DC 20057, USA

Francis X. McGuigan Department of Orthopedic Surgery, Foot and Ankle Center, Georgetown University Medical Center, 3800 Reservoir Road NW, Pasquerilla Healthcare Center (PHC), Ground Floor, Washington, DC 20007, USA

Steven C. Scherping, Jr Department of Orthopedic Surgery, Georgetown University Medical Center, 3800 Reservoir Road NW, Pasquerilla Healthcare Center (PHC), Ground Floor, Washington, DC 20057, USA

Brent B. Wiesel Department of Orthopedic Surgery, Shoulder Service, Georgetown University Medical Center, 3800 Reservoir Road NW, Pasquerilla Healthcare Center (PHC), Ground Floor, Washington, DC 20007, USA

Sam W. Wiesel Department of Orthopedic Surgery, Georgetown University Medical Center, 3800 Reservoir Road NW, Pasquerilla Healthcare Center (PHC), Ground Floor, Washington, DC 20007, USA

Mark W. Zawadsky Department of Orthopedic Surgery, Georgetown University Medical Center, 3800 Reservoir Road NW, Pasquerilla Healthcare Center (PHC), Ground Floor, Washington, DC 20007, USA

Chapter 1
Basic Science of Bone and Cartilage Metabolism

John N. Delahay

Normal Bone Growth and Development

Bone is a biphasic connective tissue consisting of an inorganic mineral phase and an organic matrix phase. The hardness of bone allows it to provide several specialized mechanical functions: the protection of internal organs, the scaffold providing points of attachment for other structural elements, and the levers needed to improve the efficiency of muscle action. In addition, bone serves two biologic functions: a site for hematopoietic activity and a reservoir of minerals needed for metabolic interchange.

Embryology

The major components of the musculoskeletal system originate from the mesoderm layer of the trilaminar embryo. This "middle layer" is populated by mesenchymal cells that are totipotent and capable of differentiating into a number of tissues. The sequence of events important in bone growth and development begins with the appearance of the limb bud around the fifth week of life. It is at that time that a tubular condensation of mesenchyme develops centrally in the limb bud. Discrete areas, called interzones, are seen between these condensations (Fig. 1.1) and represent the primitive joints.

During the sixth week, the mesenchyme differentiates into cartilage through the process of chondrification (Fig. 1.2). Interstitial and appositional growth occurs from within and from the surface, respectively. In the seventh week, the cartilage model is penetrated by a vascular spindle. This occurs coincidentally with the necrosis of the central cartilage cells. Once this vascular spindle is established, the central portion of the model is populated by osteoblasts. Matrix is secreted and this in turn is ossified, making immature (woven) bone.

J.N. Delahay (✉)
Department of Orthopedic Surgery, Georgetown University Medical Center, 3800 Reservoir Road NW, Pasquerilla Healthcare Center (PHC), Ground Floor, Washington, DC 20007, USA
e-mail: delahayj@gunet.georgetown.edu

S.W. Wiesel, J.N. Delahay (eds.), *Essentials of Orthopedic Surgery*,
DOI 10.1007/978-1-4419-1389-0_1, © Springer Science+Business Media, LLC 2010

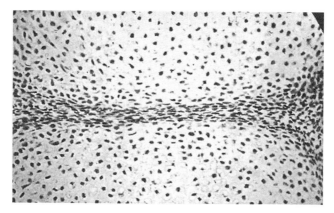

Fig. 1.1 Histologic study of fetus, approximately 6 weeks gestation, depicting early joint formation. Note the identifiable cartilage and the condensed mesenchymal tissue of the interzone destined to become the joint. (From Bogumill GP. *Orthopaedic Pathology: A Synopsis with Clinical Radiographic Correlation*. Philadelphia, PA: Saunders; 1984. Reprinted with permission)

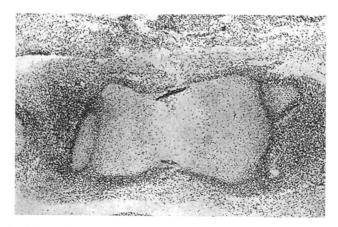

Fig. 1.2 Histologic study of fetus, approximately 8 weeks gestation. Earliest ossification is depicted here. A sleeve, or collar, of bone is present on the outer surface of the cartilage model. (From Bogumill GP. *Orthopaedic Pathology: A Synopsis with Clinical Radiographic Correlation*. Philadelphia, PA: Saunders; 1984. Reprinted with permission)

Once the central portion of the model is ossified, it is referred to as a primary ossification center (Fig. 1.3). Further ossification of the skeleton occurs via one of two mechanisms: (1) enchondral ossification within a cartilage model (i.e., long bones) and (2) intramembranous ossification within a mesenchymal model (i.e., most flat bones and the clavicle).

From the second through the sixth embryonic months, progressive changes occur in the tubular bones. First, the central (medullary) canal cavitates, leaving a hollow tube of bone with a large mass of cartilage persisting at each end (Fig. 1.4). Within

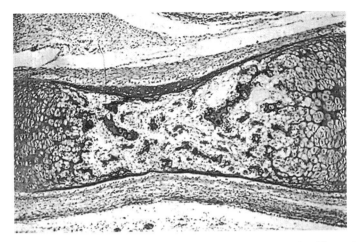

Fig. 1.3 Primary ossification center of fetus, approximately 14 weeks gestation. The cartilage cells have been removed almost entirely from the center, leaving remnants of acellular cartilage matrix. Bone deposits on the cartilage remnants will form primary trabeculae. Note that the primary sleeve, or collar, of bone has extended along both margins and is located adjacent to the hypertrophied cartilage at each epiphyseal end. (From Bogumill GP. *Orthopaedic Pathology: A Synopsis with Clinical Radiographic Correlation*. Philadelphia, PA: Saunders; 1984. Reprinted with permission)

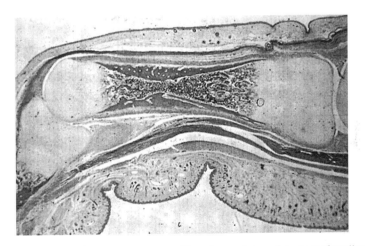

Fig. 1.4 Primary ossification center, near term. There is complete replacement of cartilage in the diaphyseal portion of the cartilage model. The remaining cartilage is confined to both epiphyseal ends of the model. Note the increasing thickness of the cortical portion of bone, which is a result of conversion of periosteum to bone. A light-staining cambium layer is identifiable. The narrowest portion of the shaft is the site of initial vascular invasion and remains identifiable throughout life in many bones, especially in hands and feet. The eccentric position of this narrowed area indicates the disproportionate contribution to growth in length from each epiphysis. (From Bogumill GP. *Orthopaedic Pathology: A Synopsis with Clinical Radiographic Correlation*. Philadelphia, PA: Saunders; 1984. Reprinted with permission)

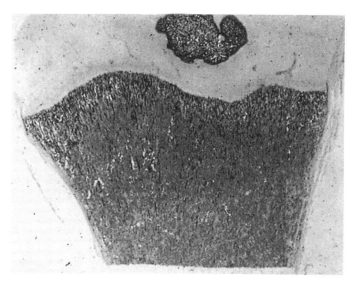

Fig. 1.5 Early secondary ossification center of mature fetus. The formation of the secondary ossification centers in the lower tibia and upper femur coincides with fetal maturity. The secondary center begins not in the center of the epiphysis, but near the growth plate. Expansion, therefore, is eccentric. (From Bogumill GP. *Orthopaedic Pathology: A Synopsis with Clinical Radiographic Correlation*. Philadelphia, PA: Saunders; 1984. Reprinted with permission)

these masses of cartilage, the secondary ossification center, or epiphysis, will form (Fig. 1.5). A cartilage plate, the physis or growth plate (Fig. 1.6), persists between the developing epiphysis and metaphysis. This structure is responsible for growth in length, whereas the covering of the bone, the periosteum, is primarily responsible for growth in girth.

Postnatal Development

The physis and the periosteum continue to function postnatally in the growth and development of the infantile skeleton. Numerous local and systemic factors impact on their activity; vascular, hormonal, and genetic effects all play important roles. In essence, the reworking or remodeling of bone that is already present occurs so that the bone can meet the mechanical and biologic demands placed on it.

Bone: The Tissue

Bone, whether it is immature or mature, consists of cells and a biphasic blend of mineral and matrix that coexist in a very exact relationship. The matrix phase consists of collagen and glycosaminoglycans, which are dimeric disaccharides. Both

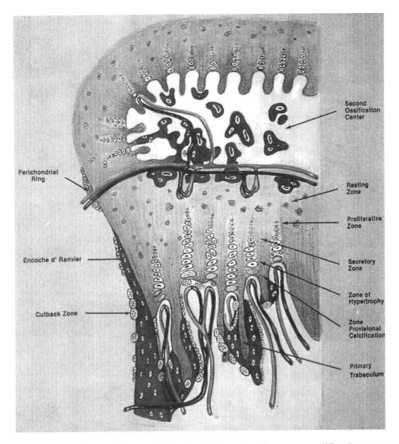

Fig. 1.6 Schematic diagram of growth plate, consisting of resting zone, proliferative zone, secretory zone, zone of hypertrophy, and zone of calcification. The cross-sectional view helps place events at the growth plate in three-dimensional perspective. (From Bogumill GP. *Orthopaedic Pathology: A Synopsis with Clinical Radiographic Correlation*. Philadelphia, PA: Saunders; 1984. Reprinted with permission)

are products of the osteoblast. Calcium hydroxyapatite is the basic mineral crystal in bone. Despite the presence of some less structured amorphous calcium phosphate, the bulk of calcium in the skeletal reservoir is bound in the crystals of hydroxyapatite.

Osteoblasts are bone-forming cells that secrete the matrix components described. As ossification progresses, the osteoblasts become trapped in the matrix they produce and are then referred to as osteocytes. These cells are rather inert, but are capable of a small degree of bone resorption. Osteoclasts are those cells whose primary function is the degradation and removal of mineralized bone. It is important to remember that the osteoclasts can remove only mineralized bone and not unmineralized matrix.

Bone Organization

Microscopically, bone is generally described as mature or immature. Mature bone (Fig. 1.7) has an ordered lamellar arrangement of Haversian systems and canalicular communications, that give it its classic histologic appearance. Immature bone (Fig. 1.8), in contrast, has a much more random appearance of collagen fibers

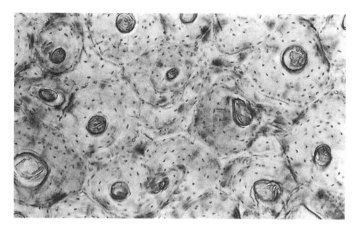

Fig. 1.7 Mature bone; osteonal structure as seen in undecalcified material. Numerous interstitial fragments (osteonal fragments without an associated Haversian canal) are readily observed. (From Bogumill GP. *Orthopaedic Pathology: A Synopsis with Clinical Radiographic Correlation.* Philadelphia, PA: Saunders; 1984. Reprinted with permission)

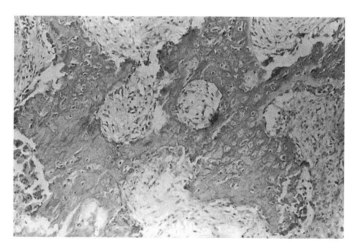

Fig. 1.8 Immature bone (early callus). Note the large number of osteoblasts and osteocytes. (From Bogumill GP. *Orthopaedic Pathology: A Synopsis with Clinical Radiographic Correlation.* Philadelphia, PA: Saunders; 1984. Reprinted with permission)

dispersed in a matrix of irregularly spaced cells. It is produced rapidly by osteoblasts and "remodeled" by the local cell population, until the mature lamellar pattern is achieved. Immature bone is seen in the adult skeleton only under pathologic conditions (i.e., fracture callus, osteogenic sarcoma, myositis, etc.). Macroscopically (Fig. 1.9), the lamellar bone is configured either as dense cortical bone or as delicate spicules called trabeculae. In both areas, the cortex and the trabecular metaphysis, the bone is histologically the same (i.e., mature lamellar bone).

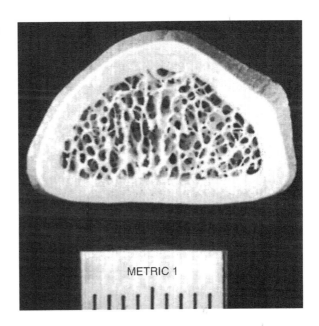

Fig. 1.9 Cross-section of the radius at the distal metaphysis. The majority of bone is cortical bone, in which the annual rate of turnover is only 2%

Turnover and Remodeling

Although the tendency is to think of adult bone as an inert tissue, nothing could be further from the truth. Throughout adult life there is a constant ebb and flow of bone formation and bone resorption. These two processes are delicately balanced and keep the skeletal mass in a state of equilibrium. A number of authors have popularized the concept of "coupling"; bone formation and bone resorption generally increase or decrease in the same direction. When one process increases, so does the other, and vice versa. It is important, however, to consider the net effect of the rate changes in these two processes. For example, in osteoporosis, both formation and bone resorption increase, but resorption increases at a much greater rate; so despite a coupled increase in bone formation, the net effect is an overall decrease in bone mass. A number of factors, systemic and local, affect these processes and hence impact on bone turnover and remodeling. Perhaps the most well-defined factor is mechanical stress, which forms the basis for the classic Wolff's law. Simply stated, trabecular, and to a lesser degree cortical, bone remodels along lines of mechanical stress. Bone forms where it is needed to meet mechanical demands and it is resorbed where the need is less. Current research suggests that bone functions as a transducer, converting mechanical energy from the applied load into electrical energy and a voltage gradient. In turn, this voltage gradient that is generated modulates cellular differentiation. Osteoblastic activity is thus seen in regions where the mechanical demands are the greatest. Osteoclastic activity predominates the pattern when those mechanical demands decrease and less bone is required. This phenomenon has been called the "piezoelectric effect." Specifically, the deformation of bone apatite crystals by superimposed load generates the voltage gradient, which in turn alters the cell population to respond to that load.

Cartilage: The Tissue

Cartilage, like bone, is a connective tissue. Its histologic organization, however, is far less structured. There are three histologic types of cartilage, each serving a different function:

1. *Hyaline cartilage* covers the ends of long bones and provides a smooth, frictionless surface for articulation in a diarthrodial (synovial lined) joint.
2. *Fibrocartilage* is typically found in certain nondiarthrodial joints such as the pubic symphysis. It is also located at the margins of certain diarthrodial joints, forming structures such as the glenoid labrum and acetabular labrum. Following injury to hyaline cartilage, repair of the chondral defect is typically accomplished in the form of fibrocartilage.
3. *Elastic cartilage* is found in certain areas where resiliency is important. Examples include the tip of the nose and the ear lobe.

The most important of the three, hyaline cartilage, is a relatively aneural, avascular, and hypocellular connective tissue. By weight, it is 70% water and 30% ground substance and cells. The ground substance of hyaline cartilage is composed primarily of type II collagen and GAG proteins (glycosaminoglycans). The collagen endows the cartilage with tensile strength and the GAGs are critical for resiliency.

The cells are called chondrocytes and are dispersed throughout the chondral layers in four zones: tangential (most superficial), transitional, radial, and calcified. These chondrocytes are found in individual lacunae, where they maintain healthy cartilage by actively synthesizing new ground substance components.

The chondral layer receives the bulk of its nutrition by diffusion from the synovial fluid above and from the vasculature at the subchondral plate below. Normal diarthrodial (synovial lined) joint function depends on the presence of normal hyaline cartilage. In its fully hydrated state, hyaline cartilage provides an almost frictionless bearing, hence minimizing wear on the articular surface.

Abnormal Bone Development and Metabolism

Most skeletal diseases are the result of disruption of normal bone growth and development, breakdown of bone once it has been normally formed or alteration of the normal mechanisms of bone formation or bone resorption. The etiologies of the pathologic states, as one would expect, are quite varied, but the final manifestations within the musculoskeletal system frequently show striking similarities.

Despite the etiology, damage to the growing skeleton will alter the overall shape of one or more bones, depending on whether the adverse process is localized or generalized. Likewise, disruption of osteoblast function will decrease the amount and/or the quality of the bone formed. Multiple factors are known to stimulate osteoclast activity, such as parathyroid hormone, the presence of particulate polyethylene, certain neoplasms, resulting in localized or generalized bone resorption.

As one considers the etiology of skeletal disease, it is helpful to first group the possible differential diagnoses by disease category. This permits one to develop a comprehensive list of possible diagnoses that may explain the findings manifested by the skeleton. The seven disease categories are best remembered using the acronym "**VITAMIN**."

V – vascular disease
I – infection
T – tumor
A – arthritis
M – metabolic bone disease
I – injury
N – neurodevelopmental causes

The remainder of this chapter will focus on these diagnostic groups and the way in which they affect the skeleton. Specific emphasis will be placed on generalized afflictions of the skeleton. In that light, certain disease categories are more likely to adversely affect the skeleton in a generalized fashion; specifically vascular, metabolic, systemic arthritis and neurodevelopmental etiologies. The others, infection, injury, and tumor, are more likely to produce localized changes and, therefore, will be considered in individual subsequent chapters.

Lastly, as a reminder, a differential diagnosis is a listing of plausible specific diagnoses that may explain observed findings such as physical and radiographic. It is not adequate to simply list a disease category since appropriate treatment of a given condition depends on identifying a specific etiology.

Metabolic Bone Disease

General Concepts

Disease processes affecting bone often can be understood as a change in the relationship of bone formation and bone resorption. It is therefore important to understand this relationship. Only by doing so can the net effect on the skeleton be appreciated.

The relationship (ratio) of mineral to matrix may be affected in abnormal metabolic states (Fig. 1.10). For example, osteoporosis is a loss of bone mass, but there is an equivalent loss of matrix and mineral; therefore, the ratio remains normal. In contrast, osteomalacia is a relative loss of mineral resulting in a predominance of matrix, hence decreasing the ratio of mineral to matrix. Serum calcium is rarely representative of skeletal activity. Considering that more than 95% of the body's calcium is stored in bone apatite, it is understandable that the 180 mg of ionized plasma calcium represents literally the "tip of the iceberg." Peripheral sampling of the serum calcium provides only a remote clue to the true content of skeletal apatite. It does, however, provide a convenient way to think about and classify metabolic bone disease.

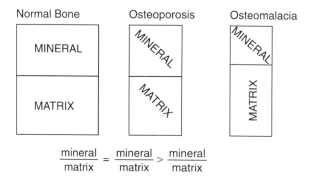

Fig. 1.10 Ration of mineral to matrix in certain disease states. In osteoporosis, the ratio remains constant despite an overall decrease in bone mass. However, in osteomalacia there is a decrease in the ratio of mineral to matrix as a result of skeletal demineralization; in addition, there is an overall decrease in bone mass

Eucalcemic States: Osteoporosis

As mentioned, osteoporosis is a predominance of bone resorption over bone formation, with the net effect being bone loss (Fig. 1.11). There is a parallel loss of mineral and matrix, so their ratio remains normal. Essentially, osteoporosis is a decrease in bone mass with an increase in cortical porosity and in diaphyseal bone diameter. This latter phenomenon is an attempt by the organism to use what limited bone there is and to disperse it as far as possible from the neutral axis of the long bone. Mechanically, this increases the torsional rigidity of the bone. Numerous etiologies

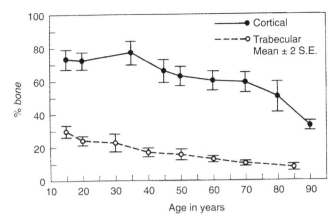

Fig. 1.11 The relative decrease in cortical and trabecular bone with age in apparently normal persons. Note the relatively rapid loss early in life in trabecular bone and comparatively little loss at this age in cortical bone. The situation is reversed after age 55. (From Jowsey J. *Metabolic Diseases of Bone*. Philadelphia, PA: Saunders; 1977. Reprinted with permission)

of osteoporosis have been identified (Table 1.1), but clinically most significant is the postmenopausal type, which occurs shortly after the withdrawal of estrogen (naturally or surgically) from the predisposed female (Table 1.2). The yearly cost in dollars, as well as pain and suffering, is overwhelming. Women with this affliction frequently sustain classic osteoporotic fractures. These fractures typically involve the vertebrae, the wrist, the proximal femur, and/or the proximal humerus. In addition to the pathologic fractures, there is frequently a loss of height as a result of the cumulative effect of multiple vertebral fractures, as well as the progressive development of a kyphotic deformity in the thoracic spine, which is referred to as a "dowager's hump" (Fig. 1.12).

Patients present with a history of pain and/or repeated fractures. Occasionally they will complain of early satiety because of some abdominal compression resulting from loss of height of the vertebral column. Similarly, the increasing kyphosis in the thoracic region may be responsible for some shortness of breath. On examination, typically one finds the prominent dowager's hump, a barrel chest, a protuberant abdomen, and generalized bone pain with percussion tenderness.

One of the most difficult problems in the past has been to determine bone mass. Typically, a crude estimate of bone density determined by plain radiograph has been used to extrapolate to the amount of bone previously lost. Classically, once osteopenia is noticeable radiographically, it has been estimated that the bone density is decreased by 30–50%.

Recently, additional diagnostic techniques have become available to more carefully estimate the amount of bone loss and, therefore, the amount of bone that remains. Isotope measurements, specifically single photon absorptiometry, using an iodine compound, or dual photon absorptiometry, using a gadolinium compound,

Table 1.1 Causes of
osteoporosis

Primary
    Involutional (postmenopausal or senile)
    Idiopathic (juvenile or adult)

Secondary
Endocrine
    Hypogonadism
    Adrenocortical hormone excess (primary or iatrogenic)
    Hyperthyroidism
    Hyperparathyroidism
    Diabetes mellitus
    Growth hormone deficiency
Nutritional
    Calcium deficiency
    Phosphate deficiency
    Phosphate excess
    Vitamin D deficiency
    Protein deficiency
    Vitamin C deficiency
    Intestinal malabsorption
Drug
    Heparin
    Anticonvulsants
    Ethanol
    Methotrexate
Genetic
    Osteogenesis imperfecta
    Homocystinuria
Miscellaneous
    Rheumatoid arthritis
    Chronic liver disease
    Chronic renal disease
Immobilization
    Malignancy (multiple myeloma)
    Metabolic acidosis
    Cigarette smoking

Source: Borenstein D, Wiesel SW. *Low Back Pain: Medical Diagnosis and Comprehensive Management.* Philadelphia, PA: Saunders; 1989:329. Reprinted with permission.

have been developed. They have significant technical limitations. The single photon technique, measuring peripheral sites, such as the forearm and heel, is rarely an adequate reflection of the true bone mineral density in the axial skeleton. The dual photon study, although providing more reliable information about the bone mineral density of the axial skeleton, continues to have some technical limitations. As of this writing, it is probably fair to say that both of these techniques have been replaced by dual-energy X-ray absorptiometry (DEXA) scanning. The DEXA technique is currently the standard, used in the evaluation of bone mineral density (BMD) in women approaching or following their menopause. This technique allows accurate and reproducible measures of density of the spine and the hip.

Table 1.2 Types of involutional osteoporosis

	Type 1 (Postmenopausal)	Type 2 (Senile)
Age (years)	50–75	Over 70
Sex ratio (M/F)	1:6	1:2
Type of bone loss	Trabecular	Trabecular and cortical
Fracture site	Vertebrae (crush)	Vertical (multiple wedge)
	Distal radius	Hip
Main causes	Menopause	Aging
Calcium absorption	Decreased	Decreased
(1,25-OH)$_2$-vitamin D synthesis from 25-(OH) Vitamin D	Secondary decrease	Primary decrease
Parathyroid function	Decreased	Increased

Source: Modified from Riggs BL, Melton LJ III. Involutional osteoporosis. *N Engl J Med.* 1986;314:1676

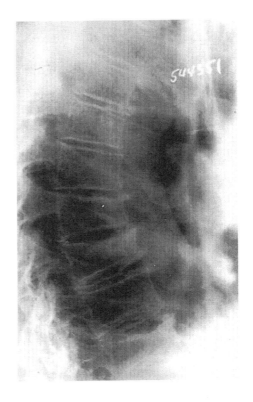

Fig. 1.12 Radiograph of spine showing osteoporosis. Cortical bone appears accentuated by contrast with osteopenic marrow. Longitudinal trabeculae also appear accentuated because smaller transverse trabeculae are absent. Anterior wedging and end plate compression are present. (From Bogumill GP. *Orthopaedic Pathology: A Synopsis with Clinical Radiographic Correlation.* Philadelphia, PA: Saunders; 1984. Reprinted with permission)

It does so with a minimal amount of radiation exposure. There are currently guidelines in place as recommended by the National Osteoporosis Foundation and the World Health Organization that allow comparison of an individual's bone density to that of healthy normals. The difference is expressed as a T score which essentially represents one standard deviation above or below ideal bone mass. The definitions based on T scores are as follows:

Normal	0 to −1
Osteopenia	−1 to −2.5
Osteoporosis	Less than −2.5

The unfortunate result of DEXA scanning, however, has been to adulterate the use of the term "osteopenia." For many years, this term was defined as a generalized decrease in radiographic bone density. As such, it was nonpejorative and did not speak to a specific metabolic bone disease. In its present accepted context, the implication of using the term "osteopenia" is to imply a mild form of postmenopausal osteoporosis. This was certainly not the original connotation of the term. Diseases other than osteoporosis, such as hyperthyroidism and multiple myeloma, are characterized by observed decreases in radiographic bone density, hence osteopenia.

Without question, the most definitive diagnostic technique is direct bone biopsy with or without tetracycline labeling. It can clearly give the most reliable information regarding the presence of osteoporosis, its degree, and whether or not a superimposed osteomalacic state exists. Once the diagnosis has been confirmed and the risk analysis carried out, a treatment protocol can be tailored for the individual patient.

Most treatment regimens are considered either prophylactic or therapeutic. Prophylactic regimens include regular weightbearing exercise, such as walking or jogging, supplemental calcium administration, and vitamin D administration with or without the administration of postmenopausal estrogen substitutes. The complications of oral estrogen administration, such as its relation to breast and cervical cancer, its relation to heart disease and the incidence of deep venous thrombosis (DVT), make its general use controversial; however, its efficacy in maintaining skeletal mass is beyond question.

Therapeutic regimens, in contrast, are much more debatable. Current therapeutic regimens include the use of any or all of several different pharmacologic agents. Selective estrogen receptor modulators (SERMs) are drugs that behave either as an agonist or as an antagonist of estrogen. They have been shown in selective populations to decrease or minimize bone loss. These drugs theoretically have an estrogen-like protective effect on bone. It has also been suggested that they have inhibitory (protective) effects on the breast and the endometrium.

Bisphosphonates are structurally similar to naturally occurring pyrophosphates. Because they have a strong chemical affinity for hydroxyapatite, they are potent inhibitors of bone resorption. They, therefore, are able to decrease the rate at which bone remodeling occurs and, as a result, reduce the amount of bone resorption. It has been said that bisphosphonates are able to "freeze the skeleton." It is hoped that the consequence of decreasing bony resorption is that there will be a coincident increase in bone mass. At the present time, the most popular bisphosphonate in current use is Fosamax, which has been approved for both the prevention and treatment of osteoporosis.

Calcitonin, a naturally occurring polypeptide hormone, is currently being administered in an effort to also decrease the rate of bony resorption by decreasing the number and activity of osteoclasts. The drug is currently being administered in the form of a nasal spray.

The current regimens used for the therapeutic management of osteoporosis include one or more of these drugs in addition to the standard prophylactic measures. Not infrequently, these agents are used cyclically or in an alternating fashion. Since the true measure of any therapeutic regimen for osteoporosis is an increase in bone density and a reduction in fracture risk or in the number of fractures, the true efficacy of these agents and various therapeutic regimens must be evaluated over the long term. As of this writing, the use of SERMs, bisphosphonates, and calcitonin all have shown early promise in this regard.

Hypercalcemic States: Hyperparathyroidism

The effect of parathormone on bone is the same whether it is released as a result of a parathyroid adenoma (primary hyperparathyroidism) or by one of several secondary causes. In essence, parathormone stimulates osteoclastic activity, causing an intense resorption of bone (Fig. 1.13). The cavities resulting from this clastic activity fill

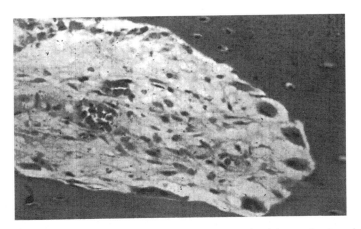

Fig. 1.13 "Cutting cone." Successive relays of osteoclasts on the right resorb a tunnel of bone, making it longer and wider with each relay. Behind the cutting cone is a "filling cone" of successive relays of osteoblasts secreting osteoid. Resorption is facilitated by high-speed flow of well-oxygenated blood in small vessels, whereas refill is accompanied by dilated sinusoidal vessels with sluggish flow and low oxygen content. (From Bogumill GP. *Orthopaedic Pathology: A Synopsis with Clinical Radiographic Correlation*. Philadelphia, PA: Saunders; 1984. Reprinted with permission)

with vascular fibrous tissue, resulting in the classic "osteitis fibrosa cystica." As the cavities coalesce, they form a single large cyst called a "brown tumor," because of the hemosiderin staining one sees within. Clinical and radiographic changes result from this cavitation as well as from the erosive changes occurring under the periosteum.

Hypocalcemic States: Rickets and Osteomalacia

The same underlying mechanism accounts for rickets and osteomalacia: there is a general failure to mineralize bony matrix resulting in the presence of unmineralized osteoid about bony trabeculae. This lack of mineral for adequate mineralization can be due to a number of different etiologies: nutritional deficiency, malabsorption states, and renal disease (Table 1.3) are some of the more common. Despite the etiology, the metabolic effects on the skeleton are similar.

Despite the etiology, if the failure of mineralization impacts the skeleton prior to physeal closure, the result is rickets. The affected child will demonstrate the characteristic hallmarks of the disease: bowlegs, frontal bossing, rickety rosary, and knobby joints (Fig. 1.14). All of these findings are due to the presence of large masses of unmineralized osteoid. In addition, abnormalities of the physis and abnormal physeal growth can be anticipated.

If the process impacts the skeleton after physeal closure, the disease that results is osteomalacia. As noted earlier, the ratio of mineral to matrix decreases as a result of the paucity of mineral available to the skeleton. In the adult, these areas of unmineralized osteoid present as radiographic lucent areas in the bone, frequently referred to a Looser's lines (Fig. 1.15). In addition, the bones themselves tend to be somewhat malleable and can bow under load. This is in contradistinction to osteoporotic bone which is very brittle.

Miscellaneous Metabolic Bone Disease: Renal Osteodystrophy

Renal osteodystrophy encompasses the skeletal changes that result from chronic, acquired renal disease. These changes are truly a "collage" of the other metabolic bone diseases. To understand the pathogenesis of renal osteodystrophy is to understand the basis of all of the metabolic afflications of the skeleton (Fig. 1.16). Chronic uremia allows a twofold drive to depress the serum calcium. First, the kidney is unable to excrete phosphate; hence the serum phosphate level rises. The serum calcium level is then of necessity driven down to maintain the fixed solubility product. Coincidentally, since the absence of a functional renal parenchyma stops the output of significant amounts of activated vitamin D, intestinal absorption of calcium is retarded, further depressing serum calcium. This dual mechanism profoundly depresses serum calcium and thus in turn mandates a parathormone response. The changes in the bone reflect the metabolic drives. The vitamin D deficiency is

Table 1.3 Diseases associated with osteomalacia

Disorder	Metabolic defect
Vitamin D	
Deficiency	Decreased generation of vitamin D_3
Dietary	
Ultraviolet light exposure	
Malabsorption	Decreased absorption of vitamins D_2 and D_3
Small intestine	
Inadequate bile salts	
Pancreatic insufficiency	
Abnormal metabolism	
Hereditary enzyme deficiency	Decreased 1-alpha-hydroxylation of 25-(OH)-vitamin D
D-dependent rickets (type I)	Decreased 25-hydroxylation of vitamin D
Chronic renal failure	
Mesenchymal tumors	
Systemic acidosis	
Hepatic failure	
Anticonvulsant drugs	
Peripheral resistance	Absent or abnormal 1,25-$(OH)_2$-vitamin D receptors
Vitamin D-dependent rickets (type II)	
Phosphate depletion	
Dietary	Inadequate bone mineralization secondary to low serum concentrations
Malnutrition (rare)?	
Aluminum hydroxide ingestion	
Renal tubular wasting	
Hereditary	Decreased serum phosphate concentrations
X-linked hypophos-phatemic osteomalacia	
Acquired	
Hypophosphatemic osteomalacia	
Renal disorders	
Fanconi's syndrome	
Mesenchymal tumors	
Fibrous dysplasia	
Mineralization defects	
Hereditary	Abnormal alkaline phosphatase activity
Hypophosphatasia	
Acquired	Inhibition of bone mineralization
Sodium fluoride	
Disodium etidronate	
Miscellaneous	
Osteopetrosis	Abnormal osteoclast activity
Fibrogenesis imperfecta	Unknown
Axial osteomalacia	Unknown
Calcium deficiency	Inadequate bone mineralization secondary to low serum calcium concentration

Source: From Borenstein D, Wiesel SW. *Low Back Pain: Medical Diagnosis and Comprehensive Management*. Philadelphia, PA: Saunders; 1989:339. Reprinted with permission

Fig. 1.14 Radiograph of wrist of child with active rickets exhibiting the irregular widened zone of provisional calcification that is replaced by abnormal osteoid. The cartilage masses are not visible, but the widened epiphyseal growth plate and irregular calcification are readily seen. Note pathologic fracture of radial shaft. (From Bogumill GP. *Orthopaedic Pathology: A Synopsis with Clinical Radiographic Correlation*. Philadelphia, PA: Saunders; 1984. Reprinted with permission)

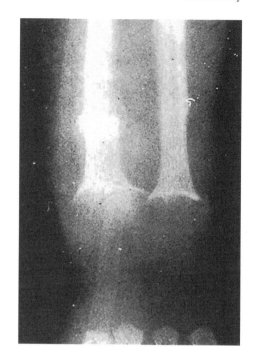

Fig. 1.15 Radiograph of osteomalacia showing Looser's transformation zone. These lines appear at sites in which stress fractures would occur. Stress of normal use incites remodeling with removal of bone. In normal individuals, the removed bone is replaced by normal osteons. In persons with osteomalacia, the removed bone is replaced with abnormal osteoid, which fails to mineralize and leaves a linear radiolucency that may persist for years. (From Bogumill GP. *Orthopaedic Pathology: A Synopsis with Clinical Radiographic Correlation*. Philadelphia, PA: Saunders; 1984. Reprinted with permission)

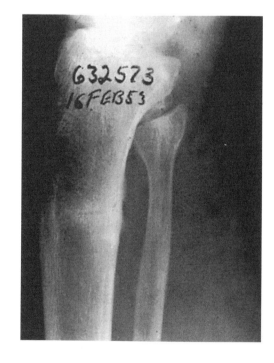

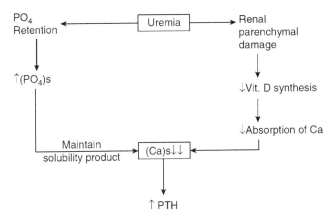

Fig. 1.16 Pathogenesis of renal osteodystrophy

demonstrated by the presence of unmineralized osteoid (Fig. 1.17). The elevated levels of parathormone cause osteitis fibrosis cystica. Unique to this syndrome, the hyperphosphatemia results in a diffuse osteosclerosis. The latter finding causes one of the most pathognomic radiographic findings (Fig. 1.18), the "rugger jersey" spine.

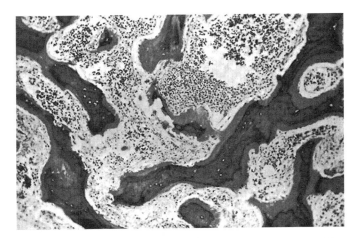

Fig. 1.17 Renal osteodystrophy. Histologic section of bone exhibiting wide osteoid seams. These seams are seen in patients with primary renal disease, but they are not present in patients with primary hyperparathyroidism because the osteoid produced in primary hyperparathyroidism is normal. (From Bogumill GP. *Orthopaedic Pathology: A Synopsis with Clinical Radiographic Correlation.* Philadelphia, PA: Saunders; 1984. Reprinted with permission)

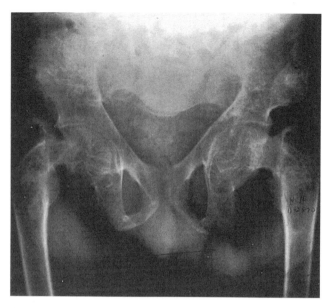

Fig. 1.18 Radiograph of patient with long-standing renal osteodystrophy. Marked osteoporosis attributable to secondary hyperparathyroidism is evident. There is bowing of the proximal femurs, marked lordosis, and pelvic tilt. The deformity of the pelvis is commonly seen in osteomalacia, but it does not usually occur in primary hyperparathyroidism. (From Bogumill GP. *Orthopaedic Pathology: A Synopsis with Clinical Radiographic Correlation*. Philadelphia, PA: Saunders; 1984. Reprinted with permission)

Sick Cell Syndromes: Osteogenesis Imperfecta and Osteopetrosis

The underlying mechanism seen in these conditions is a qualitative, functional deficit in a specific cell population – despite the fact that the population is quantitatively normal.

Osteogenesis imperfecta (Fig. 1.19) is typified by the impotence of the osteoblasts; they are unable to manufacture and secrete normal collagen. Ossification is, therefore, abnormal and results in inferior quality bone. Clinically and radiographically, there is marked cortical thinning and attenuation of the diaphyseal caliber. The long bones, because of their altered anatomy, are at very high risk for fracture (Fig. 1.20). This bone fragility is the hallmark feature of osteogenesis imperfecta.

Since osteogenesis imperfecta is due to a genetic mutation in the normal coding for type I collagen, there is significant phenotypic heterogeneity. In an effort to accommodate the variations in phenotype, the Sillence classification has been adopted by most authors. Four specific types are described in this classification:

Type I is the most common form and the mildest clinically and is transmitted as an autosomal dominant. These patients demonstrate the classic findings of blue sclera, long bone fractures after the age of walking and a relatively normal life expectancy.

Type II is the lethal form of the disease. These children are usually stillborn or die shortly after birth, usually due to respiratory failure or intracranial hemorrhage.

Type III is the severe nonlethal form, characterized by sclera of normal color, multiple birth fractures, and significant long-term deformity and disability

Type IV is the intermediate form, with variable manifestations and the least common.

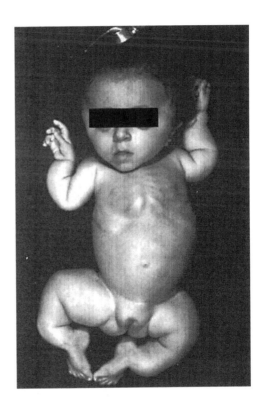

Fig. 1.19 Deformity in a child with severe osteogenesis imperfecta. Note the prominence of the ribs in the abnormally shaped thoracic cage, the flattening of the skull with frontal bulging, and the malformed ribs. (From Gertner JM, Root L. Osteogenesis imperfecta. *Orthop Clin North Am.* 1990;21(1):153. Reprinted with permission)

Osteopetrosis is similarly considered a sick cell syndrome resulting from the failure of the osteoclasts to remove primary spongiosa bone. This latter osseous material then "piles up" in the skeleton, making it appear very dense radiographically (Fig. 1.21). Despite the fact that the bones look extremely dense and, indeed, lack a medullary canal, they are biomechanically very weak. This results in frequent pathologic fractures. An additional complication is the displacement of marrow elements

Fig. 1.20 Radiograph of the lower extremities of a child with osteogenesis imperfecta. The bones are slender and the cortices excessively thin; both femurs have incurred fractures that are partially healed, although deformity still exists. (From Jowsey J. *Metabolic Diseases of Bone*. Philadelphia, PA: Saunders, 1977. Reprinted with permission)

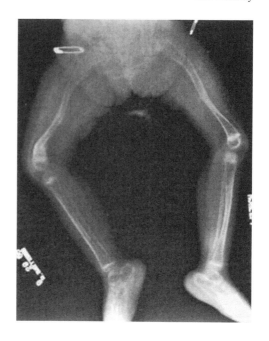

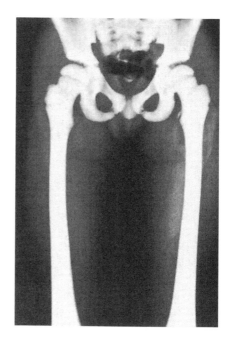

Fig. 1.21 Radiologic appearance of the femurs and pelvic girdle of a patient with osteopetrosis. There is almost complete absence of the marrow cavity and lack of remodeling of the femoral neck and acetabulum. (From Jowsey J. *Metabolic Diseases of Bone*. Philadelphia, PA: Saunders; 1977. Reprinted with permission)

from the long bones. This results in a myelophthisic anemia. This in turn generates extramedullary hematopoiesis and the clinical finding of hepatosplenomegaly usually seen in these patients.

Paget's Disease

Sir James Paget described a syndrome of unknown etiology that bears his name. The initial description referred to the condition as "ostetitis deformans." The syndrome is most common in individuals of European descent and in patients typically over the age of 55. Men tend to be more affected than women.

There is strong evidence, specifically the finding of radiodense viral-like particles in the osteoclasts (Fig. 1.22), pointing to a slow virus as the cause of Paget's disease. It is basically a disease of bone turnover wherein bone formation and bone resorption dramatically increase. The two processes occur alternately rather than simultaneously in any given bone. The net effect is bones of increased density with marked trabecular thickening (Fig. 1.23). The skull, pelvis, spine, tibia, and femur are the favorite targets of this process. Sadly, and not unlike osteopetrosis, the pagetic bones are mechanically weak, making pathologic fracture a frequent complication. Despite the presence of abundant quantities of bone, it is poorly formed and the minimal and matrix are poorly integrated. Bone pain, spinal stenosis, and

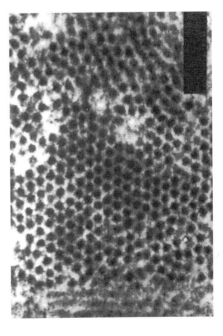

Fig. 1.22 Viral particles located in osteoclasts within pagetoid bone have been implicated as a causal factor in Paget's disease. (From Merkow RL, Lane JM. Paget's disease of bone. *Orthop Clin North Am.* 1990;21(1):172. Reprinted with permission)

Fig. 1.23 Example of pagetoid bone demonstrating deformity and thickening of the cortex of the hip. The neck shaft angle has developed varus deformity. (From Merkow RL, Lane JM. Paget's disease of bone. *Orthop Clin North Am.* 1990;21(1):172. Reprinted with permission)

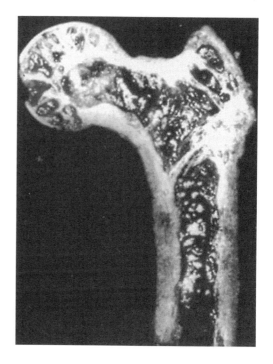

hearing defects resulting from disease in the skull base compromising the eighth nerve are frequent problems in these patients.

Several different therapeutic approaches have been attempted. Currently, bisphosphonates and calcitonin are frequently employed therapeutic agents. Much like in osteoporosis, they are used in an attempt to inhibit bone resorption and also to a lesser degree to block bone mineralization. The rationale is to "freeze the skeleton" and thereby decrease bone turnover. Cyclic treatment regimens are currently being employed in hopes of allowing new bone to become mineralized while decreasing the osteoclastic activity. The serum alkaline phosphatase level provides a reliable way of monitoring the response to treatment, since it is elevated in the presence of active bone turnover.

Arthritis

Since any significant discussion on this subject is well beyond the scope of this chapter, it is hoped that presentation of some basic concepts will allow consideration of this diagnosis in the scheme of differential diagnosis. It is important to recall that a diarthrodial joint includes three tissues: bone, cartilage, and synovium. Each of the arthritic diseases tends to impact one of these tissues, with changes in the other two resulting as secondary phenomena. The radiographic and microscopic changes encountered represent a composite of the result of the initial injury and the organism's attempt at repair of that injury.

Noninflammatory Arthritis: Osteoarthritis

Osteoarthritis can be primary or secondary, if one considers the degenerative joint disease that can follow trauma or other primary events. The process itself targets the articular cartilage. Whether the initial event is mechanical or biochemical remains controversial. The net result is progressive damage to the articular surface. The secondary bone changes that occur are reparative in nature. Joint space narrowing, subchondral sclerosis, osteophytes, and subchondral cysts, therefore, are the classic radiographic changes. Since this is most typically a disease of weight-bearing joints, the hip and knee are the joints that usually require orthopedic care. Total joint arthroplasty has become the mainstay of surgical management in these patients, producing reliable long-term results.

Inflammatory Arthritis: Rheumatoid Arthritis

Rheumatoid arthritis, and to some degree its variants, target the synovial membrane as the site for the immunologic process that is the root mechanism of this disease. As the synovium hosts this inflammatory process, it becomes hyperplastic and hypertrophic. The thickened synovium destroys the articular cartilage by enzymatic degradation and destroys the underlying bone by pressure necrosis and erosion (Fig. 1.24). Unlike osteoarthritis, repair changes are, for the most part, abortive. The radiograph reflects this overall atrophic process. Soft tissue swelling, osteopenia on both sides of the joint, and bone erosions are the standard findings (Fig. 1.25). Joint destruction is generally symmetric and much more global than with osteoarthritis. Extensive alterations in normal anatomy usually necessitate multiple joint arthroplasties.

Metabolic Arthritides: Crystalline Arthropathy

The common denominator of the metabolic arthritides is the deposition of crystals or metabolic by-products in or around joints. Destructive changes in these joints necessitate rheumatologic and frequently orthopedic care.

In gout, sodium urate crystals are deposited in and around the joints. Finding these crystals in joint fluid is the diagnostic sine qua non of this metabolic imbalance. An intense chemical synovitis and bony erosions can occur. Typically, the first metatarsophalangeal joint is the classic site, but certainly the process can present in any joint, including the spine. The acute onset and signs of acute inflammation

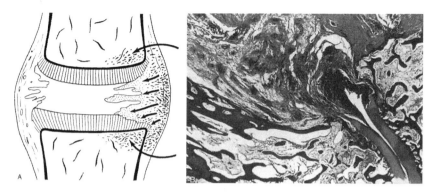

Fig. 1.24 Diagram (**a**) and section (**b**) of a finger joint of a patient with rheumatoid arthritis. The marked synovitis is evident in the synovial recesses with erosions into the bone on both sides of the articular surface (*long curved arrows*). The pannus is beginning to encroach on margins of the joint (*short arrows*). Although the cartilage retains its normal appearance in the center of the joint, the proteoglycan structure is affected by the altered synovial fluid. It is susceptible to rapid removal by wear and tear as well as by the encroaching pannus. Since the pannus grows in from the margins, the earliest radiographic erosions are seen at the margins, and the contract surfaces are spared until relatively late. (From Bogumill GP. *Orthopaedic Pathology: A Synopsis with Clinical Radiographic Correlation*. Philadelphia, PA: Saunders Company; 1984. Reprinted with permission)

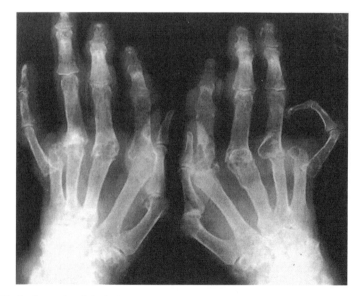

Fig. 1.25 Radiograph of both hands of a patient with long-standing rheumatic arthritis. Osteoporosis in all bones is marked. The wrist joints show advanced destruction. There is dislocation of the metacarpophalangeal joints of all fingers. Steroid therapy causes expansion of metacarpals and phalanges secondary to changes in the marrow fat (steroid lipomatosis). (From Bogumill GP. *Orthopaedic Pathology: A Synopsis with Clinical Radiographic Correlation*. Philadelphia, PA: Saunders; 1984. Reprinted with permission)

should suggest the diagnosis, which is best confirmed by arthrocentesis. The finding of needle-like, negatively birefringent crystals under polarized light confirms the diagnosis. The treatment is usually medical. However, in the presence of late destructive changes, surgical intervention can be considered.

Pseudogout is one of the many causes of chondrocalcinosis and should not be considered synonymous with it. The presence of weakly positively birefringent crystals, rhomboid in shape, attests to the diagnosis. The calcium pyrophosphate crystals are radiopaque and, as such, can be viewed on standard radiographs as calcification of cartilage, including the menisci and articular surfaces. The condition rarely mandates surgical intervention, and treatment frequently revolves around nonsteroidal antiinflammatory drugs or intraarticular steroid injections.

Ochronosis is an inborn error of metabolism. The error is an absence of homogentisic acid oxidase. As a result, homogentisic acid accumulates and targets articular cartilage for its deposition. The articular cartilage is stiffened by the presence of this by-product and loses its resiliency. The net result is fissuring and fibrillation of the articular surface; these changes radiographically and pathologically mimic osteoarthritis. The unique feature of this condition is the fact that this material pigments and stains the cartilage black (Fig. 1.26), thereby accounting for the blackish tinge of the earlobes and the tips of the nose seen in these patients.

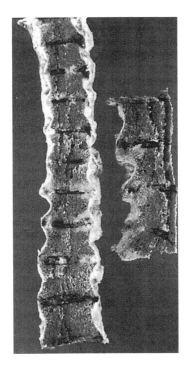

Fig. 1.26 Gross appearance of vertebral bodies in a patient with ochronosis. Notice the diminution of the intervertebral discs, black discoloration of the cartilage components, virtual disappearance of all joint spaces, and bony bridging. (From Bogumill GP. *Orthopaedic Pathology: A Synopsis with Clinical Radiographic Correlation.* Philadelphia, PA: Saunders; 1984. Reprinted with permission)

Vascular Disease

This diagnostic category is a somewhat diverse grouping of clinical entities that are best considered under this heading lest they be overlooked.

Circulatory Disease: Avascular Necrosis

Afflictions of the vascular tree, especially the arterial side, tend to produce similar lesions in bone, despite the etiology. Bone deprived of a portion of its blood supply becomes necrotic, like all other tissues (Fig. 1.27). Depending on the extent of the vascular involvement, the infarcts can range from small areas of bony necrosis in the metaphysis (Fig. 1.28), which are clinically inconsequential, to extensive involvement at the ends of the long bones that progresses to significant degenerative joint disease.

The radiographic appearance of dead bone is essentially that of sclerosis. In truth, the dead tissue is incapable of changing its density since no viable cells exist. Rather, the viable bone adjacent to the necrotic segment develops a reactive hyperemia and resorbs. The necrotic bone then appears to be more dense on the radiograph – so-called relative radiodensity. There is also some compaction of dead trabeculae, as

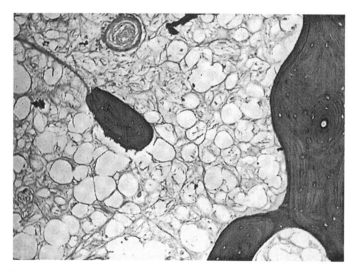

Fig. 1.27 Bone from central area of infarction, exhibiting infarcted fatty tissue, obliterated vessels, and infarcted bone. Note absence of either osteoclastic or osteoblastic activity. The trabeculae in this zone have retained their original density. (From Bogumill GP. *Orthopaedic Pathology: A Synopsis with Clinical Radiographic Correlation*. Philadelphia, PA: Saunders; 1984. Reprinted with permission)

Fig. 1.28 Radiograph of humerus of patient with history of deep-sea diving. The sclerotic area represents infarction of the marrow cavity with formation of calcium soaps and new bone from the reparative margins. (From Bogumill GP. *Orthopaedic Pathology: A Synopsis with Clinical Radiographic Correlation.* Philadelphia, PA: Saunders; 1984. Reprinted with permission)

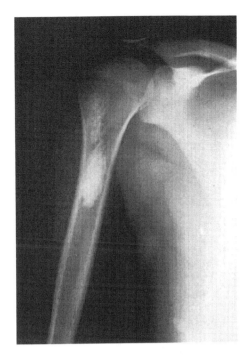

well as marrow necrosis with subsequent saponification and calcification of the dead fat to additionally explain the sclerotic changes seen on radiographs.

A number of vaso-occlusive phenomena can cause avascular (aseptic) necrosis (AVN). Although AVN can involve any number of different sites, the femoral head is by far the most typical (Fig. 1.29).

Etiologies of AVN can be grouped by causation:

1. *Trauma*: damage to vessels supplying the segment of the bone in question (i.e., fractures of the femoral neck and scaphoid).
2. *Occlusive phenomenon*:

    a. Emboli: such as fat in alcoholism and pancreatitis; nitrogen as in Caisson's disease
    b. Stasis: coagulopathies and hemaglobinopathies
    c. External constriction: vasculitis such as systemic lupus erythematosus (SLE) and inflammatory bowel disease
    d. External compression: typical of storage diseases (Gaucher's and Fabry's) where stored material compresses intraosseous arterioles

3. *Idiopathic*: the causative factor is unknown, as in steroid-induced osteonecrosis and Chandler's disease.

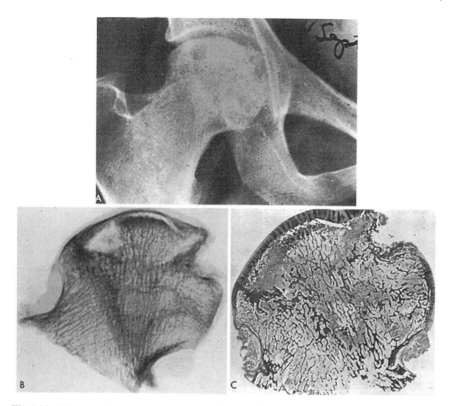

Fig. 1.29 Clinical radiograph (**a**), specimen radiograph (**b**), and corresponding macrospecimen (**c**) of femoral head from a 26-year-old patient on long-term steroid therapy for idiopathic thrombocytopenic purpura with progressive pain and disability of both hips. Note the crescent sign, a cleft beneath the articular cartilage resulting from compression fractures of dead trabeculae. Also note the lytic areas in lateral aspect of the femoral head caused by revascularization with removal of dead trabeculae and replacement with viable fibrous tissue. Zones of increased density are also evident. (From Bogumill GP. *Orthopaedic Pathology: A Synopsis with Clinical Radiographic Correlation.* Philadelphia, PA: Saunders; 1984. Reprinted with permission)

Hematologic Syndromes

The genetic hemoglobinopathies, although not truly circulatory diseases, are best remembered in this group. Sickle cell disease and to a lesser degree thalassemia produce skeletal changes primarily through two mechanisms: myeloid hyperplasia and vaso-occlusive phenomena. Because of the anemia these patients suffer, there is a drive to increase medullary hematopoiesis, and this results in dilation of bony contours to accommodate a marrow driven to produce more blood. Widening of the diploe of the skull, dilation of the small bones of the hands and feet, and increased trabecular markings are all radiographic hallmarks of this process. The vaso-occlusive effect of these distorted red cells causes bone infarcts similar to those previously discussed (Fig. 1.30).

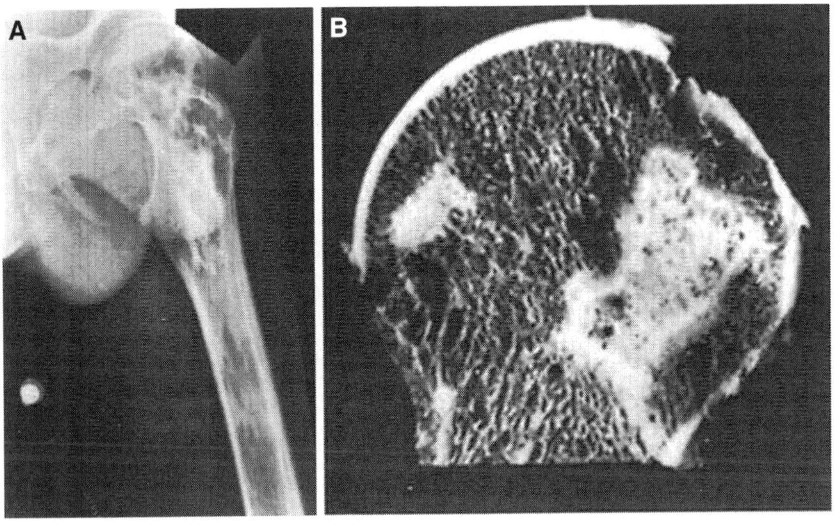

Fig. 1.30 (a) Radiograph of hip and proximal femur of a 25-year-old male with sickle cell anemia. Areas of mottling and sclerosis are seen, suggestive of bone infarction. Evidence of sequestrum formation is seen in the lateral femoral cortex (bone within a bone). (b) Gross specimen of the femoral head taken from the same patient. Light necrotic areas are well demarcated from viable bone. (From Johanson NA. Musculoskeletal problems in hemoglobinopathy. *Orthop Clin North Am.* 1990;21(1):196. Reprinted with permission)

However, in a select group of patients the infarcts are frequently painful and a component of the "painful crisis." The stasis, sludging, and dead bone create a comfortable environment for bacterial invasion, accounting for the increased incidence of osteomyelitis in these patients.

Neurodevelopmental Disorders

The final diagnostic category discussed in this chapter is the most heterogeneous of all. There are a few common threads that can be found to tie this eclectic mix of clinical states together. Clearly, they all have an impact on the musculoskeletal system. An attempt is made to describe them generically and use an example in each category to underscore their impact on the skeleton.

Neurologic Diseases

The deficit produced by neurologic diseases can be either sensory, motor, or central in origin. The level of involvement will determine the skeletal changes. Central nervous system deficits are typified by cerebral palsy. Prenatal anoxia can cause damage to the cerebral cortex. This includes damage to neural tissue that normally inhibits or damps muscular tone and keeps it at an acceptable level. Without normal inhibitory influences, these muscles become spastic. Muscle spasticity existing over a protracted period results in muscle imbalance around joints. Ultimately contractures and chronic joint deformities, such as subluxations and dislocations, will follow. The hip, for example, is of particular concern in the spastic child.

Poliomyelitis is an example of a motor deficit disease. Viral damage to anterior horn cells results in focal motor weakness in various muscle groups in the extremities. Bone deprived of normal muscle loading tends to become osteopenic. In addition, the variable nature of the involvement again causes muscle imbalance around joints, with its subsequent deformities.

Sensory deficits may result in neuropathic arthritis. Joints deprived of proprioception are rapidly destroyed. The aggressive sequence of microtrauma, repeated effusions, ligamentous incompetence, articular damage, and severe degenerative joint disease is the fate of patients with tertiary lues, diabetes, pernicious anemia, leprosy, and heavy metal intoxications. Although proprioception is the initial sensory component lost, pain fiber deficit usually follows, resulting in destroyed, but painless joints.

Spina bifida, or myelodysplasia, may result in mixed deficits. This congenital defect combines motor and sensory deficits to produce skeletal changes that parallel both. Osteopenia, joint deformity, and joint destruction may all be found. The joints, as expected, are insensate, a fact that only compounds the clinical problems.

Developmental/Congenital Defects

It is important to remember that congenital defects (present at birth) need not be genetic, and vice versa. However, any process that impacts on the growing skeleton, whether it be congenital or developmental, can be expected to produce changes. These changes can generally be expected to be alterations in the configuration of the bone itself. Shortening, bowing, or angular deformities may be seen. Changes in bone density may or may not be seen.

Achondroplasia is the most common dwarfing syndrome. It follows an autosomal dominant inheritance pattern (Fig. 1.31). This syndrome disrupts normal enchondral bone growth and, therefore, results in shortening of all bones that depend on this mechanism for their growth (Fig. 1.32).

Bone dysplasias (intrinsic defects of bone growth) are, as a general rule, genetic in origin despite the fact that some of the milder (tarda) forms may not be apparent until the child begins growing.

Chromosomal defects, such as Down syndrome, are often characterized by severe ligamentous laxity. This is the basis for the numerous orthopedic conditions that are typical in this group. Atlanto-axial instability, flat feet, patellar subluxation, bunions, and subluxation of the hips all point to the inability of the ligamentous structure to

Fig. 1.31 (**a**) Posterior photograph of achondroplastic dwarf showing distorted growth of long bones. The proximal limb segments are proportionately shorter than the distal, with the hands reaching only to the hip region. The legs are bowed, and the scapulae and pelvis are smaller than normal. Scoliosis is uncommon. (**b**) Lateral photograph of child with achondroplasia. Note marked lumbar lordosis with prominent buttocks as a result of pelvic tilt. The lordosis is due in part to differential growth of vertebral body versus posterior elements. (From Bogumill GP. *Orthopaedic Pathology: A Synopsis with Clinical Radiographic Correlation.* Philadelphia, PA: Saunders; 1984. Reprinted with permission)

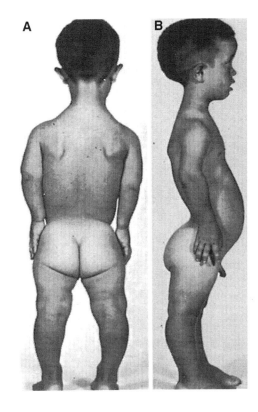

Fig. 1.32 Radiographic appearance of lower limbs in a patient with achondroplasia. Note the narrow sciatic notch and flat broad acetabulum resulting from inadequate growth of "Y" cartilage in acetabulum. Shortened, thick femurs, fibias, and fibulas are bowed. Bone density is normal. Epiphyses do not yet exhibit secondary ossification centers. (From Bogumill GP. *Orthopaedic Pathology: A Synopsis with Clinical Radiographic Correlation.* Philadelphia, PA: Saunders; 1984. Reprinted with permission)

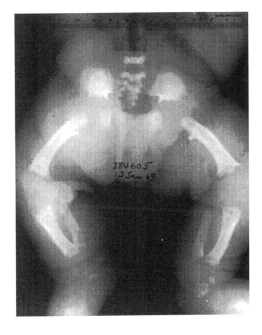

stabilize joints. Many of the chromosomal abnormalities involve defects in meso-derm development. This accounts for the common coincidence of musculoskeletal, genitourinary, and cardiac abnormalities.

The clubfoot deformity is probably multifactorial in its etiology. The interplay of heredity and environment is accepted, although poorly understood. Clubfoot, like developmental dysplasia of the hip and scoliosis, is a defect that is considered to be a reflection of this interplay. Usually identified at birth, clubfoot is a generalized dysplasia of the mesenchymal structures (bone, ligament, muscle) of the foot and perhaps the entire lower extremity. Genetic as well as environmental (intrauterine position) factors have been implicated, but their exact interaction remains unknown.

Summary

Many different pathologic states have impact on the skeletal system, whether they are primary or secondary. Bone has a limited number of ways of responding to abnormal stimuli whether they are chemical, mechanical, infectious, circulatory, etc. In general, one can expect to see either bone resorption or bone formation, either locally or systemically, dominate the pattern. A working knowledge of the normal usually allows the observer to anticipate the response to many of these pathologic processes.

In this regard, observing the changes that one sees on standard imaging stud-ies will often permit the development of a working differential diagnosis. Using the basic seven disease categories and expanding each into a plausible list of diag-noses should lead, given more data, to a definitive diagnosis and hence appropriate treatment.

Suggested Reading

1. Bernstein J, ed. *Musculoskeletal Medicine.* Rosemont, IL: American Academy of Orthopaedic Surgeons; 2003.
2. Bogumill GP, Schwamm HA. *Orthopaedic Pathology: A Synopsis with Clinical and Radiographic Correlation.* Philadelphia, PA: Saunders; 1984.
3. Buckwalter JA. Einhorn TA, Simon SR, eds. *Orthopaedic Basic Science: Biology and Biomechanics of the Musculoskeletal System.* 2nd ed. Rosemont, IL: American Academy of Orthopaedic Surgeons; 2000.

Chapter 2
Skeletal Trauma

Francis X. McGuigan

Skeletal trauma can be divided into three major groups of injuries to the musculoskeletal system: fractures, dislocations, and fracture/dislocations. A fracture is a disruption in the continuity of cortical and/or cancellous bone. A dislocation is a disruption of the normal articulating anatomy of a joint. Dislocations can be either a complete disruption of the normal anatomy or a partial dislocation, termed a subluxation. A fracture/dislocation is a fracture occurring in or near a joint that results in a subluxation or dislocation of the joint.

Fractures

Fracture Descriptors

A number of different terms are used to describe the configuration and features of any given fracture. These general descriptors are as follows:

1. Open versus closed: A closed fracture is one in which the skin is intact over the fracture site and an open fracture is one in which the skin is disrupted.
2. Simple versus comminuted: A simple fracture is one in which there are only two major fragments and one fracture line. A comminuted fracture is one in which there are multiple fragments of bone and multiple fracture lines.
3. Complete versus incomplete: A complete fracture is one in which the fracture line goes completely across the bone. Incomplete fractures, most typically seen in children, have a fracture line that only crosses one cortex of the bone involved.

F.X. McGuigan (✉)
Department of Orthopedic Surgery, Foot and Ankle Center, Georgetown University Medical Center, 3800 Reservoir Road NW, Pasquerilla Healthcare Center (PHC), Ground Floor, Washington, DC 20007, USA
e-mail: fxm122@gunet.georgetown.edu

S.W. Wiesel, J.N. Delahay (eds.), *Essentials of Orthopedic Surgery*,
DOI 10.1007/978-1-4419-1389-0_2, © Springer Science+Business Media, LLC 2010

Fracture Deformities

A fracture can be deformed in any one of three possible planes. Traditionally, the deformity is described by the relative position of the distal fragment in relation to the proximal fragment. Classic deformations are described as follows (Fig. 2.1):

1. Displacement is the amount of translation of the distal fragment in relation to the proximal fragment in either the anterior/posterior or the medial/lateral planes. Displacement is the opposite of apposition.
2. Angulation occurs when two fracture fragments are not aligned and an angular deformity is present in either the anterior/posterior or the medial/lateral planes.

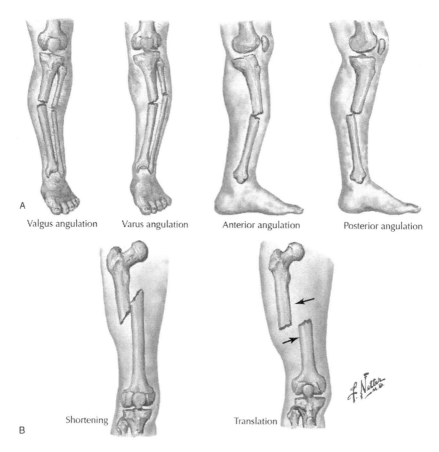

Fig. 2.1 (**a**) Angulation is described by the direction in which the apex of the fracture is pointing. (**b**) Displacement (*arrows*) is defined by the position of the distal fragment in relation to the proximal fragment. (Netter images reprinted with permission from Elsevier. All rights reserved)

Alignment means that the axes of the proximal and distal fragments are parallel to each other and the joint above and below are in the normal (anatomic) relationship. Angulation is typically described by the direction in which the apex of the angle points – medial, lateral, dorsal, volar, etc.

3. Rotation occurs when there is an axial change between the two fractured fragments in the transverse plane.
4. Shortening or lengthening occurs when the distal fragment is positioned in relation to the proximal fragment to either decrease or increase the overall length of the fractured bone.

Fracture Patterns

A number of basic fracture patterns have been described (Figs. 2.2–2.4). They include:

1. Transverse
2. Spiral
3. Oblique
4. Impacted or compressed
5. Avulsion
6. Torus (buckle)
7. Complex (multiple patterns)
8. Segmental

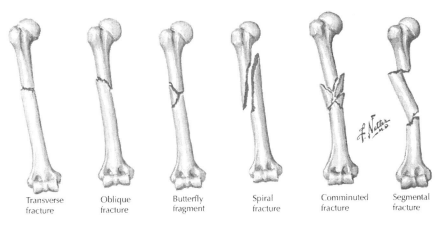

Transverse fracture | Oblique fracture | Butterfly fragment | Spiral fracture | Comminuted fracture | Segmental fracture

Fig. 2.2 Fracture patterns. (Netter images reprinted with permission from Elsevier. All rights reserved)

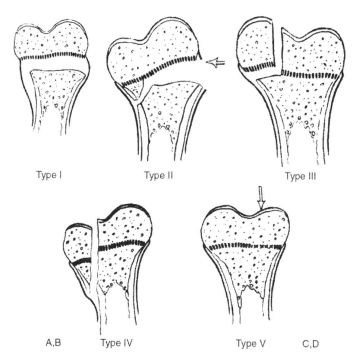

Fig. 2.3 Salter classification of epiphyseal plate fractures. Type I: separation of epiphysis. Type II: fracture-separation of epiphysis. Type III: fracture of part of epiphysis. Type IV: (**a**) fracture of epiphysis and epiphyseal plate; (**b**) bony union causing premature closure of plate. Type V: (**c**) crushing of epiphyseal plate; (**d**) premature closure of plate on one side with resultant angular deformity. (From Gartland J. *Fundamentals of Orthopaedics*, 3rd ed. Philadelphia, PA: Saunders; 1987. Reprinted with permission)

Fracture Mode of Loading

The biomechanics that create a fracture offer a great deal of information as to the mechanism of injury and the extent of that injury. For that reason, biomechanical analyses have been performed to elucidate the specific modes of loading that create certain fracture patterns such as the following:

1. Bending loading produces a transverse fracture
2. Torsional loading produces a spiral fracture
3. Axial loading produces a compression or impacted fracture
4. Tensile loading produces an avulsion fracture
5. Combined loading such as bending and axial loading, which together produce an oblique fracture.

Taken together with the degree of fracture displacement and comminution, the fracture pattern suggests the direction and amount of force applied during the injury. From the degree of injury an extrapolation can be made that predicts the amount of soft tissue damage associated with the fracture.

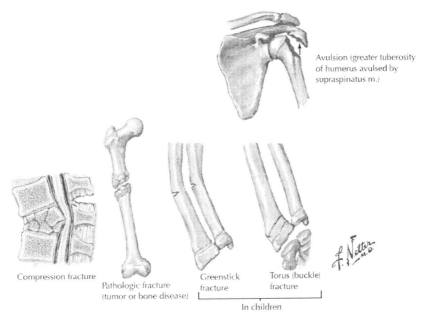

Avulsion (greater tuberosity of humerus avulsed by supraspinatus m.)

Compression fracture

Pathologic fracture (tumor or bone disease)

Greenstick fracture

Torus (buckle) fracture

In children

Fig. 2.4 Descriptive terms for typical fracture patterns. (Netter images reprinted with permission from Elsevier. All rights reserved)

Soft Tissues

As mentioned above, a number of soft tissues can be damaged. They include the periosteum, blood vessels, nerves, muscles, tendons, and ligaments. The types of injury involving them are covered in the following sections.

Vascular Injury

Vascular injuries associated with fractures are relatively rare. When arterial injuries occur, it is always an emergent situation. Injury to arterial vessels is uncommon because these vessels are elastic and mobile. The vessels can be damaged when they are either inelastic as in atherosclerosis or fixed by soft tissue structures. The most frequent arterial injury is an intramural hematoma in which signs of arterial disruption are present. Injury to the artery is classically associated with several specific fractures involving injuries such as clavicle fractures, supracondylar humerus fractures (especially in children), and knee dislocations. Because of the irreparable damage to the vessel wall, a vein graft or prosthesis is usually required for repair.

The most common form of a vascular injury is a compartment syndrome. Increased pressure within a fascial compartment can cause muscle necrosis in a relatively short period of time. In the front of the leg, for example, the anterior compartment is bounded by the tibia, the syndesmotic membrane, the fibula, and the fascia overlying the tibialis anterior muscle. Since none of these four bound-aries can be stretched, the contents of the compartment – that is, the tibialis anterior muscle among others – will necrose from increased pressure due to accumulated fluid occurring after trauma. This can cause muscle necrosis and nerve damage in a relatively short period of time. Early diagnosis is essential. Clinical findings and evaluation methods, such as compartmental pressure monitoring, assist in the diagnosis of a compartment syndrome. The earliest and most reliable diagnostic indicator of compartment syndrome is pain out of proportion on exam, particularly with passive stretch of the muscles in the involved compartment. Once the diagno-sis is confirmed, immediate surgical release of the compartment via fasciotomy is required.

Nerve Damage

Typically, a nerve is compressed, contused, or stretched due to a fracture or other injury. Classic examples include radial nerve injury secondary to fractures of the distal humerus and sciatic nerve injury following posterior fracture dislocations of the hip. The types of neural injuries are as follows:

1. Neuropraxia. Death of the axon does not occur. The most common mechanism is nerve stretch and usually improves by itself in weeks to months. The nerve is anatomically intact and physiologically nonfunctional.
2. Axonotmesis. Axonotmesis is an anatomic disruption of the axon in its sheath. Improvement follows regeneration, the axon growing at a rate of 1 mm a day along the existing axonal sheath.
3. Neurotmesis. This is an anatomic disruption of the nerve including the sheath. Surgical repair is required if recovery is to occur.

Muscle Injury

In any fracture or dislocation there is always some associated muscle damage. The extent of this damage and the effects vary depending on the direction of force and the amount of energy imparted to the limb during fracture. Rarely complete transection of the muscle belly can occur. More often a partial tear or contusion occurs. Myositis ossificans is a specific complication of muscle contusion in which heterotopic bone forms within the damaged muscle or in normal muscle after traumatic brain or spinal cord injuries. The quadriceps and brachialis are specifically predisposed to develop this complication.

Ligament Tears

Ligaments regulate the movements of bones that form a joint. Damage to these structures are called sprains. Complete disruption can result in a joint dislocation in the acute setting and instability of the joint in the long term. The strength of ligaments is constant throughout life.

Age is an important determinant of the injury type that results from the application of a traumatic force. At any given age, the "weak link," or the first structure to fail, varies; it could be bone, ligament, or cartilage growth plates. Once growth plates close, ligaments are the most likely structures to fail in an injury. Ligamentous strength is relatively constant throughout life. With aging, there is a decrease in cancellous bone volume and an increase in cortical bone porosity. With increasing age, therefore, bone becomes weaker; hence, ligament and cartilage injuries are less likely than bone injuries. Thus the same mode of loading can produce different injury patterns depending on the age of the patient. A lateral force, such as a tackle in football or a blow by an automobile on the outer side of the knee, is likely to cause a fracture through the distal femoral growth plate in a 12-year-old, a tear of the medial and anterior cruciate ligaments in a college football player, and a compression fracture of the lateral tibial plateau in a 70-year-old man.

Classic Fractures

A number of classic fracture types have been described in the literature. They are defined in the sections below.

Incomplete Fractures

An incomplete fracture, typical in a child, is one that traverses only a portion of the bone. Two variations have been described. A "greenstick" fracture occurs in the diaphyseal portion of a long bone. Separation of the cortex only occurs on the tension side of the bone. The compression side of a greenstick fracture remains intact. The other common type of incomplete fracture is the torus or buckle fracture. This type of fracture occurs in the metaphyseal region of a bone. In a torus fracture, the compression side of bone fails and the tension side remains intact, creating impaction of the cancellous bone.

Stress Fractures

These are fractures resulting from repetitive loading – each load being below the endurance limit, but through accumulated stress creates a level of force that causes a bone to fail. These injuries are typical in the proximal tibia, the second metatarsal, and the femoral neck. They may heal if the cause of the force ceases soon enough – that is, if the patient stops the repetitive activity for a period of time. Stress fractures of the femoral neck especially those located on the tension side of the bone are predisposed to displacement and are usually treated with surgical stabilization. They usually present as complaints of groin pain in runners. A high index of suspicion in evaluating these patients can avoid catastrophic complications.

Pathologic Fracture

These are fractures that occur through abnormal or diseased bone. Among the more common examples are those that occur due to tumors, osteomyelitis, or osteoporosis.

Physeal Fractures

In children, a fracture through the cartilaginous growth plate is a common event. The Salter-Harris classification system precisely characterizes these injuries. Physeal fractures heal very rapidly. They may be complicated by complete or incomplete growth arrest, producing shortening or angular deformity of the limb.

Intraarticular Fractures

Intraarticular fractures disrupt the joint surface and articular cartilage. Intraarticular fractures can specifically be complicated by joint stiffness and/or the development of posttraumatic arthritis. The basic tenets of intraarticular fracture treatment are anatomic reduction, rigid fixation, early motion, and progressive weightbearing.

Fracture Healing

The biology of fracture healing is not particularly complex and parallels that of any non-ossified tissue. Essentially, fracture healing occurs in three phases (Fig. 2.5):

1. Vascular phase. This begins at the time of the injury and proceeds through the development of a soft callus. Following an injury, a hematoma forms. The hematoma is infiltrated by cellular elements, which in turn lay down collagen and cause hematoma organization. This is followed by a vascularization, in which the organized hematoma is vascularized by small arterial extensions. The end result of the vascular phase is the development of a soft callus.
2. Metabolic phase. This stage begins about 4–6 weeks after the injury. During this period, the soft callus is reworked by a number of specific cellular elements to produce a firm, hard callus satisfactory for meeting some mechanical demands. There are biochemical changes in pH and oxygen tension during this phase that direct fracture healing.
3. Mechanical phase. This phase begins once a hard callus is present, which is then manipulated according to the rules of Wolff's law. Essentially, mechanical stress is required to produce skeletal remodeling during this phase and ultimately to produce a solid, mechanically strong bone.

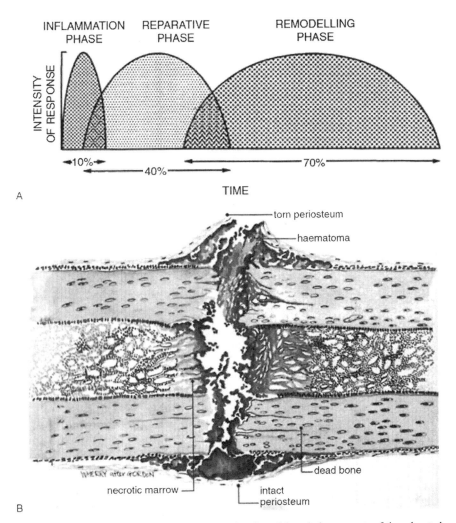

Fig. 2.5 Phases of fracture healing. (**a**) An approximation of the relative amounts of time devoted to inflammation, reparative, and remodeling phases in fracture healing. (**b**) The initial events involved in fracture healing of long bone. The periosteum is torn opposite the point of impact and, in many instances, is intact on the other side. There is an accumulation of hematoma beneath the periosteum and between the fracture ends. There is necrotic marrow and dead bone close to the fracture line. (**c**) Early repair. There is organization of the hematoma, early primary new bone formation in subperiosteal regions, and cartilage formation in other areas. (**d**) At a later stage in the repair, early immature fiber bone is bridging the fracture gap. Persistent cartilage is seen at points most distant from ingrowing capillary buds. In many instances, these are surrounded by young new bone. (From Cruess RL. Healing of bone, tendon, and ligament. In: Rockwood CA Jr, Green DP, eds. *Fractures in Adults*, 2nd ed, vol 1. Philadelphia, PA: Lippincott; 1984. Reprinted with permission)

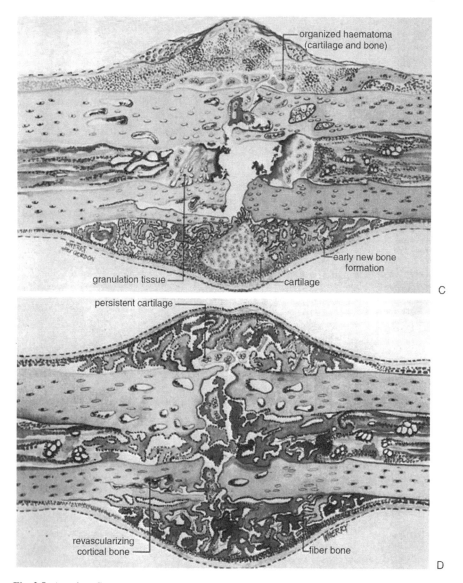

Fig. 2.5 (continued)

Evaluation of the Patient with Skeletal Trauma

The complete evaluation of a trauma patient is complex and beyond the scope of this chapter. A number of specific points germane to the orthopedic trauma patient are listed below:

1. History of injury. The mechanism and severity of trauma are important to focus the physical exam and identify commonly associated injuries.
2. Occupation and activity level of the patient. Taking these into account is frequently helpful in determining surgical versus nonsurgical treatment, as well as subsequent rehabilitation.
3. Deformity and swelling. These must be carefully evaluated to identify fractures, joint dislocations, or soft tissue injuries.
4. Joint motion. Pain on motion may indicate intraarticular joint involvement.
5. Neurovascular status. It is imperative that the neurovascular status of the extremity be carefully evaluated to document neurologic deficits and to identify surgical emergencies such as compartment syndrome or arterial disruption.
6. Integrity of the skin. This is an absolute. Great care needs to be taken to be sure that there is no violation of the skin over the area of the fracture site. An open fracture requires urgent surgical care.

Fractures: The Principles of Treatment

All fracture treatments require that two basic goals be accomplished: (1) reduction of the fracture and (2) maintenance of that reduction. Different techniques may be used for achieving these two goals. Reduction of a fracture can be accomplished by

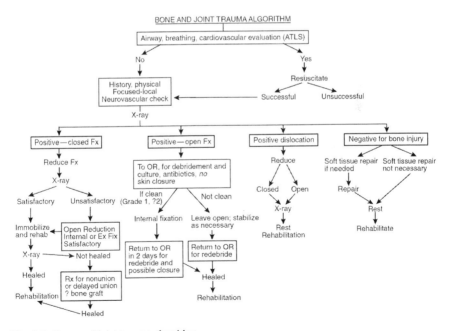

Fig. 2.6 Bone and joint trauma algorithm

closed manipulation, skeletal traction, or surgical fixation. Following reduction, the fracture site must be immobilized so that the fracture will heal in the optimum position. Immobilization can be achieved with external methods such as casts, splints, and external fixators; with internal methods, using various devices such as screws, plates, and intramedullary rods; or through the maintenance of the patient in traction (Fig. 2.6).

Orthopedic Emergencies

There are relatively few orthopedic problems that mandate immediate intervention. However, those that do exist truly represent emergent situations. They are open fractures, dislocations of major joints, and fractures associated with vascular injury, including compartment syndrome.

Complications of Fractures

There are a number of complications that can occur following fractures and joint dislocations. These include the following:

1. Problems of union

    a. Malunion: a bone that heals in poor functional position.
    b. Delayed union: a fracture that does not heal within the usual time frame.
    c. Nonunion: a fracture that has not healed and will not heal because it has lost the "biological drive" to heal. In some instances a pseudarthrosis, or "false joint," develops as a result of a nonunion.

    A number of reasons can be found for why fractures do not heal. Excessive motion, infection, steroids, radiation, age, nutritional status, and devascularization locally are all causes of delayed healing. The two most common types are hypertrophic and atrophic nonunions. Hypertrophic nonunions possess the biology but lack the stability to unite. On the other hand, atrophic nonunions lack the biology to heal. Recognizing the type of nonunion is important to establish a treatment plan. Hypertrophic nonunions generally require more stable fixation, whereas atrophic nonunions may require bone grafting or other modalities, such as electrical or ultrasound stimulation.
2. Stiffness and loss of motion. These commonly occur following many types of fractures – especially intraarticular fractures, in which arthrofibrosis is known to occur. Additional problems such as bony blocks, loose bodies in the joints, nerve palsies, and posttraumatic arthritis may exacerbate this problem.

3. Infection. Open fractures increase the risk of subsequent sepsis. Closed fractures treated operatively are also at risk. The use of implants increases the risk of infection simply because they provide a substrate for the microcolonization of certain bacteria. Some bacteria have the unique ability to sequester themselves under a slime layer called a glycocalyx, which protects the bacteria from immune attack and antibiotics and makes cultures difficult to obtain. In addition, the presence of necrotic bone contributes to infection risk.

4. Myositis ossificans. This problem, previously mentioned under the heading of muscle injury, is the development of bone in an abnormal location, usually as the result of muscle trauma.

5. Avascular necrosis. Certain bones are predisposed to this complication due to a tenuous or retrograde blood supply. The bones most at risk are the head of the femur, the talus, and the scaphoid.

6. Implant failure. This is more a complication of treatment rather than of the fracture itself. Placed under enough load or repetitions of load (termed fatigue), any implant will eventually fail. Fixation of fractures begins a race between fracture healing and implant failure. Implant failure may lead to a fracture nonunion and frequently leads to revision surgery.

7. Chronic Regional Pain Syndrome (reflex sympathetic dystrophy). This unusual and disastrous complication is typically seen following trivial trauma that causes the development of abnormal sympathetic tone. The mechanism is unknown, but may be associated with a partial nerve injury or contusion. The patient develops an exquisitely painful, tender extremity with erythema, bone resorption, and loss of motion. Prognosis depends on early recognition of the syndrome and timely initiation of countermeasures such as sympathetic blocks and aggressive physical therapy. Stellate ganglion blocks are used for involvement of the upper extremity, whereas epidural blocks and lumbar sympathetic blocks are used in the lower extremity.

Fractures and Dislocations by Region: The Upper Extremity

The Shoulder Region

The physician must keep in mind that the purpose of the bones and joints of the upper extremity is primarily that of putting the hand where the patient needs it – that is, allowing the hand to do its work.

Fractures of the Clavicle

The clavicle is the first bone to ossify, and it does so by intramembranous ossification. Fractures of the clavicle are very common in children and occur either by direct trauma or a fall on the outstretched hand. Fractures of the clavicle in children heal reliably. The usual treatment consists of a figure-of-eight brace or bandage that holds the shoulders back and tends to reduce the clavicle. Anatomic reduction is unnecessary and impractical. A sling is also a treatment option. In a child, a callus sufficient to provide pain free activity will develop in 2–3 weeks. The biggest dangers are over-treatment with prolonged immobilization or a rigid bandage that interferes with the circulation of the extremity.

In adults, fractures of the clavicle require greater trauma than they do in children. Therefore, significant soft tissue injuries occur more often. Because of the proximity of the subclavian vessel behind the clavicle and the proximity of the brachial plexus, a careful neurovascular evaluation is imperative. Treatment is usually conservative, using the figure-of-eight brace or a sling. The patient must be told at the time of the fracture that a "bump" or swelling may be noticed after healing has occurred. Not all clavicular fractures heal primarily. If a nonunion develops, it is treated with internal fixation and bone grafting. Complete healing of a fractured clavicle in the adult will frequently take 3 months or more. Open fracture requires operative debridement. Occasionally, the skin is "tented" over a spike of bone and surgical treatment is undertaken to prevent skin compromise. Fractures of the clavicle occurring lateral to the coracoclavicular ligaments may require open reduction and internal fixation if displaced due to the high rate of nonunion (Fig. 2.7).

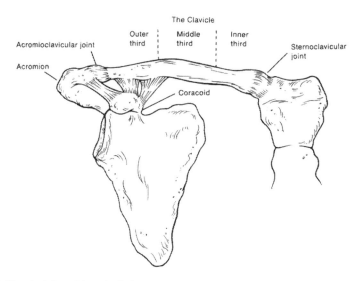

Fig. 2.7 The clavicle and its articulations

Fractures of the Proximal Humerus

Fractures just distal to the head of the humerus, through the area called the surgical neck, are extremely common in elderly osteoporotic bone. Healing of these fractures, even with some displacement, is rarely a problem. Shoulder stiffness following treatment of this injury may severely impair function in the older patient. Therefore, treatment of this fracture includes early mobilization after a short period of immobilization. Codman's exercises are usually begun after the first week. Immobilization is commonly accomplished with a collar and cuff or sling, using the weight of the arm itself as a traction mechanism. Codman's exercises are performed by the patient holding onto a table or other steady object with the good hand, and bending 90 degrees at the waist while allowing the injured extremity to hang straight down – hence employing the pull of gravity. Circular motions of the extremity in this position (also known as pendulum exercises) are frequently adequate to minimize shoulder stiffness.

An entirely different injury is seen in the younger patient. Although the fracture pattern may be the same, the mechanism and force vary greatly. The high-energy fractures of the proximal humerus seen in younger adults are due to contact sports, motor vehicle accidents, or high-velocity falls. These injuries are often combined with dislocations of the shoulder (described below). Intraarticular fractures of the head of the humerus present a significant problem. The Neer classification (Fig. 2.8) can guide treatment of these injuries. The classification defines four segments of the proximal humerus: (1) the articular cartilage covered head, (2) the shaft, (3) the greater tuberosity, and (4) the lesser tuberosity. Any fragment separated more than a centimeter or angulated more than $40°$ is considered as a separate part. Generally speaking, if conservative treatment cannot reduce a two- or three-part fracture, open reduction with internal fixation is performed. A four-part fracture, or one in which the head fragment is split, is most often treated by the insertion of a humeral head prosthesis replacing the broken segments (Fig. 2.9). Inherent to all treatment protocols is an aggressive rehabilitation program to regain shoulder motion. Therefore, fixation must be rigid enough to allow early motion.

Glenohumeral Dislocation

Dislocation of the shoulder is a common event. The vast majority of dislocations are anterior, with the humeral head displacing anterior to the glenoid. Dislocations result when the arm is forcefully abducted and externally rotated – a frequent position, unfortunately, in contact sports. This is an extremely painful condition requiring early reduction of the dislocation. If a fracture, such as the greater tuberosity, coexists with the dislocation, reduction is even more urgent. The patient presents in the emergency room with an obvious "squared" silhouette of the upper arm (the normal contour of the deltoid being altered). A careful neurologic and vascular exam is required to ensure that the axillary nerve and radial pulse are intact. The so-called autonomous zone of the axillary nerve, sensation over the lateral shoulder, must be documented in this neurological check. The trauma series of shoulder radiographs includes a true anteroposterior glenohumeral projection, a scapular lateral, and an axillary lateral. Reduction is accomplished by one of several techniques, most of which employ traction and counter-traction with the patient relaxed. Relaxation

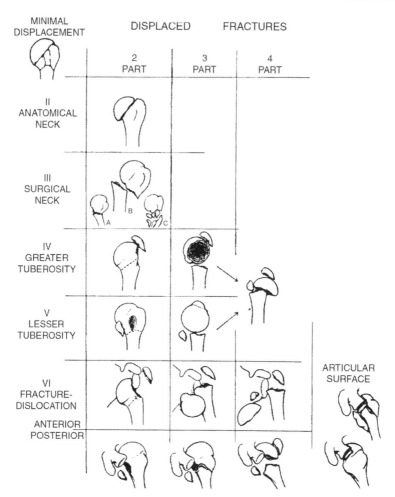

Fig. 2.8 The Neer classification of proximal humeral fractures. (From Neer CS II: Displaced proximal humeral fractures. I. Classification and evaluation. *J Bone Joint Surg.* 1970;52A: 1077–1089. Reprinted with permission)

is usually obtained in the emergency room by the intravenous administration of sedatives and narcotics. There is an immediate and dramatic decrease in pain once the shoulder is reduced. Once reduced, the neurological and vascular exams are repeated. A sling and swathe are generally adequate to immobilize and rest the shoulder; post-reduction X-rays should be taken.

Posterior shoulder dislocations account for only 4% of all dislocations and usually occur in patients during seizures or from electrocution, though occasionally they may occur in sporting events such as wrestling.

The duration of immobilization is not generally agreed upon. The classic thought that a month of immobilization will decrease the likelihood of a recurrent dislocation

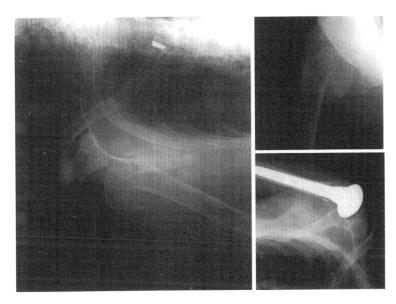

Fig. 2.9 Four-part humeral fracture

has unfortunately not proven to be the case. The percentage of shoulder dislocations that recur after the first dislocation depends on the age at which the first event
occurs. In the late teens and early twenties, the likelihood of a recurrence is very high
(80–90%). In patients over 50 years old, the likelihood of a recurrence is lower
(30–40%). Shoulder stiffness is of a greater concern in this age group; therefore,
shoulder motion should be instituted early.

In the case of recurrent dislocations in a young person, surgical reconstruction
is best performed on an elective basis. Repair of the anterior shoulder capsule and
glenoid labrum is usually required. Rotator cuff tears may occur as part of dislocations or fracture/dislocations of the shoulder, especially in the elderly. Rotator cuff
structural integrity is imperative for good shoulder function. More will be discussed
on tears of the rotator cuff in Chapter 9, The Shoulder.

Acromioclavicular Separation

An acromioclavicular (AC) separation is a ligamentous injury involving a dislocation between the distal clavicle and the acromion. Such separations are frequently
sports injuries sustained in a fall on the "point of the shoulder" and can be divided
into six classes. Type I is a sprain of the acromioclavicular ligaments without displacement. There is tenderness in that joint on palpation. A type II injury is a more
pronounced deformity of the joint, with some prominence of the distal clavicle
felt above the level of the acromion. A complete rupture of the acromioclavicular
ligament is present. The X-ray, taken with the patient standing and the arm hanging down with or without weight on it, shows the clavicle to be riding higher, but

still in continuity with the acromion. Type III acromioclavicular separations occur with rupture of both the acromioclavicular ligaments and coracoclavicular ligaments (conoid and trapezoid ligaments). The muscles that insert on the clavicle tend to pull it up superiorly, resulting in an obvious deformity. Type IV injuries involve a posterior displacement of the clavicle from the acromion. These injuries are difficult to reduce because they may protrude through the fascia of the trapezius. A type V injury is a dislocation of the AC joint, with superior displacement of the clavicle greater than twice the normal coracoclavicular distance. Type VI injuries are rare and involve an inferior dislocation of the AC joint. Type I and II injuries are treated conservatively with a sling until pain subsides enough to undergo gentle range of motion exercises and then physical therapy. Treatment of type III injuries remains controversial, with the current trend toward operative treatment. Type IV, V, and VI injuries are almost always treated operatively, with surgical stabilization of the AC joint.

Fractures of the Shaft of the Humerus

Humeral shaft fractures are common, and their patterns vary. Displacement is generally due to eccentric muscular pull with action of the supraspinatus, pectoralis major, and the deltoid determining the displacement of the proximal fragment (Fig. 2.10). The long muscles determine the displacement if the fracture is below the deltoid insertion. Treatment of the humeral shaft fracture has traditionally been conservative. Options include coaptation plaster splints, hanging arm casts, and functional braces, as popularized by Sarmiento. The functional brace is a plastic, prefabricated

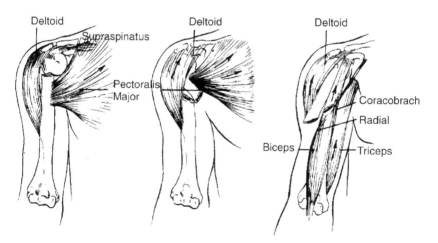

Fig. 2.10 The deformity of the humeral shaft fracture is dependent on the muscles that insert above and below the fracture. (From Epps CH Jr. Fractures of the shaft of the humerus. In: Rockwood CA Jr, Green DP, eds. *Fractures in Adults*, 2nd ed, vol 1. Philadelphia, PA: Lippincott; 1984. Reprinted with permission)

device, usually worn 6–10 weeks. It permits function of the hand while healing progresses.

In fractures at the junction of the middle and distal third of the humerus, the radial nerve is vulnerable to injury. Radial nerve function must be assessed during the physical examination. Fortunately, most of these nerve injuries are neuropraxias; hence if a radial nerve deficit is present excellent recovery can be expected. The use of plates versus intramedullary locked rods for fixation is a current controversy. Comminuted fractures of the humeral shaft are best treated with open reduction and internal fixation.

Elbow and Forearm

Supracondylar Fractures in Children

This notorious fracture in children presents a "minefield" for the orthopedic surgeon. On initial evaluation, one must be vigilant in evaluating the child for vascular compromise, specifically compartment syndrome. Missed compartment syndrome can result in a forearm muscular contracture, called a Volkmann's contracture. Angular deformities can result from inadequate reduction or growth plate injury. Because of cartilaginous growth centers (physes, epiphyses, and apophyses) around the child's elbow, diagnosis may be difficult. The inexperienced clinician may benefit from review of comparison views of the normal elbow. In an effort to minimize deformity, closed reduction and percutaneous pinning are the treatment of choice. Alternatives such as open reduction or overhead traction are less desirable options.

Closed reduction is best accomplished in the operating room with adequate anesthesia. Considering the risk of vascular compromise, these should be treated emergently. With the C-arm (fluoroscopy) in place, a closed reduction is performed and two Kirschner wires are driven across the fracture site percutaneously. A plaster splint is then used to hold the elbow initially, with cast application in several days. In 3 weeks, the pins are generally removed, and in 3 more weeks the cast is discontinued. It is normal for a good deal of stiffness to be present after initial treatment. The key to postoperative management is to tell the parents not to make the child move the elbow. If the child is left alone, a good deal of elbow motion is automatically regained in a reasonably short time. There should be no passive manipulation of the child's elbow.

Distal Humeral Fractures in Adults

These intraarticular fractures are difficult to treat and are often followed by stiffness and arthritis. Open reduction with anatomic restoration of the articular surfaces and rigid fixation of the fragments to the shaft of the humerus yields the best functional results. The ulnar nerve, because of its location, is at risk during surgery and generally has to be moved from the cubital tunnel and transposed anteriorly. It is generally agreed that if a traumatized elbow is immobilized for 3 weeks or more a

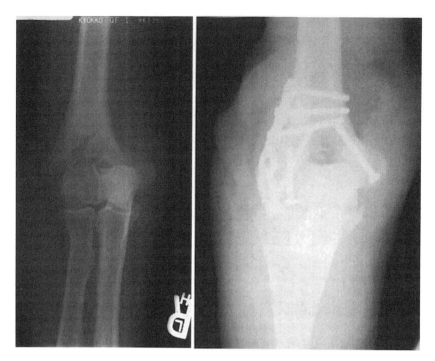

Fig. 2.11 Distal humerus fracture

poor result will follow, as the elbow is particularly prone to develop both stiffness and heterotopic ossification. A functional range of elbow motion is approximately 30–110°. This allows the hand to reach the mouth (Fig. 2.11).

Dislocation of the Elbow

Most elbow dislocations occur in a fall on the outstretched extremity. The ulna dislocates posterior to the humerus. Reduction of a posterior elbow dislocation is easily accomplished by closed means using manual traction and manipulation. Intravenous sedation and augmentation with local anesthetic injected into the joint is usually adequate for reduction. Radiographs must confirm the reduction. Short-term immobilization for comfort is all that is required. Following this, active flexion and extension are essential to regain motion. Any elbow trauma in an adult should be accompanied by a warning that a few degrees of full extension are normally lost, but that this loss will present no functional disability.

Two specific forearm/elbow injuries are often seen. The Monteggia fracture–dislocation is a fracture of the proximal ulna with a dislocation of the radial head. It requires not only alignment of the ulna but also reduction of the radial head. While closed reduction is possible in children, in adults the ulna is almost always treated by open reduction and internal fixation with a plate and screws. Radial head position must be assured with X-rays (Fig. 2.12). The Galeazzi fracture–dislocation is a fracture of the distal radius with a dislocation of the distal radio-ulnar joint. This radial fracture is treated by open reduction and internal fixation with plate and screws. The ulnar dislocation usually requires positioning of the forearm in supination to achieve reduction (Fig. 2.13).

Fig. 2.12 The Monteggia fracture–dislocation (type 1, anterior)

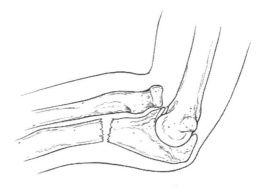

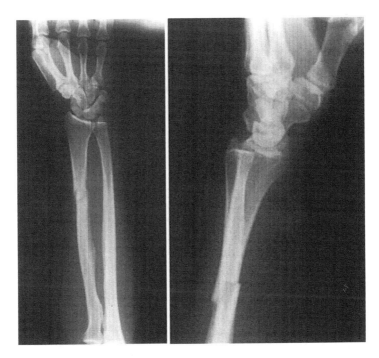

Fig. 2.13 The Galeazzi fracture

Fracture of Both Bones of the Forearm

In children, this fracture is almost always treated nonsurgically by closed reduction and immobilization in a long arm cast. Anatomic reduction is not necessary because of the excellent remodeling potential in children. Six to eight weeks of immobilization is necessary in a child. In adults, because of the concern over loss of pronation and supination and delayed union, operative treatment is indicated. Open reduction of both the radius and the ulna, done through two separate incisions and fixation with plates, is the standard treatment.

Fractures of the Olecranon

The triceps muscle inserts into the olecranon process, providing extension of the elbow joint. While nondisplaced fractures of the olecranon may be treated closed, displaced fractures are routinely opened and fixed by means of a tension band technique. Early motion is allowed after such a procedure, but lifting must await early bone consolidation, which takes at least 6 weeks (Fig. 2.14).

Fracture of the Head of the Radius (Elbow)

This common intraarticular injury usually occurs from a fall on the outstretched hand. When there is little displacement and comminution, and as long as there is no mechanical block to pronation and supination, early active motion is encouraged. For fractures with large amounts of displacement and significant comminution, or for those with mechanical blocks to motion, open reduction and internal fixation may be required. For highly comminuted, non-reconstructible radial head fractures, radial head replacement is the best option. Currently, radial head resection alone is not recommended for acute trauma.

Wrists and Hands

Wrist Fractures (Distal Radius)

Wrist fractures in children are commonly of the torus or buckle type. Reduction is occasionally necessary followed by cast immobilization for 4–6 weeks, depending on the age of the child. Another frequent fracture type, usually occurring in older children, traverses the open and actively growing physis. Typically, this is a Salter-Harris II fracture (Fig. 2.3). Reduction by closed means can be readily accomplished, and a cast is applied until healing occurs. Fractures of both bones of the distal forearm are fairly common. Closed reduction under local hematoma block anesthesia with intravenous sedatives works well. Perfect reduction is not needed because of the excellent remodeling potential of the child.

In the adult, the most frequent fracture about the wrist is the classic Colles fracture. The description in 1894 by Abraham Colles of Ireland predated the discovery of X-rays. This is a fracture of the distal radius usually seen in elderly patients, in

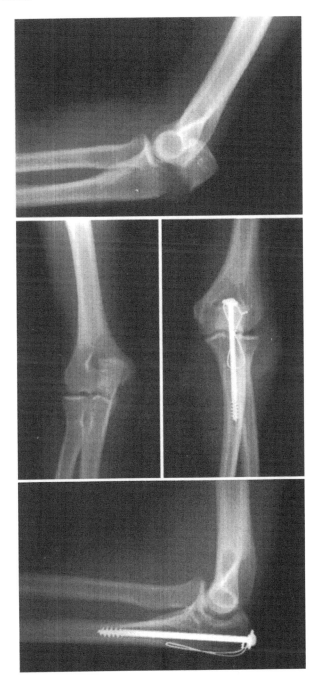

Fig. 2.14 Olecranon fracture

whom osteoporosis is common. The three classic deformities are (1) dorsal displacement of the distal fragment, (2) apex volar angulation, and (3) radial shortening. It is the latter that presents the most significant functional problem if not corrected. Although traditionally closed reduction and cast application was the treatment of choice and is frequently still employed, improvements in the contour of plating systems and the use of locking screw holes have made surgical repair a more frequent option, especially if the wrist injured is in the dominant extremity. Since these fractures usually occur with a fall on the outstretched hand, comminution is frequently encountered. A particular type of comminution is the so-called die-punch injury in which the lunate depresses a portion of the distal radius articular surface. This injury usually requires open reduction and fixation for an anatomic reduction. After elevation of the depressed fragment the construct is often supplemented with autogenous bone graft and held with a locking buttress plate. An alternative treatment method is the use of percutaneous pins to reduce the joint surface and an external fixator to hold the bone out to length. The external fixator spans the joint with two pins anchored in the metacarpals and two pins in the radius connected by an external carbon fiber bar. It is, however, quite usual for people in their upper seventies and eighties to prefer not to have an extensive operation. They will usually be satisfied with a simple closed reduction and cast immobilization. Even though the cosmetic result may not be perfect, the functional result can be quite good.

Scaphoid (Navicular) Fractures

Active young adults are vulnerable to scaphoid injury. This fracture, like many other upper extremity injuries, results from a fall on the outstretched hand. Patients often feel that they have had a sprained wrist, but a true "sprained" wrist is rare. Any patient who gives this history and has tenderness in the anatomic snuffbox of the wrist should be considered to have a scaphoid fracture and have a full series of wrist radiographs. The anatomic snuffbox is the area just distal to the radial styloid and bordered by the extensor pollicis longus dorsally and by the extensor pollicis brevis and abductor pollicis longus volarly. Radiographs of the wrist taken soon after the injury frequently may fail to reveal a fractured scaphoid. Because of the danger of nonunion at the site, it is generally accepted to treat such this fracture initially with a thumb spica cast and remove this cast 10–14 days later. At that time, clinical examination and new radiographs can confirm the presence of a fracture. A bone scan, computed tomography, or magnetic resonance imaging occasionally may be needed, if uncertainty remains. Open reduction is recommended for displaced fractures because of the high risk of malunion, nonunion, and avascular necrosis of the proximal pole of the scaphoid. Other carpal bones are usually treated simply by immobilization in a cast and generally do well.

Lunate dislocation and perilunate dislocation are uncommon injuries and require significant trauma. Aggressive operative treatment is usually required to produce a satisfactory result.

Phalangeal Fractures

In treating finger fractures, it is critical to remember to evaluate the patient for rotational malalignment. This deformity is frequently subtle so the fingers are examined in the flexed position so that the fingernails can be compared for rotational alignment. Once reduced, the hand should be immobilized in the intrinsic plus position, never in full extension. The intrinsic plus position is 20° of wrist extension, 90° of metacarpal phalangeal flexion, and full extension of all interphalangeal joints. This immobilizes the intrinsic ligaments of the hand and fingers in their longest position, preventing contractures that may restrict motion. Fractures involving articular surfaces must be openly reduced and internally fixed if any displacement is present. Otherwise severe stiffness and arthritis can result.

Gamekeeper's/Skier's Thumb

This is a common and frequently missed injury. The injury is a tear of the ulnar collateral ligament of the metacarpophalangeal joint at the base of the thumb. Typically, it occurs during a fall with a valgus stress is applied to the thumb. This injury frequently results when a skier falls with a ski pole in the hand. The result, if overlooked, can be significant instability with impairment of the thumb for pinching. While partial injuries are treated with a thumb spica cast, complete injuries are best treated by surgical repair.

Fractures and Dislocations by Region: The Spine

Injuries to the spine are best understood by considering the anatomy of the spine. For descriptive purposes, the spinal column is divided into anterior, middle, and posterior columns. The anterior column includes the anterior half of the body of the vertebrae and the anterior longitudinal ligament. The middle column includes the posterior half of the body and the posterior longitudinal ligament. The posterior column includes the pedicles and the lamina (Fig. 2.15). If only one column is involved, the injury usually can be considered stable and is often treated conservatively. If two or more columns are involved, then the injury is considered unstable. Injury encompasses ligament tears as well as bone fractures. Another important consideration in treatment is the presence of neurologic compromise. Plain radiographs will reveal much of the bone damage to the columns of the spine. Computed tomography (CT) scans can reveal the impingement of bone fragments on the spinal canal. The spinal cord ends at the upper border of the second lumbar vertebra. Below this level, the cauda equina occupies the spinal canal. Magnetic resonance imaging is best used to study additional soft tissue injury.

Simple compression fractures of the anterior column of the spine are usually considered stable if the vertebral height is compressed less than 50%. If they are more than 50%, it is felt that the middle column is involved, which makes the

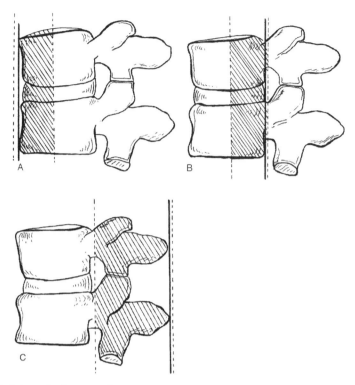

Fig. 2.15 Schematic diagrams of the three columns of the thoracolumbar spine. (**a**) Anterior column: anterior longitudinal ligament, anterior half of the body, and anterior half of the disk. (**b**)
Middle column: posterior longitudinal ligament, posterior half of the body, and posterior half of
the disk. (**c**) Posterior column: neural arch, ligamentum flavum, facet joint capsules, and the inter-
spinous ligaments. (From Bucholz RW, Gill K. Classification of injuries of the thoracolumbar
spine. *Orthop Clin North Am*. 1986;17(1):70. Reprinted with permission)

fractures unstable. Similarly, burst fractures characterized by fragments of the
vertebral body being displaced posteriorly into the spinal canal may significantly
encroach on the spinal cord. A CT scan will show the extent of encroachment.
Patients without neurological symptoms or fracture collapse on standing X-rays may
be treated with early mobilization and bracing. Patients with significant kyphosis,
neurological deficits, fracture collapse than 50%, or intractable pain may be treated
with operative fixation. Fractures of the facets and dislocations of the facets are also
encountered. Generally speaking, these are reduced and, if unstable, treated with
fixation or fusion. The first and second cervical vertebrae have unique anatomic
characteristics and are prone to specific fracture patterns. The Jefferson fracture,
Hangman's fracture, and the various odontoid fractures (Fig. 2.16) involve the
C1/C2 complex. Rigid immobilization is required for satisfactory results. Treatment
options include application of a halo brace and various open surgical techniques.

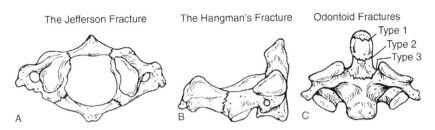

The Jefferson Fracture   The Hangman's Fracture   Odontoid Fractures

Fig. 2.16 Fractures of the atlas and axis. (**a**) The Jefferson fracture. (**b**) The Hangman's fracture. (**c**) Odontoid fractures

Fractures and Dislocations by Region: Pelvis

The unique anatomy of the pelvis presents a challenge in management when it is disrupted. The pelvis is a ring structure of three bones: two innominate bones and the sacrum. They are joined by dense, strong ligamentous structures. Each innominate bone is formed from three bones: an ilium, an ischium, and the pubis, which fuse at the triradiate cartilage at skeletal maturity. The juncture between the two innominate bones anteriorly is called the symphysis pubis. Posteriorly the innomiate bones join the sacrum through the two sacroiliac joints which are secured by dense sacroiliac ligaments.

There are two completely different types of pelvic fractures. In elderly and osteoporotic patients, minor trauma, such as a fall from a standing position, may cause a crack of the ischium or pubis. If this is the only fracture in the pelvic ring, the pelvis is considered stable. Bed rest for a few days for pain control is followed by early full weightbearing mobilization. The patient usually becomes asymptomatic within a few weeks and fully functional in a matter of 6–8 weeks.

The other type of pelvic fracture occurs following high-energy trauma. In these injuries, blood loss is often excessive and should be anticipated. These patients typically sustain multiple injures and frequently present with hemo-dynamic compromise. Mortality approaches 50% for the most severely injured patients. Initial management consists of maintaining ABCs: airway, breathing, and circulation. A multidisciplinary approach to care is coordinated by the general trauma surgeon. Early treatment in these severe life-threatening pelvic injuries centers on control of hemorrhage, which occurs following disruption of the vast pelvic venus plexus. Pelvic binders, circumferential sheets, exter-nal fixation, pelvic packing, and angiographic embolization (in cases of arterial laceration) may be employed to decrease pelvic volume, tamponade retroperi-toneal bleeding, and coagulate bleeding arteries. Once initial stabilization of the patient has occurred, definitive fixation of the pelvic ring is undertaken after 3–7 days. This is best performed by a surgeon familiar with the operative treatment of pelvic fractures. Stabilization is achieved through the use of per-cutaneous screws or open plating. Fractures of the ilium involving disruption of the acetabular articular surface with or without a dislocation of the hip are best managed by surgical acetabular reconstruction. These injuries carry a high incidence of late onset of osteoarthritis, often requiring early conversion to total hip replacement.

Fractures and Dislocations by Region: The Lower Extremity Femur

Femoral Neck Fractures

The neck of the femur is surrounded by the joint capsule. The capsule contains the veins and arteries that are the blood supply to the femoral head. The blood supply to the head is tenuous. It originates from the medial and lateral femoral circumflex arteries at the base of the femoral neck and the extracapsular arterial ring. These vessels nourish the head of the femur. Any disruption of the femoral neck is likely to interfere with the blood supply of the head of the femur. This makes fractures of the neck of the femur subject to two problems: avascular necrosis of the femoral head and nonunion. Avascular necrosis occurs in more than one-third of displaced femoral neck fractures. Nonunion, the other complication of femoral neck trauma, is related to the compromised blood supply and the instability of some femoral neck fracture patterns.

Patients with femoral neck fractures present with a shortened, externally rotated limb and have severe pain with log rolling of the limb and with axial loading. Similar to pelvic fractures, femoral neck fractures result from two broad types of injuries: those occurring in young people after high-energy trauma and those in elderly patients after simple falls. Femoral neck fractures in young patients are an orthopedic emergency. Immediate anatomic reduction and fixation help decrease the likelihood of osteonecrosis. The location and displacement of these fractures help to determine their proper treatment (Fig. 2.17). The goal is to preserve the young patient's native femoral head.

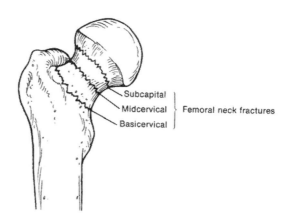

Fig. 2.17 Locations of femoral neck fractures. Displacement is important to note

In elderly patients, nondisplaced fractures are typically treated with percutaneous screw fixation and restricted weightbearing. Displaced fractures are typically treated with hemiarthroplasty or total hip arthroplasty. The decision for total hip arthroplasty is controversial as the risk of postoperative dislocation is high. The indications for total hip arthroplasty in patients with hip fractures include preexisting hip osteoarthritis and an active lifestyle. Nonoperative treatment of femoral neck fractures in elderly patients is reserved for only those special circumstances where the patient is too sick for surgery. Nonoperative treatment carries a 1-year mortality of up to 80% due to the complications of prolonged bed rest including: urinary tract sepsis, pneumonia, deep vein thrombosis, pulmonary embolism, and decubitus ulcers. Even with operative treatment in ideal candidates, in-hospital mortality after femoral neck fracture approaches 3%, and 1-year mortality may reach 20%.

Intertrochanteric Fractures

These femoral fractures occur between the greater and lesser trochanter and lie *outside* the hip joint capsule (Fig. 2.18). The blood supply to the femoral head is therefore not jeopardized by the fracture. On physical examination in the emergency room, these patients, similar to those with displaced femoral neck fractures, will manifest with shortening and external rotation of the limb. Operative fixation is the norm, and multiple options are available. The compression hip screw with side plate (Fig. 2.19) and the cephalomedullary nail are the most

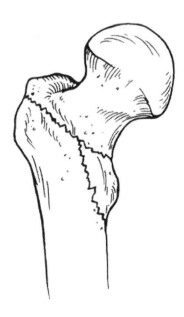

Fig. 2.18 Intertrochanteric femoral fracture. Involvement of the lesser trochanter defines an unstable fracture pattern

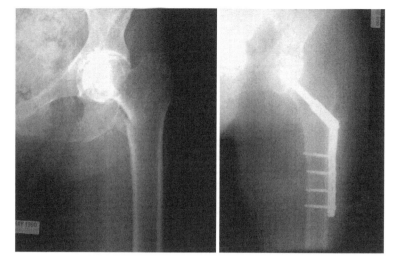

Fig. 2.19 Intertrochanteric fracture

common devices. Healing of intertrochanteric fractures is usually not a problem, as large areas of cancellous bone are loaded in compression by the fracture anatomy.

Subtrochanteric Fractures

These fractures occur distal to the lesser trochanter. They are characterized by their typical deformation pattern, which includes flexion and abduction of the proximal fragment, with adduction and shortening of the distal fragment. The pull of the iliopsoas and abductors deform the proximal fragment, while the adductors displace the distal fragment. In the younger population, subtrochanteric fractures usually follow the severe trauma of motor vehicle accidents. In the elderly, they are due to osteoporosis or a pathologic process in the subtrochanteric area. With low-energy mechanisms, transverse subtrochanteric fractures should be considered pathologic until proven otherwise. Fixation is generally accomplished using an intramedullary nail with proximal and distal locking screws.

Femoral Shaft Fractures

These injuries usually follow significant trauma. In children, they are treated based upon age. Infants can be treated in a Pavlik harness, young children in spica casts, and older children and teenagers with flexible intramedullary nails. In adults, these fractures are almost always treated with intramedullary nails locked at both ends. These are inserted using minimally open techniques. While the fractures do not heal

Fig. 2.20 Femoral shaft
fracture

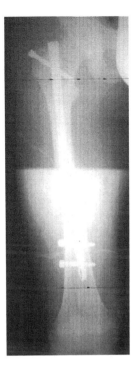

faster with this treatment, the devices share load with the bone, thereby stimulating biologic drive for fracture healing and allowing the patient to bear weight as
tolerated (Fig 2.20).

Dislocation of the Hip

Typically, this occurs from the impact between the dashboard and the knee in a
motor vehicle accident. This impact drives the hip out posteriorly and, as expected,
will often damage the blood supply to the head of the femur as well as the sciatic
nerve. The sciatic nerve lies directly posterior to the femoral head. Dislocations of
the hip are surgical emergencies. Reduction within 6–8 h decreases the incidence of
osteonecrosis. An associated PCL tear in the knee can be seen with this injury.

Fractures About the Knee

Distal Femoral Fractures

Fractures of the lower end of the femur in the region of the condyles may be supracondylar or Y- or T-shaped, the latter types entering the joint. If displaced, these

fractures are treated surgically, with the goal being to obtain an anatomic reduction of the articular surfaces. The reconstructed articular surface is then affixed to the distal femoral shaft. Anatomic restoration is necessary to prevent significant traumatic arthritis of the knee. Rigid fixation is necessary to allow early motion. Weightbearing is delayed for 3 months, but early motion begins within a couple of days of the fixation process. Frequently, a continuous passive motion (cpm) machine is valuable in the early stages to maximize motion.

Fractures of the Tibial Plateau

These intraarticular fractures typically occur on the lateral side of the tibia after a valgus load, for example, when a pedestrian is struck by the bumper of a car. Treatment depends on the degree of displacement and comminution. Nondisplaced fractures may be treated by restricting weightbearing and initiating early motion. Displaced fractures are best treated surgically, including anatomic reduction of the articular surface and stable fixation to the shaft of the tibia. Early motion is begun, but full weightbearing should be delayed for 8–12 weeks.

Fractures of the Patella

The patella is a sesamoid bone that gives the quadriceps mechanism a mechanical advantage in knee extension. If the fracture is nondisplaced, closed treatment in a cast for up to 6 weeks is preferred. However, for displaced fractures open reduction and internal fixation is the treatment of choice. As in the fracture of the olecranon (Fig. 2.21), a tension-banding procedure achieves reliable fixation. In extremely comminuted fractures, a patellectomy may be the only option to avoid an irregular patellar surface that would result in painful traumatic arthritis of the patellofemoral joint.

Dislocation of the Knee

This injury is the result of very severe trauma. When a patient gives a history that the "knee came out of place," the injury is usually not a knee dislocation, but rather a patella dislocation or anterior cruciate ligament tear. True dislocation of the knee is a very serious injury notable for producing arterial damage to the popliteal vessels. The popliteal artery is fixed anatomically at the level of the proximal tibia by the interosseous membrane and, therefore, is at great risk when the knee dislocates. Arteriography can be performed following immediate closed reduction of the dislocation if vascular compromise is suspected. The results of angiography will then determine whether arterial repair is necessary. If gross instability is present following this injury, an external fixator bridging the knee may be necessary until definitive ligament repair is performed. Multiple ligament injuries are the norm after knee dislocations. Ligamentous repair is usually necessary after early emergent reduction, external fixation, and vascular management have been accomplished.

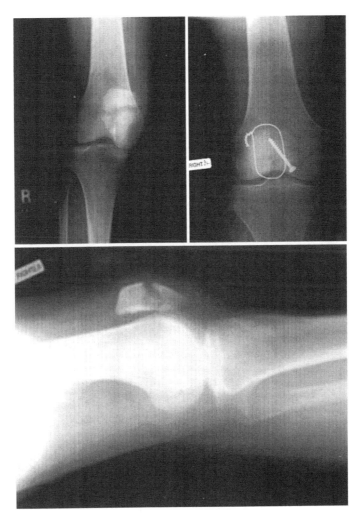

Fig. 2.21 Patella fracture

Fracture of the Tibial Shaft

Diaphyseal fractures of the tibia are predisposed to nonunion. The blood supply of the tibial shaft is less than robust, especially at the junction of the middle and distal thirds where a vascular watershed exists and the muscle envelope is deficient over the anteriomedial surface of the bone. The time to fracture union is prolonged, generally taking 20 weeks. Nondisplaced or minimally displaced tibial fractures are generally treated by the application of a long leg cast. When early healing has occurred, a shorter, so-called patella tendon bearing cast may be applied. Operative treatment options include percutaneous or open plating for proximal or distal fractures, external fixation for open shaft fractures or comminuted metaphyseal fractures, and intramedullary nailing with locking screws for displaced and comminuted shaft fractures. As with long bone fractures in other locations, intramedullary nailing allows relatively early weightbearing and functional return.

Ligamentous Injuries to the Knee

The knee is a relatively incongruous joint that is stabilized through an elaborate system of ligaments. The major contributors are the medial and lateral collateral ligaments and anterior and posterior cruciate ligaments. Sports-related ligament injuries of the knee are common, especially the anterior cruciate ligament. Generally speaking, ligament tears are first treated conservatively with a period of immobilization, followed by physical rehabilition. After 6 weeks of rehabilitation, emphasizing muscle strengthening and return of motion, repair of the torn ligaments is usually considered (see Chapter 6, Sports Medicine).

Fractures Around the Ankle

Fractures of the malleoli are termed "ankle" fractures by convention and involve the distal end of the fibula (lateral malleolus), the medial malleolus, and the posterior malleolus of the tibia. The most commonly used classification system for ankle fractures is the Lauge-Hansen (Fig. 2.22) classification system. The first word in each category describes the position of foot at the time the force was applied. The second word denotes the anatomic direction of the load. This system is based on cadaver study and likely does not apply adequately to all ankle fractures. It also has limited value in directing treatment. However, its use is nearly ubiquitous in practice and serves as a common basis of communication between surgeons.

While a nondisplaced fracture of the lateral malleolus with a stable ankle joint may be treated by a simple below-the-knee cast, displaced ankle fractures with an unstable ankle joint are typically treated with open reduction and internal fixation. The primary goal of treatment for ankle fractures is anatomic restoration and maintenance of reduction of the mortise of the ankle. Following operative fixation, patients are generally kept non-weightbearing for 6 weeks, followed by gradual return to weightbearing and initiation of range of motion and strengthening exercises.

Fractures of the distal articular surface of the tibia are categorized separately from common ankle fractures. They typically result from axial loading injuries and involve a significant amount of articular cartilage damage. They are termed pilon (French for "pestle") fractures and represent a difficult management problem. They are frequently complicated by posttraumatic arthritis of the ankle, nonunion, and infection. The posttraumatic arthritis that can develop following these injuries may necessitate an ankle fusion for pain relief.

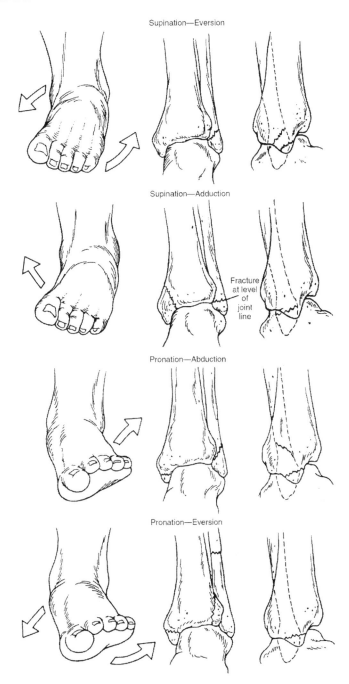

Supination—Eversion

Supination—Adduction

Fracture
at level
of
joint
line

Pronation—Abduction

Pronation—Eversion

Fig. 2.22 Lauge-Hansen classification of ankle fractures

Fractures and Soft Tissue Injuries of the Foot

Fractures of the Calcaneus

This calcaneus is unique in that it is predominately a cancellous bone (not unlike the vertebral body) that is nevertheless ideally adapted to withstand a great deal of load. If that load is applied vertically and quickly, however, crushing of the calcaneus can occur as the talus impacts down into the calcaneus. This produces injury to the subtalar joint and ultimately results in subtalar stiffness and arthritis no matter what type of treatment is provided. Concurrent fractures of the lumbar spine are not infrequent and should be considered in all patients presenting with calcaneus fractures. Treatment of the calcaneus fracture is often nonsurgical with early range of motion and restricted weightbearing. In expert hands, open reduction and fixation may give a better result for fractures involving the articular surface of the subtalar joint in a high demand and highly motivated patient.

Fractures of the Talar Neck

Like the scaphoid bone of the wrist, the talus in the ankle is unusual in that it has a retrograde blood flow. As such, fractures through the neck of the talus are frequently complicated by osteonecrosis of the talar dome. Historically, this injury was called "aviator's astragalus" due to its nearly exclusive occurrence in downed pilots during World War I. In an effort to minimize complications, emergent open reduction and internal fixation with delayed weightbearing are usually recommended for displaced fractures.

Ankle Sprains

Ankle sprains are the most common of all orthopedic injuries. The anterior talofibular ligament, calcaneofibular ligament, the deltoid ligament, and the syndesmotic ligaments are the major ligaments involved in ankle stability. The anterior talofibular ligament is the most commonly injured ligament. Rest, ice, compression, and elevation (RICE regimen) is the standard treatment for a few days following a sprain. The use of a walking cast or fracture boot with the foot in slight dorsiflexion often allows patients to assume their normal activities much faster than without support. Formal casting may predispose to muscular atrophy of the calf and stiffness. Early motion and rehabilitation begin as the pain and swelling begin to subside. Immediate open suturing of torn ligaments, even in athletes, is controversial. Various braces are commonly used to prevent reinjury during activities of daily living in the first several weeks following injury and during athletic activities for a period of 2–3 months. Pain, swelling, and/or disability lasting more than 2 months after a significant ankle sprain is rare and other pathologic processes should be considered, such as an osteochondral defect of the talus.

Achilles Tendon Rupture

Often occurring in the middle-aged athlete, Achilles tendon ruptures result from push-off sports. Patients often describe a loud pop and a feeling that they were hit in the back of the leg during a jump. Typically patients are able to bear weight on the leg, but have posterior pain and swelling and calf weakness. The Thompson test, performed on a prone patient, consists of squeezing the calf with the knee flexed. Normally the foot should plantarflex with this maneuver when an Achilles tendon is intact. These injuries may be treated by conservative means using a cast in plantar flexion; surgical repair is more common.

Lisfranc Dislocation of the Tarsometarsal Joints

The Lisfranc joint, which is the joint between the tarsal bones and the second metatarsal, can commonly be injured by trauma resulting in forced dorsiflexion or abduction of the forefoot. Football players and drivers stepping on the brake in motor vehicle collisions are common examples. This injury, unfortunately, is frequently missed, with significant consequences. If the examiner is unsure that the pain and tenderness are located in the midfoot rather than the ankle or hindfoot, comparison foot X-rays with weightbearing may be useful. These injuries usually result in lateral dislocation or subluxation of one or more of the metatarsal bones, and if not treated (thus restoring anatomical congruity of the joint), midfoot arthritis may result.

Distal Foot Fractures

Most fractures of the metatarsals and phalanges are treated conservatively. Metatarsal fractures may be immobilized in a walking boot or treated with a hard-soled shoe. Fractured toes generally are treated by "buddy" taping the toe gently to its neighbor for support. Fifth metatarsal fractures represent different clinical entities and are treated according to fracture location. Specifically, fractures of the fifth metatarsal base (proximal) at the level of the 4–5 metatarsal articulation are prone to nonunion because this area represents a vascular watershed. These Jones fractures are treated with a non-weightbearing until clinically healed. This typically requires 6–8 weeks of casting. In high-performance athletes, intramedullary screw fixation is an alternative method of treatment.

Summary and Conclusions

Orthopedic trauma can range from an isolated soft tissue or bony injury to multiple musculoskeletal injuries in a patient with life-threatening injuries to many organ systems. Knowledge of anatomy and common orthopedic injuries is important to ensure optimal treatment. A basic understanding of musculoskeletal radiology of the axial and appendicular is a key part of the evaluation. Most important is a systematic approach to examining every orthopedic patient to make the diagnosis so that an appropriate and timely referral for treatment is instituted.

Operative Technique: Femoral Intramedullary Nailing

Intramedullary nailing has become the fixation of choice for most orthopedic trauma surgeons for a wide variety of fractures of the femur. Depending upon the specific device design and insertion point used, intramedullary nails can be used to treat femoral neck, intertrochanteric, subtrochanteric, midshaft, and distal femur fractures. A general technique guide for antegrade insertion of a femoral intramedullary nail is described here. The femur is a curved bone, and most femoral nails are manufactured with a certain amount of curve to more closely approximate the anatomy of an average adult femur. However, considerable anatomic variation is present in a normal population and can cause a variety of intraoperative problems.

The patient is positioned in a manner to allow access to the entire involved thigh and flank, at least from the level of the ipsilateral iliac crest to the knee joint line. Additionally, the patient should be positioned in a way to allow intraoperative fluoroscopy in both the anteroposterior and lateral planes, from the femoral neck down to the knee. The procedure can be performed in a supine or lateral position on a variety of different surgical tables with the leg draped free or in traction.

The subcutaneous border of the femur is palpated along the lateral thigh, and the outline of the greater trochanter is marked on the skin. A skin incision, inline with the femoral shaft, approximately 4–5 cm proximal to the tip of the trochanter, is made down to fascia. Blunt dissection is then carried down to the greater trochanter and superior neck of the femur. Next, either a guidewire or a sharp trocar is used to define the entry point of the nail, which for standard nails is located in the piriformis fossa. This is a small recess at the postero-superior border of the femoral neck at its junction with the greater trochanter. Nail entry at this point allows direct targeting down the femoral shaft. Correct insertion point should be verified using fluoroscopy.

Once the entry point is obtained, the proximal femur is reamed with a large drill over the guidewire down to the level of the lesser trochanter in order to prepare a canal large enough to accept the nail. A long guidewire is then placed down the length of the femoral shaft across the reduced fracture site. Reduction of the fracture is often the most difficult and time-consuming portion of the case. Various methods and tools are available to aid in reduction. The appropriate nail length is measured from the guidewire. A series of reamers of increasing size are inserted over the guidewire to increase the inside diameter of the femoral canal, allowing for insertion of a larger, stiffer nail, and to facilitate nail passage. Biofeedback from the sound and feel of the reamers is used to determine the appropriate nail diameter; generally this is 1.5–2 mm less than the reamed diameter.

The nail is inserted over the guidewire and appropriate position is verified using fluoroscopy. Strict attention is paid to the rotation of the nail as it is inserted to facilitate the placement of interlocking screws later in the procedure. Ideally the nail will be flush with the superior neck surface and extend to the level of the distal physeal scar.

The nail is now locked into position with proximal and distal transverse screws. This is accomplished by predrilling and percutaneously inserting screws through holes in the nail in the coronal plane at the proximal and distal ends. Most nail designs are inserted using an attached jig which allow for accurate targeting of proximal locking holes. Distal locking holes, however, must be targeted by using accurate intraoperative fluoroscopy and precise technique. Once proximal and distal locking screws are inserted, fluoroscopy is used to verify position of all hardware and the wounds are irrigated and closed.

At the completion of every femoral nailing procedure, the femoral neck must be imaged in multiple planes (especially internal rotation) to ensure that an intra-operative femoral neck fracture has not occurred. Additionally, the limb should be compared to the contralateral side for length and rotation. Malreduction is a common problem in comminuted fracture patterns where it is difficult to determine the correct length and rotation of the bone. Finally, a thorough knee exam should be performed to rule out ligamentous injury. Many femur fractures occur by mechanisms that involve knee injuries, such as the knee striking the dashboard in a motor vehicle collision, and should be suspected in any femur fracture.

Suggested Reading

1. Beaty JH, Kasser JR, eds. *Rockwood and Wilkins' Fractures in Children.* 5th ed. Philadelphia, PA: Lippincott; 2002.
2. Bucholz RW, Heckman JD, eds. *Rockwood and Green's Fractures in Adults.* 5th ed. Philadelphia, PA: Lippincott; 2002.

Chapter 3
Orthopedic Infections

Mark W. Zawadsky and Steven C. Scherping, Jr.

Introduction

Musculoskeletal infections can prove to be extremely difficult to diagnose and treat due to the wide variation in clinical presentation, which often mimics other diagnoses such as trauma, and due to the potential for serious complications that can have lifelong implications for the patient. Unrecognized infections can destroy normal joint anatomy and function, threaten limb viability, and potentially be fatal if not recognized and treated appropriately. The most important aspect of caring for patients with a musculoskeletal infection is to come to an early and accurate diagnosis. When proper treatment is administered in a timely manner, most musculoskeletal infections can be effectively treated and the morbidity minimized with an excellent outcome for the patient. A missed infection can lead to irreversible impairment and loss of mobility for the individual, along with significant costs for society due to loss of productivity and requirements for medical care.

Pathophysiology of Osteomyelitis

The pathogenesis of osteomyelitis, although conceptually similar in all cases, may vary depending upon the age of the host, duration of infection, etiology of infection, and type of host response to the infection. Osteomyelitis is often classified using these parameters which can assist in defining the severity of infection, identifying a mode of treatment, and assessing the potential for recovery. Duration of infections is often divided into either acute or chronic osteomyelitis. This also applies to infections involving the joints, such as a septic arthritis. Although the distinction is somewhat arbitrary, acute osteomyelitis is usually considered to occur within the first 6 weeks following inoculation, with chronic osteomyelitis being greater than 6 weeks.

M.W. Zawadsky (✉)
Department of Orthopedic Surgery, Georgetown University Medical Center, 3800 Reservoir Road NW, Pasquerilla Healthcare Center (PHC), Ground Floor, Washington, DC 20007, USA
e-mail: mark.w.zawadsky@gunet.georgetown.edu; mwzl@hotmail.com

S.W. Wiesel, J.N. Delahay (eds.), *Essentials of Orthopedic Surgery*,
DOI 10.1007/978-1-4419-1389-0_3, © Springer Science+Business Media, LLC 2010

The development of bone and joint infections takes place via one of two basic mechanisms involving either exogenous or hematogenous pathways. Exogenous delivery involves direct inoculation of the bone from either trauma, surgery, or a contiguous focus of infection. Hematogenous delivery is via the vascular system into either osseous or synovial tissue producing a localized focus of infection. Local tissue compromise (i.e., surgery or fracture) or systemic tissue compromise (i.e., diabetes or chronic disease) is often associated with an increased risk of bone infection by either method.

Two patterns of response are noted and are often dependent on the infecting organism. Pyogenic organisms elicit a rapidly progressive course of pain, swelling, abscess formation, and aggressive bone destruction. A gram-positive staphylococci is a classic example of an organism that may produce a pyogenic response. In contrast, less aggressive nonpyogenic organisms invoke a more insidious granulomatous reaction, classically seen with acid-fast bacilli. Age of the host is important in that differences in bone vascular anatomy between adults and children slightly alter the mechanism of hematogenous delivery. In addition, children are susceptible to different organisms depending upon their age.

Exogenous osteomyelitis usually involves a clearly identified anatomic site, is usually inoculated with pyogenic organisms, and is often polymicrobial – frequently in association with foreign debris. This is often caused by trauma, such as open fractures or puncture wounds, or through direct inoculation during surgery due to a compromise in sterile technique. The bacteria are inoculated into a compromised local environment, with bone and soft tissue disruption providing ample amounts of necrotic and devascularized material favorable for bacterial growth. In addition, tissue devascularization prevents host response mechanisms from reaching bacterial colonies, thereby permitting unchecked proliferation.

Once a bone infection is recognized by the host, several steps are undertaken. Initial host response to both the injury and infection includes an acute inflammatory reaction with activation of inflammatory and immunological pathways. Inflammatory elements serve to destroy bacteria and remove nonviable material. Humoral and cellular immunologic mechanisms act to recognize specific bacteria and subsequently confer immunity to prevent further bacterial dissemination. The inflammatory response is initiated with increases in blood flow and vascular permeability, with the delivery of polymorphonuclear leukocytes responding by chemotaxis. The leukocytes phagocytize and destroy bacteria and nonviable tissue. Mononuclear cells arrive within 24–48 h and assist in eradication of bacteria and removal of necrotic bone. As a large number of these cells arrive and die, pus can be formed, with an abscess often being clinically appreciable.

Eventually, granulation tissue surrounds the infected area in an attempt to wall off the infection. Further isolation is achieved as chronic avascular fibrous tissue is produced around the infected area. Finally, reactive bone formation can occur to further sequester the infection from the host. Within the infected region, dead bone is often prominent, and this is commonly termed the "sequestrum," while the reactive bone is known as the "involucrum." Unfortunately, this sequestered area is isolated from host defense mechanisms due to the avascular fibrous tissue and can permit the continued proliferation of bacteria, leading to a chronic infection.

Pivotal to treatment of osteomyelitis is obtaining a better understanding of how bacteria achieve a foothold in either damaged tissues or on surgical implants. Adhesion to the surface of tissue cells and implants depends on the physical characteristics of the bacteria, the fluid interface, and the substratum. Initially, bacteria arrive at random near a damaged tissue or implant surface by direct contamination, contiguous spreading, or hematogenous seeding. All surfaces, regardless of whether they are tissue- or implant-derived, acquire a glycoproteinaceous conditioning film when exposed to a biological environment. This surface is anionic and initially repels bacteria, whose surface is also anionic. However, attractive forces (van der Waals) in conjunction with hydrophobic molecules on the exposed substrate and the bacteria increase the duration of bacterial juxtaposition to permit the formation of irreversible cross-links between bacteria and host surfaces. Following anchorage of the bacteria, proliferation occurs with formation of a polysaccharide slime layer. The biofilm or slime layer is comprised of bacterial extracapsular exopolysaccharides that bind to surfaces, thereby promoting cell-to-cell adhesion, microcolony formation, and layering of the microorganisms. Additional species of bacteria may attach to the surface of the biofilm, resulting in syntropic interactions between differing bacteria. Thriving bacterial colonies may be dispersed by sheer force, enabling a localized colony to establish secondary sites of infection (Fig. 3.1).

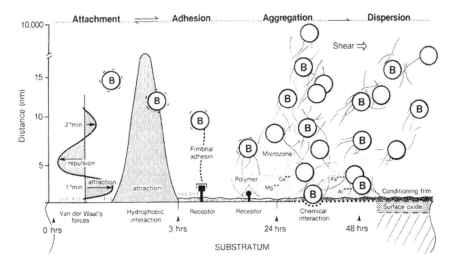

Fig. 3.1 Molecular sequence in bacterial (*B*) attachment, adhesion, aggregation, and dispersion at substratum surface. A number of possible interactions may occur depending on the specificities of the bacteria or substratum system (graphics, nutrients, contaminants, macromolecules, species, and materials). (From Gristina AG, Naylor PT, Myrvik QN: Mechanisms of musculoskeletal sepsis. *Orthop Clin North Am.* 1991;22(3):363–371. Reprinted with permission)

Bacterial attachment in production of biofilms can lead to antibiotic resistance. Initially felt to be due to problems of antibiotic diffusion through the biofilm, more current theories center on decreased metabolic rates and phenotypic changes in surface-adherent bacteria. Therefore, bacteria on surfaces or within microcolonies appear to be physiologically different from free-floating organisms, which may, in part, convey antibiotic resistance. Treatment of osteomyelitis involves the disruption of these bacterial colonies. This is best achieved with aggressive debridement of nonviable tissues such as dead muscle and necrotic bone, and with the disruption and dilution of bacterial colonies and their associated biofilm by means of extensive surgical irrigation. In the case of osteomyelitis involving a prosthesis or fracture implant, it is often necessary to remove either the prosthesis or implant to eradicate the infection.

Pediatric Infections

Acute Hematogenous Osteomyelitis

The most common etiology for acute osteomyelitis in the pediatric population is via hematogenous inoculation. The vascular anatomy of children's long bones can predispose them to hematogenous inoculation and proliferation of bacteria. The nutrient artery of long bones enters through the cortical bone to divide within the medullary canal, ending in small arterioles that ascend toward the physis (Fig. 3.2). Just beneath the physis, these arterioles bend away from the physis and empty into venous lakes within the medullary cavity. The acute bend in these arterial loops serves as points of diminished blood velocity promoting sludging of bacteria directly under the physis. In addition, phagocytic capability and reticuloendothelial function may be depressed in these vascular loops, promoting the establishment of bacterial colonies. Trauma, often associated with the emergence of osteomyelitis in children, may actually promote bacterial seating and proliferation in metaphyseal sites.

As previously discussed, an established infection will result in the delivery of inflammatory cells and, if the infection remains untreated, purulent material will be produced. This pus can spread in one of three ways: through the physis, toward the diaphysis, or through the adjacent bony cortex (Fig. 3.3). This purulent material tends to seek the path of least resistance through the metaphyseal cortex to form a collection of subperiosteal pus. Though this is the most common route of egress, younger children (less than 1 year) with intact transphyseal vessels may demonstrate epiphyseal spread with the development of epiphyseal abscesses.

In older children, the developmental of a subperiosteal abscess results in devascularization of the bone both from thrombosis of the endosteal blood supply and from the stripping away of the overlying periosteum. The periosteum, which is extremely thick and loosely adherent in children, is not easily penetrated. In the devascularization process, it is lifted off of the bone, with the inner cambium layer producing a layer of new bone. In this case, the devascularized bone is termed the "sequestrum," with the reactive periosteal bone being the "involucrum" (Fig. 3.4). A cellulitic phase precedes abscess formation, with medical management alone being successful

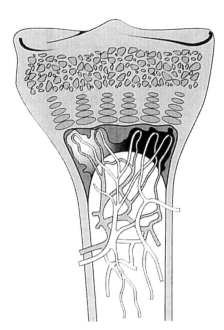

Fig. 3.2 The location of hematogenous osteomyelitis is explained by the bone anatomy in the metaphysis of the long bone. Nonanastomosing capillary ends of the nutrient artery make sharp loops under the growth plate and enter a system of large venous sinusoid, where the blood flow becomes slow and turbulent. A localized abscess can develop and the microenvironment is altered leading to spread of the infection throughout the metaphysis. (From Mader J, Kumar R, Simmons D, Calhoun. Atlas of Infectious Diseases: Skin, Soft Tissue, Bone, and Joint Infections. Edited by Gerald Mandell (series editor), Thomas P. Bleck. ©1995 Current Medicine Group LLC)

to cure the infection. Once an abscess forms, surgical debridement and irrigation is necessary to remove the nonviable bone, reduce the bacterial population, and provide for a vascularized tissue bed for antibiotic delivery. As the majority of pediatric infections emanate via hematogenous seeding from other sites, the specific organisms may differ depending upon the child's age. The vast majority of osteomyelitis in children is secondary to *Staphylococcus aureus* (90%). In neonates, the most common organisms include *S. aureus*, group B Streptococcus, and gram-negative organisms.

Diagnosis and Treatment

A careful history and physical examination combined with an index of suspicion is necessary to diagnose osteomyelitis. Invariably, patients present with pain from one to several days' duration, with the typical onset of pain being fairly rapid. The pain is generally severe enough to limit or entirely restrict movement and use of the involved extremity. Older patients may be able to assist in localization of the pain, although the clinician must be capable of identifying potential sites of referred

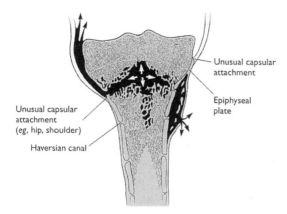

Fig. 3.3 The infection may proceed from the metaphysis laterally through the Haversian and Volkmann canal systems, perforate the bony cortex, and separate the periosteum from the surface of the bone. When this occurs in the presence of medullary extension, both the periosteal and endosteal circulations are lost and large segments of dead cortical and cancellous bone, termed sequestrum, are formed. The infection may also spread down the intramedullary canal. Because of the anatomy, the joint is usually spared unless the metaphysis is intracapsular such as in the hip or shoulder. Cortical perforation at the proximal radius, humerus, or femur infects the elbow, shoulder, or hip joint, respectively, regardless of the age of the patient. (From Mader J, Kumar R, Simmons D, Calhoun J. Atlas of Infectious of Diseases: Skin, Soft Tissue, Bone, and Joint Infections. Edited by Gerald Mandell (series editor), Thomas P. Bleck. ©1995 Current Medicine Group LLC)

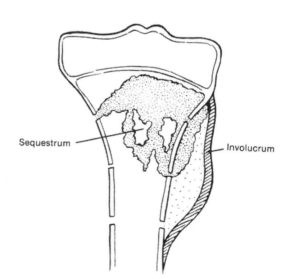

Fig. 3.4 Sequestered fragments of dead bone and periosteal new bone, or involucrum, may be seen on radiographs

pain such as knee pain in the presence of hip osteomyelitis. Children are usually irritable and febrile and often give a history of generalized malaise. Uncovering a potential site of a concomitant infection, such as a recent upper respiratory or ear infection, may provide the clinician with an etiology for hematogenous spread. Physical examination is extremely important, with localized swelling and tenderness often characterizing the physical exam. Care must be taken to gain the child's confidence and to proceed in a slow, nonthreatening manner when examining the patient. Examination of an uncooperative and agitated child can be extremely frustrating for both the clinician and the patient, making interpretation of physical findings difficult at best.

Laboratory results are extremely important in diagnosing and treating osteomyelitis; however, they do not replace a complete history and physical examination. A complete blood count with differential, an erythrocyte sedimentation rate (ESR), and a c-reactive protein study is imperative, as these are typically elevated. It must be emphasized that not all patients suffering from osteomyelitis present with a classic clinical history, physical findings, and laboratory values. Presentation at early onset may preclude a large amount of soft tissue swelling and pain or an elevated sedimentation rate or white blood cell (WBC) count. An elevation of the c-reactive protein value may occur early in the process, but it is nonspecific. Notably, a normal WBC count in the presence of an osteomyelitis is not unusual and therefore must be interpreted in the context of the entire clinical setting. Diagnosis in neonates may be especially problematic due to the immaturity of their immune system, which may not be able to mount an identifiable host response.

Plain radiographs should be obtained of all involved areas and include adjacent joints to accommodate for referred pain. Unfortunately, initial radiographs may be negative, except for soft tissue swelling, since the characteristic changes of osteomyelitis require 10–14 days to be appreciated. After 2 weeks, increasing radiolucency and a periosteal reaction are generally visible, with bone sclerosis, sequestra, and involucrum formation occurring much later (6 weeks or more).

Bone scanning can serve as a valuable tool in the identification of osteomyelitis. Technetium (Tc^{99}), coupled with methylene diphosphonate, is attracted to areas of rapid bone turnover. Though nonspecific, it exhibits sensitivity for identifying areas of accelerated bone formation or destruction. Unfortunately, it is less than 80% accurate when used to evaluate acute hematogenous osteomyelitis. This may be due, in part, to local thrombosis of vascular channels or devascularization of bone cortices, thereby preventing delivery of the isotope to these surfaces. In fact, a cold scan, in the face of an aggressive bone infection, is indicative of a high degree of bone necrosis and is a poor prognostic indicator for recovery. Bone scanning may be helpful in cases of multifocal infection found in neonates or when the exact site is not readily identifiable such as seen in the pelvis. It must be remembered that bone scanning does not obviate a good clinical and physical examination.

The use of magnetic resonance imaging (MRI) in osteomyelitis continues to evolve and has become an important diagnostic tool. This modality is an excellent means of diagnosing osteomyelitis even in its early phases. It does, however, have the distinct drawback that many children will require intravenous (IV) sedation or anesthesia in order to obtain an adequate study and has high costs.

Bone aspiration is the best means of clinically identifying the presence of a bone or joint infection as well as any organisms associated with it. Aspiration should be performed immediately following the diagnosis or strong suspicion of osteomyelitis and directed toward the area of maximal swelling and tenderness. A large bore stiletted needle (18- or 16-gauge spinal needle) should be used to prevent plugging of soft tissue, bone, or thickened purulent material in the tip. Both subperiosteal and intramedullary sites must be aspirated. In addition, using a second needle, one should consider aspirating the adjacent joint if clinically indicated. Local anesthesia is given, with the needle being easily drilled through the soft metaphyseal cortex. If purulent material is obtained, the fluid is sent for immediate gram stain and culture. The presence of pus necessitates that the patient undergo an operative irrigation and debridement. However, antibiotics should be started immediately following aspiration with these initial cultures serving to direct later modifications to organism-specific antibiotic coverage. The initial antibiotic choice is often based upon the "best guess" of the infecting organism. In patients who are not allergic to penicillin, a semisynthetic penicillin that is beta-lactamase-resistant should be chosen. Good initial choices include oxacillin or nafcillin, with penicillin-allergic patients often being treated with cefazolin. The optimal length of therapy is still under debate, with a regimen of 3 weeks of IV antibiotics, followed by 3 weeks of oral therapy often being acceptable. In the event that purulent material is not aspirated, sterile saline can be injected, aspirated, and sent for culture in the hope of identifying an organism. Bacteriostatic saline should not be used as this may inhibit bacterial growth. In cases in which no frank purulent material is aspirated, surgery is usually not indicated, as there is no pus to decompress or necrotic bone to debride. In this setting the administration of antibiotics is the mainstay of treatment. In the face of a negative aspirate, MRI and bone scans may provide more useful information in delineating the cause for bone pain.

Chronic infections are uncommon in children, as patients usually present early in the course of the disease. These patients almost invariably require surgical intervention to debride sequestrated tissues. Complications are high in this setting, from both the disease process and the surgical procedure, and include pathological fracture and physeal arrest.

Pediatric Septic Arthritis

Acute septic arthritis may develop from hematogenous sources or more commonly from extension of adjacent foci of osteomyelitis into the joint. Susceptible joints are those in which the metaphysis is intraarticular, such as seen in the hip and shoulder where bacteria are afforded an avenue for dissemination (Fig. 3.5). Though relatively uncommon, septic arthritis can rapidly destroy articular surfaces and,

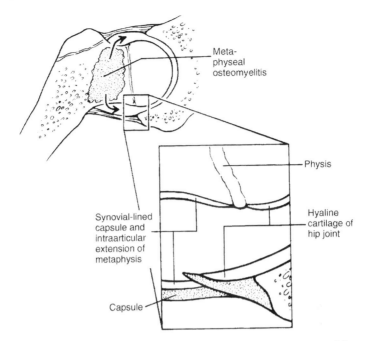

Fig. 3.5 Schematic representation of the immature hip. Metaphyseal osteomyelitis spreads by direct extension into the hip joint

Table 3.1 Common pathogens and recommended treatment for septic arthritis

Age group	Probable organisms	Initial antibiotic choice
Neonate	Group B strep, *S. aureus*, gram-negative coliforms	Penicillin, oxacillin, and gentamicin
Infants and children (4 weeks–4 years)	*S. aureus*, *H. influenzae*, group B strep, group A strep	Cefuroxime
Children (>4 years)	*S. aureus*	Oxacillin or cefazolin
Adolescent	*N. gonorrhoeae*	

therefore, must be definitively excluded at symptom onset. Depending upon the age of the patient different organisms prevail as likely pathogens (Table 3.1).

Diagnosis and Treatment

Clinical presentation and physical findings are often similar to those seen with acute osteomyelitis (Fig. 3.6). However, patients tend to be sicker with higher temperatures, more pain, and an extremely high ESR. Patients are extremely reluctant to move the involved extremity or infected joint, often positioning the joint so as to

Fig. 3.6 Acute osteomyelitis
and septic arthritis
management algorithm

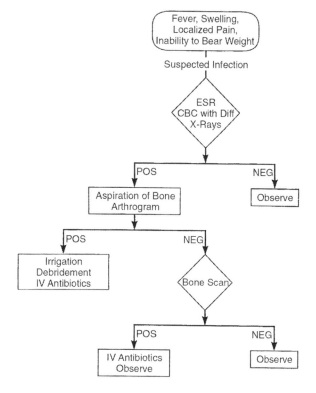

maximally relax the surrounding joint capsule. For the hip, this is usually flexion abduction and external rotation. For the knee, this tends to be roughly 30° of flexion. Radiographs will demonstrate a joint effusion and associated soft tissue swelling. Occasionally, adjacent bone involvement may be appreciable.

Joint aspiration is mandatory for diagnosis, with immediate gram stains and cultures being obtained of the joint fluid. The fluid should be analyzed for cell count and differential, for protein and glucose levels, and for the presence of crystals. In addition, the adjacent metaphysis and subperiosteum should also undergo aspiration, as these are often sites of contiguous spread to the joint. In the majority of cases the joint aspiration will demonstrate a WBC count in excess of 50,000 and may often exceed 100,000 in severe cases. The white blood cell population is usually comprised of polymorphonuclear leukocytes, comprising up to 90–95% of the cells in fulminant cases. On occasion, circumstances may require the clinician to inform the laboratory of the possible organism as special techniques may be necessary to obtain bacterial growth. Haemophilus influenza is difficult to culture and must be incubated in a CO_2 environment. Because the percentage of organism retrieval has been reported by some series to be between 70 and 85%, blood cultures should also be obtained. Additional clues to possible infection include an elevated protein or a decreased glucose level in the joint aspirate.

Aspiration of accessible joints, such as the knee, shoulder, and ankle, can usually be performed at the bedside using appropriate analgesia and sterile techniques. However, inaccessible sites, such as the hip, may require that the patient undergo fluoroscopically directed aspiration. Requiring the patient to be sedated, this procedure is performed either in the radiology or in the operating room setting. If a septic arthritis is suspected, the initial aspiration can be performed in the operating room under general anesthesia, to be followed by immediate open debridement and irrigation upon confirmation of the presence of pus or organisms. It is important to be assured that joint fluid has been sampled, with an arthrogram being necessary in the case of hip aspiration to confirm needle position. As with osteomyelitis, a negative aspiration can be followed by sterile saline flushing to obtain an adequate sample for culture.

As a joint is considered a closed cavity and a joint infection an abscess, drainage of the joint is mandatory. Some controversy still persists as to whether septic arthritis can be adequately decompressed with serial aspirations, thus avoiding surgery. Despite the controversy, open surgical drainage is favored in most instances given the disadvantages of serial joint aspiration, including repeated trauma to the joint, higher risk for inadequate decompression, and repeated exposure of the surrounding bony structures. In addition, the joint must be readily accessible, which precludes the hip from being treated with serial aspirations. An infected hip joint is considered an operative emergency. The risk of avascular necrosis is especially high in the hip, as the blood supply is intracapsular and can be disrupted by intraarticular fluid secondary to a high intracapsular pressure. Reexamination of the joint is necessary following surgery or aspiration to be assured a purulent material has not reaccumulated.

Another more recent trend has been the use of arthroscopic debridement techniques. The minimal soft tissue trauma with arthroscopic debridements has led to widespread use in acute infections. The role of these techniques in subacute or chronic infections in which a more aggressive synovectomy may be necessary is less clear. Regardless of the method employed, the goals of treatment still hold true – namely, adequate decompression of all purulent material, irrigation of both bacteria and host lysozymes from the joint, and debridement of nonviable tissues.

Intravenous antibiotics are initiated immediately following acquisition of joint fluid. Again, antibiotic choice is based upon the suspected pathogens. Compared to treatment of osteomyelitis, the antibiotic course for septic arthritis is usually shorter (4 weeks), with 2 weeks of IV antibiotics followed by an additional 2 weeks of oral therapy.

Figures 3.7–3.10 show the plain radiographs and MRIs of a child who presented with right hip pain after a minor fall and skin abrasion. He had a subtle limp but was able to bear weight on his right leg. He was afebrile and his lab values only showed a mild elevation of his ESR with a normal white count. The hip pain was attributed to the trauma since the initial radiographs were negative (Fig. 3.7). A repeat radiograph (Fig. 3.8) taken several days later shows a subtle lucency in the metaphyseal region just below the physis. The MRI (Fig. 3.9) shows extensive osteomyelitis in

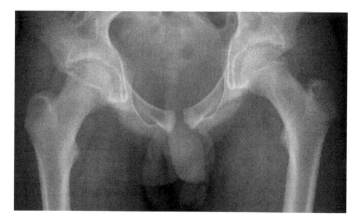

Fig. 3.7 Radiograph at presentation showing no significant bony changes

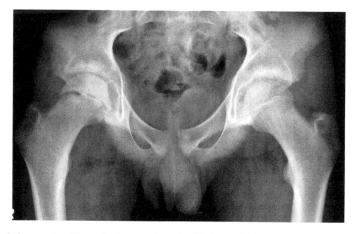

Fig. 3.8 Subsequent radiograph at approximately 10 days which now shows a lucency in the metaphyseal region just below the physis

the metaphyseal region with extension into the hip joint itself after penetrating the cortex, leading to a large effusion and damage of the articular cartilage. A radiograph (Fig. 3.10) taken after several surgical irrigation and debridement procedures shows significant destruction of the joint itself leading to a painful and abnormal hip joint with significant disability at a young age. This tragic case points out the need for a high level of clinical suspicion for an infectious process even when the classic presentation is not present.

Fig. 3.9 An MRI image which shows extensive osteomyelitis throughout the metaphyseal region and a large joint effusion indicating that the infection has penetrated the intracapsular portion of the cortex and entered the joint itself

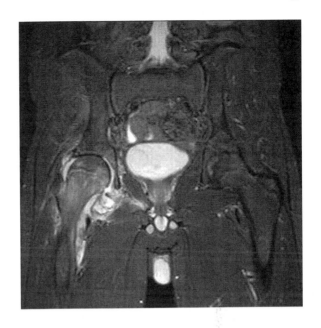

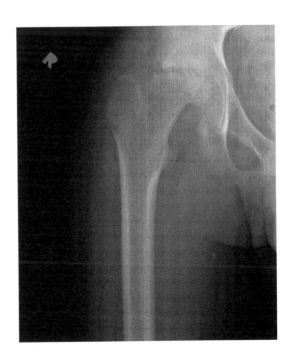

Fig. 3.10 A follow-up radiograph demonstrating extensive damage to the joint with bony collapse

Adult Osteomyelitis

Management of osteomyelitis involves consideration of several patient variables: physiologic, anatomic, and psychosocial. It is important to weigh all of these variables to assess and classify the patient's level of infection, and thereby formulate a treatment plan with reasonable goals. At the initiation of treatment it must be determined whether the infection is simple or complex, whether the goal of therapy is palliative or curative, and whether the patient would be better served by an amputation as opposed to a limb-sparing procedure. Host factors may adversely affect wound healing in cases of malnutrition, immune deficiency, malignancy, and diabetes, amongst others. Local factors, such as chronic lymphedema, venous stasis, major vessel disease, or extensive scarring, may also play a role. The Cierny–Mader classification has been developed to assist surgeons in classifying and selecting various modalities of treatment and to assist in predicting outcomes (Fig. 3.11). Local extent of disease is classified as medullary, superficial, localized, or diffuse osteomyelitis. Medullary involvement is entirely endosteal and does not require bone stabilization following debridement. Superficial osteomyelitis only involves the outer cortex and again does not require bone reconstruction following local excision of infected material. Localized osteomyelitis combines types I and II, thereby necessitating full thickness cortical resection to effectively debride the bone. Though segmental instability is avoided, bone grafting techniques may need to be employed to reestablish bone continuity and subsequent stability. Type IV osteomyelitis results in widespread cortical and endosteal involvement, requiring a segmental resection to eradicate the infection. Diffuse osteomyelitis is mechanically unstable both before and after debridement and requires bone reconstruction to attain stability.

Host variables are stratified with regard to physiologic capacity to withstand infection, treatment, and disease morbidity. A-hosts are normal healthy patients. The B-host has a local (B^L), a systemic (B^S), or a combined local and systemic ($B^{L/S}$) compromise. The C-host, because of severe systemic problems, is not a treatment candidate. Treatment of C-hosts may potentially result in greater patient morbidity following treatment than it would prior to intervention.

Surgical treatment of osteomyelitis involves three main facets: (1) extensive debridement, (2) vascular soft tissue coverage, and (3) bone stabilization. An aggressive debridement is crucial to achieving successful eradication of osteomyelitis. All nonviable tissue must be removed to prevent residual bacteria from persistently reinfecting the bone. Removal of all adherent scar tissue and skin grafts should be undertaken. In addition, a high-speed burr can be used to debride the cortical bone edges until punctate bleeding can be appreciated, demonstrating a healthy vascular supply. Multiple cultures of all debrided material should be obtained in order to identify the infecting organisms. The patient may require several debridements until the wound is considered to be clean enough to accept soft tissue coverage. Soft tissue reconstitution may involve a simple skin graft, but often requires a local transposition of muscular tissue or vascularized free tissue transfers to effectively cover the debrided bone segment. These muscle flaps provide a fresh bed of vascularized tissue to assist in bone healing and antibiotic delivery. Finally, bone stability must

Stage I
(Medullary osteomyelitis)

Necrosis limited to medullary contents
    and endosteal surfaces
Etiology: Hematogeneous
Treatment:
    Early: Antibiotics/host alteration
    Late: Unroofing, intramedullary reaming

Stage II
(Superficial osteomyelitis)

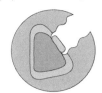

Necrosis limited to exposed surfaces
Treatment:
    Early: Antibiotics/host alteration
    Late: Superficial debridement/coverage,
        possible ablation

Stage III
(Localized osteomyelitis)

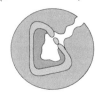

Well marginated and stable before and
    after debridement
Etiology: Trauma, evolving stages I and II,
    iatrogenic
Treatment:
    Antibiotics/host alteration
    Debridement, dead space management
    Temporary stabilization, bone graft optional

Stage IV
(Diffuse osteomyelitis)

Circumferential and/or permeative
Unstable prior to or after debridement
Etiology: Trauma, evolving stages I and II
    and III, iatrogenic
Treatment:
    Antibiotics/host alteration
    Stabilization-ORIF, external fixation (Ilsizarov)
    Debridement, dead space management
    Possible ablation

Fig. 3.11 Treatment summary of the Cierny–Mader classification system in osteomyelitis. (Mader J, Kumar R, Simmons D, Calhoun J. Atlas of Infectious Diseases: Skin, Soft Tissue, Bone, and Joint Infections. Edited by Gerald Mandell (series editor), Thomas P. Bleck. ©1995 Current Medicine Group LLC)

be achieved, with bone grafting being undertaken when necessary to bridge osseous gaps. Cancellous and cortical autografts are commonly used, with vascularized bone transfer (vascularized free fibular, iliac, and rib grafts) being occasionally necessary. Though technically demanding, vascularized bone grafts can provide a fresh source of blood flow into previously devascularized areas of bone.

The recent advent of bone distraction has been used in lieu of bone grafting or complex soft tissue procedures. Application of a small pin (Ilizarov) or half-pin external fixator with sequential bone distraction following a cortical osteotomy can produce columns of bone that fill segmental defects. As distraction is carried out, the soft tissues regenerate along with the bone to cover the newly generated tissue. Recent results appear to be encouraging, as these patients appear to achieve greater success rates for limb sparing as compared to patients undergoing more conventional bone replacement techniques.

Septic Arthritis

As with children, septic arthritis can develop from hematogenous sources, direct inoculation, contiguous soft tissue infection, or periarticular osteomyelitis. Several factors may predispose patients to septic arthritis including trauma, systemic corti-costeroid use, preexisting arthritis, and joint aspiration. As with children, *S. aureus* is the most common pathogen isolated from infected adult joints (44%). *Neisseria gonorrhoeae* is another common adult pathogen, with a reported incidence of 11%. The most commonly involved joints are the knee (40–50%), the hip (20–25%), and the shoulder and ankle (10–15%). In IV drug abusers, the sternoclavicular, sacroil-iac, and manubriosternal joints are common sites, with *Pseudomonas aeruginosa* often being isolated.

Adult patients present in a manner similar to children in that pain, swelling, and a decreased range of motion are frequent complaints. Workup involves rou-tine laboratory tests, blood cultures, and joint aspirations. The appearance of the synovial fluid, as well as the white blood cell count and the percentage of polymorphonuclear cells, can assist in the diagnosis, with cultures of the fluid being mandatory (Table 3.2). In adults, it is even important to carefully evaluate the

Table 3.2 Synovial fluid

Examination	Normal	Noninflammatory	Inflammatory	Septic
Appearance	Transparent	Transparent	Opaque Translucent	Opaque Yellow to green
Viscosity	High	High	Low	Variable
White cells/mm^3	<200	<200	5000–75,000	>50,000
Polymorphonuclear cells (%)	<25%	<25%	>50%	>75%
Culture	–	–	–	Often positive
Associated conditions	–	Degenerative joint disease Trauma Neuropathic Pigmented villonodular synovitis Systemic lupus erythematosus Acute rheumatic fever	Rheumatoid arthritis Crystal-induced arthritis Seronegative arthritis Systemic lupus erythematosus Acute rheumatic fever	Bacterial infections Compromised immunity

Source: Esterhai JL, Gelb I: Adult septic arthritis. *Orthop Clin North Am.* 1991;18:503–514; Reprinted with permission

joint aspirate for crystals associated with gout and pseudogout, as a crystal-induced arthropathy can appear quite similar to a septic arthritis.

Treatment of an adult with a septic arthritis requires aggressive irrigation and debridement utilizing either arthroscopic techniques or an open arthrotomy. Antibiotics are often delivered initially via parenteral routes, with patients being switched to oral therapy when demonstrating clinical improvement in conjunction with maintaining high bactericidal titers of at least 1:8.

Open Fractures

By definition an open fracture involves exposure of fractured bone to the extracorporeal environment, thus increasing the risk of bone contamination from foreign debris and bacteria. In addition, open fractures are often associated with severe soft tissue damage, devascularization, and devitalization of bone fragments, further increasing the susceptibility of the bone to infection. Open fractures are often graded on the degree of fracture comminution and the degree of soft tissue disruption. Though not universally accepted, the Gustilo–Anderson classification is widely used due to ease of application and prognostic ability. It is divided into three grades based upon the size of the soft tissue wound, with grade III fractures being further subdivided. Other factors that place fractures into the grade III category include severe contamination, such as farm or barnyard injuries, or shotgun wounds. The three grades are defined as follows:

Grade I: Less than 1 cm soft tissue wound
Grade II: Between a 1- and 10 cm soft tissue wound
Grade III: Greater than 10 cm soft tissue wound and further subdivided into A (soft tissue wound with sufficient remaining tissues to provide bony coverage), B (severe soft tissue compromise such that either a rotational or a free flap will be necessary to provide for bony coverage), and C (arterial laceration requiring surgical repair).

Open fractures are considered operative emergencies and need to be taken to the operating room as soon as the patient is considered medically stable enough to tolerate surgical intervention. With rare exception, patients should be taken to the operating room within 6 h of injury. Wounds should not be explored in the emergency room, as further soft tissue damage may be incurred. Active bleeding can almost always be controlled with local compression prior to surgical exploration. Cultures taken in the emergency room setting have proven to be of little value in dictating treatment. Wounds should be assessed, gently irrigated with sterile saline while removing gross contamination, and dressed with a sterile dressing in the emergency department. Fractures should be gently aligned and stabilized with splints, although the reduction of severely contaminated fractures should be avoided in the emergency room to prevent the drawing in of foreign debris into the wound.

In addition, IV antibiotics should be given immediately upon admittance to the emergency room. A general rule with regard to antibiotic therapy is first-generation cephalosporins are given for grade I and grade II fractures. For patients with grade III fractures, a first-generation cephalosporin is given in conjunction with an aminoglycoside. If the fracture is grossly contaminated, such as in a barnyard injury, then a penicillin is added to this regimen (Fig. 3.12).

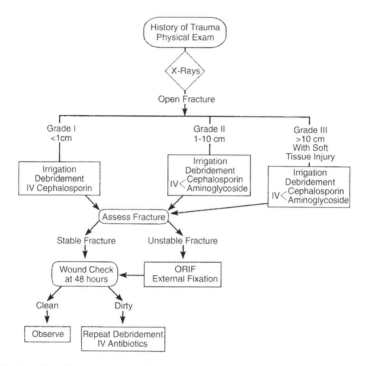

Fig. 3.12 Algorithm for management of open fractures

Assessment of the injury extent and aggressive debridement should be undertaken in the operating room in an emergent manner. Wounds should be addressed sequentially with removal of devitalized skin and subcutaneous fat followed by debridement of necrotic muscle, fascia, and devascularized bone. This prevents external contamination from being carried beyond the skin to the deeper tissues.

Another important concept is "the zone of injury." This refers to the area around the wound that has been traumatized, but can recover with appropriate management of the soft tissues and bone. Though an initial debridement should aggressively remove necrotic or devitalized tissues, marginal tissue may be preserved to permit potential recovery. If this decision is made at the initial procedure, then a second assessment and debridement should be carried out 48–72 h later. Tissues that have demonstrated local recovery can be preserved, while other tissues which have continued to remain ischemic and demonstrate evidence of necrosis should be widely excised. One cardinal rule is to never close the soft tissue laceration of an open fracture. This is potentially disastrous in that an open drainage system is converted to a closed cavity, with a greater susceptibility to develop an abscess. All open fractures should be covered with moist sterile dressings that prevent bone and soft tissue desiccation.

The principles of wound management are undisputed when dealing with open fractures, with the majority of controversies surrounding when and what to use for bone stabilization. Suffice it to say that early bone stabilization via intramedullary nailing, plate and screw fixation, or external fixation optimizes soft tissue healing and access to the extremity for examination and treatment. By preventing continued soft tissue shearing forces, with a resultant further devascularization of soft tissue, further extension of the zone of injury can be minimized. Soft tissue coverage of the fracture should be achieved within the first 5–7 days of injury. A delayed primary closure after swelling has subsided may be all that is required in grade I and grade II fractures, whereas skin grafting or soft tissue transfers may be necessary for grade III fractures. Options for soft tissue coverage should be individualized for the patient and the degree of injury.

Systemic factors play a pivotal role in promoting wound healing. It has been estimated that 50% of metropolitan medical and surgical patients have overt or subclinical protein and calorie malnutrition. Multiple injuries or even isolated fractures result in a large increase in a patient's metabolic demand needed to assist in healing. Systemic parameters that have been shown to impede soft tissue healing include a serum albumin less than 3.5 mg/dL or a total lymphocyte count less than 1500 cells/mL. Patients presenting with or developing malnutrition following multiple traumatic injuries are at increased risk of infection, delayed union, or nonunion of open fractures. Aggressive nutritional resuscitation is necessary with either oral or feeding tube supplementation or, in extreme cases, parenteral nutrition.

If osteomyelitis develops following an open fracture, then the principles of treatment for adult osteomyelitis apply with one important exception – namely, the retention of implants for fixation of the fracture. In patients who present with an infection surrounding an intramedullary nail or plate, the wound should be aggressively debrided and the implant maintained if fracture stability is being achieved. Loose implants should be removed and either replaced or substituted by another implant type; for example, an external fixator can replace a loose plate and screws. Intravenous antibiotics should be administered and directed toward isolated organisms for at least 6 weeks. Once a fracture has healed, the implant can be removed and further debridement performed as necessary. This approach reduces the complexity of treatment from an infected nonunion to an infected united bone with a better prognosis for successful healing and eradication of the infection.

Infections Associated with Joint Arthroplasty

As previously discussed, the presence of a foreign substrate, such as the surface of a total joint replacement, can provide bacteria with an excellent opportunity for binding and colonization. Unfortunately, the diagnosis of an infected joint arthroplasty can be extremely difficult. While radiographs can demonstrate subtle or even profound bone resorption surrounding implants suspected of being infected, similar changes can be seen with aseptic loosening without an associated infection. Laboratory values, though often abnormal, are also not specific for infection. However, an elevation of the WBC, ESR, and C-reactive protein is highly suspicious for infection. Aspiration still remains the best single test to identify a subclinical infection, with a sensitivity of 90%, specificity of 80%, and an accuracy of 78%. Fluoroscopy or ultrasound should be used to confirm needle localization within the joint. The use of radionuclide scanning can be utilized to diagnose joint arthroplasty infections. Studies have varied in reporting the accuracy of indium-labeled WBC and gallium scanning. At best, the accuracy of either an indium-labeled WBC scan or a combined gallium–technetium scan is approximately 80% for identifying an infected arthroplasty.

The treatment of an infected total joint arthroplasty depends on the timing of the infection. If an infection is diagnosed in the early peri-operative period, an irrigation and debridement with a poly-exchange followed by extended intravenous antibiotic treatment can successfully treat the infection while retaining the prosthesis. If the infection is acquired at a later time frame, has been present for an extended period of time (usually greater than 3–4 weeks), or involves resistant bacteria or is a multi-microbial infection, a two-stage explantation procedure is necessary. This involves the removal of the implant, including all of the cement, aggressive irrigation and debridement, placement of an antibiotic-loaded cement spacer, and at least 6 weeks of antibiotics followed by reaspiration once the patient has been off of antibiotics for at least 2 weeks. Patients with cultures negative for bacteria may undergo reimplantation at a later date. Positive cultures necessitate redebridement and another course of antibiotics prior to reimplantation. Figures 3.13–3.15 show an infected left total hip with lysis and loosening of the implant, along with a bone scan that demonstrates extensive osteomyelitis. This was treated successfully by a two-stage explantation procedure, which included a temporary antibiotic spacer placement to help maintain mobility and alignment, along with an extended course of intravenous antibiotics.

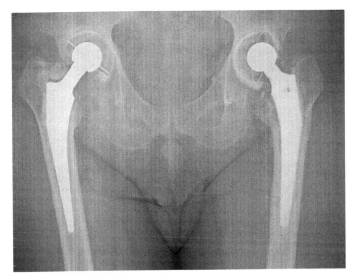

Fig. 3.13 Radiograph demonstrating extensive peri-prosthetic lysis and loosening of the implant in the left hip

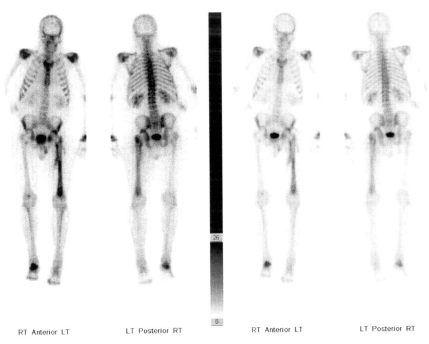

RT Anterior LT   LT Posterior RT   RT Anterior LT   LT Posterior RT

Fig. 3.14 Bone scan demonstrating uptake surrounding the prosthesis and widespread osteomyelitis

Fig. 3.15 Radiograph
following the removal
of the infected prosthesis
and cement with the
placement
of an antibiotic-loaded
cement spacer

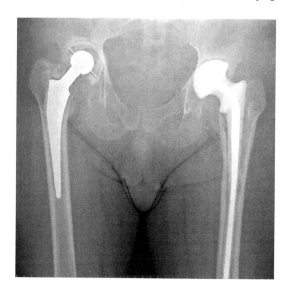

Summary and Conclusions

The timely diagnosis of a musculoskeletal infection is the most critical factor in the successful management of the condition. Though the diagnosis may be difficult due to the ability to mimic many other conditions and the variety of presentation patterns, a high index of suspicion usually leads to the appropriate diagnosis and treatment. It cannot be emphasized enough that the treatment of musculoskeletal infection in the early acute stage is orders of magnitude simpler that that of a chronic infection. A missed diagnosis can be devastating to the patient often leading to permanent disability and impaired function.

In general, infections that do not involve a joint or a significant abscess may be effectively treated with proper diagnosis and antibiotic therapy. In instances in which there is an intraarticular infection or the formation of an abscess, prompt surgical debridement and subsequent intravenous antibiotic therapy is typically necessary. In the proper host with early and effective therapy, the long-term sequelae of an infection can be minimized. It is for this reason that all clinicians should be able to recognize and initiate treatment, even if only to make the proper referral, for all patients suspected of having a musculoskeletal infection.

Suggested Reading

1. Cierny G 3rd. Chronic osteomyelitis: results of treatment. *Inst Course Lect.* 1990;39: 495–508.
2. Cierny G 3rd, DiPasquale D. Treatment of chronic infection. *J Am Acad Orthop Surg.* 2006;14(10)(suppl):S105–S110.

3. Conterno LO, da Silva Filho CR. Antibiotics for treating chronic osteomyelitis in adults. *Cochrane Database Syst Rev.* 2009 Jul 8;(3):CD004439.
4. Copley LA. Pediatric musculoskeletal infection: trends and antibiotic recommendations. *J Am Acad Orthop Surg.* 2009;17(10):618–626.
5. Fletcher N, Sofianos D, Berkes MB, Obremskey WT. Prevention of perioperative infection. *J Bone Joint Surg Am.* 2007;89(7):1605–1618.
6. Gardner GC, Kadel NJ. Ordering and interpreting rheumatologic laboratory tests. *J Am Acad Orthop Surg.* 2003;11(1):60–67.
7. Song KM, Sloboda JF. Acute hematogenous osteomyelitis in children. *J Am Acad Orthop Surg.* 2001;9(3):166–175.
8. Gristina AG. Biomaterial-centered infection: microbial adhesion versus tissue integration. *Science.* 1987;237(4822):1588–1595.

Chapter 4
Tumors of the Musculoskeletal System

Martin M. Malawer and Kristen L. Kellar-Graney

Overview

Both benign and malignant tumors (neoplasms) may arise from any mesenchymal soft tissue or bony tissue of the extremities, pelvis, shoulder girdle, or the axial skeleton. All tumors arise from one of the different histological types of tissue that comprise the musculoskeletal system: bone (osteoid forming tumors), cartilage (chondroid forming tumors), muscle, and the fibrous connective tissue (soft-tissue tumors). Only rarely do tumors arise from the arteries or nerves.

In general, most tumors are benign, but malignant tumors may also occur. Malignant mesenchymal tumors are termed sarcomas. Sarcomas rank among the least-common malignant diagnoses. There are only 8,000 new cases (6,000 soft tissue and 2,000 bone) of sarcoma out of the 1.2 million new patients that will be diagnosed with cancer each year in the United States. This accounts for less than 1% of malignant tumor occurrences.

Most bone sarcomas (osteosarcoma and Ewing's sarcoma) occur during childhood or adolescence, unlike most malignancies (carcinomas) that occur in the older decades of life (greater than 40 years of age). Soft-tissue sarcomas tend to occur in young adults and the risk of development increases with each decade of life. Bone tumors usually present with pain, in contrast to soft-tissue tumors that often present as a painless mass (usually greater than 5 cm in size).

Orthopedic surgeons are often the first physicians to see these patients and are called upon to make a correct diagnosis and/or to determine if an individual should be referred to a specialist (orthopedic oncologist). To emphasize the rarity of these entities, the average orthopedic surgeon will see one to two tumors every 5–10 years of practice.

M.M. Malawer (✉)
Departments of Orthopedic Surgery, Orthopedic Oncology, Georgetown University School of Medicine, 913 Frome Lane, McLean, VA 22102, USA
e-mail: mmalawer1@aol.com

S.W. Wiesel, J.N. Delahay (eds.), *Essentials of Orthopedic Surgery*,
DOI 10.1007/978-1-4419-1389-0_4, © Springer Science+Business Media, LLC 2010

A high degree of clinical suspicion, necessary for early diagnosis, is ever more important as fundamental changes in health care delivery alter patient access to specialists and to expensive imaging studies. Early detection, combined with proper techniques of diagnosis and treatment, can dramatically improve the chances of achieving functional limb salvage and survival. Continued progress in radiographic imaging, chemotherapy, radiation therapy, and biotechnology, coupled with a better understanding of the biological behavior of mesenchymal neoplasms, has led to a rational basis of diagnosis, staging, and surgical treatment (Figs. 4.1 and 4.2).

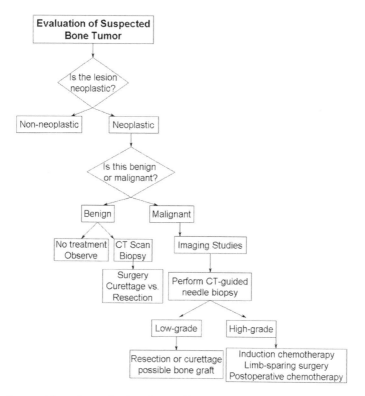

Fig. 4.1 Process taken when evaluating abnormal bone radiographs

This chapter reviews the common benign as well as malignant tumors arising from bone and soft tissues of the extremities, shoulder girdle, and pelvis. The biologic basis of tumor growth, staging, and radiographic determination is emphasized. Radiographic characteristics are accentuated and evaluation with the use of staging studies, such as computed tomography (CT) and magnetic resonance imaging (MRI), is described. An overview of the basic surgical procedures utilized by orthopedic oncologists is also presented.

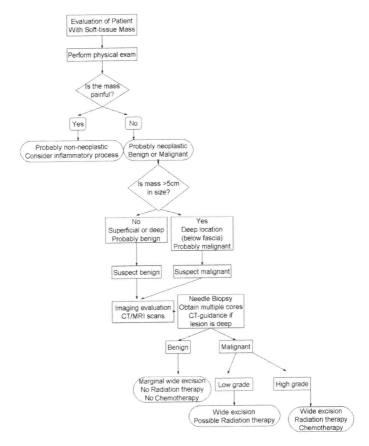

Fig. 4.2   Process taken when evaluating suspected soft-tissue tumor

Natural History of Bone and Soft-Tissue Tumors

Mesenchymal neoplasms have characteristic patterns of behavior and growth that distinguish them from other malignancies. These patterns form the basis of a staging system and provide a focus for current treatment strategies.

Biology and Growth

Spindle cell sarcomas form solid lesions through circumferential growth, in which the periphery of each lesion is composed of the least mature cells. In contradistinction to benign lesions, which are surrounded by a true capsule composed of compressed normal cells, malignant tumors are generally enclosed by a pseudocapsule consisting of viable tumor cells and a fibrovascular zone of reactive tissue with a variable inflammatory component that interdigitates with the normal tissue adjacent and beyond the lesion. The thickness of the reactive zone varies with the degree of malignancy and histogenetic type.

High-grade sarcomas characteristically have a poorly defined reactive zone that may be locally invaded and destroyed by the tumor. In addition, tumor nodules not in continuity with the main tumor may be present in tissue that appears to be normal. Low-grade sarcomas rarely form tumor nodules beyond the reactive zone.

Local anatomy influences the growth of sarcomas by setting natural barriers to extension. In general, bone sarcomas take the path of least resistance. The three mechanisms of growth and extension of bone tumors are compression of normal tissue, resorption of bone by reactive osteoclasts, and direct destruction of normal tissue. Benign tumors grow and expand by the first two mechanisms; direct tissue destruction is characteristic of malignant bone tumors. Most benign bone tumors are unicompartmental; they remain confined and may expand the bone in which they arise. Most malignant bone tumors are bicompartmental; they destroy the overlying cortex and push directly into the adjacent soft tissue. Soft-tissue tumors may start in one compartment (intracompartmental) or between compartments (extracompartmental). The determination of anatomic compartment involvement has become more important with the advent of limb-preservation surgery. In general, most benign and malignant bone and soft-tissue tumors grow like a ball, pushing normal tissue away as they expand.

The Five Basic Patterns of Sarcoma Behavior

On the basis of biological considerations and natural history, all bone and soft-tissue tumors, benign and malignant, may be classified into five categories, each of which shares certain clinical characteristics and radiographic patterns and requires similar surgical procedures. These five categories and the associated tumor behavior are as follows (Table 4.1):

1. *Benign/latent*: Lesions whose natural history is to grow slowly during normal growth of the individual and then to stop, with a tendency to heal spontaneously. They never become malignant and heal rapidly if treated by curettage (i.e., lipomas and unicameral bone cysts).
2. *Benign/active*: Lesions whose natural history is progressive growth. Excision leaves a reactive zone with some tumor (i.e., chondroblastoma of bone).
3. *Benign/aggressive*: Lesions that are locally aggressive but do not metastasize. Tumor extends through the capsule into the reactive zone. Local control can be obtained only by removing the lesion with a margin of normal tissue beyond the reactive zone (i.e., giant cell tumors of bone or fibromatosis of soft tissues).
4. *Malignant, low grade*: Lesions that have a low potential to metastasize. Histologically, there is no true capsule but a pseudocapsule. Tumor nodules exist within the reactive zone but rarely beyond. Local control can be accomplished only by removal of all tumor and reactive tissue with a margin of normal bone.

These lesions can be treated successfully by surgery alone; systemic therapy is not required (i.e., myxoid chondrosarcoma of bone and low-grade soft-tissue sarcomas).

5. *Malignant, high grade*: Lesions whose natural history is to grow rapidly and to metastasize early. Tumor nodules are usually found within and beyond the reactive zone and at some distance in the normal tissue. Surgery is necessary for local control, and systemic therapy is warranted to prevent metastasis (i.e., osteosarcoma. Ewing's sarcoma of bone, and high-grade malignant fibrous histiocytoma of soft tissues).

Table 4.1 Behavioral classification of bone and soft-tissue tumors

Classification	Bone	Soft tissue
Benign/latent	Nonossifying fibroma	Lipoma
Benign/active	Aneurysmal bone cyst	Angiolipoma
Benign/aggressive	Giant cell tumor	Aggressive fibromatosis
Malignant/low grade	Parosteal osteosarcoma	Myxoid liposarcoma
Malignant/high grade	Classic osteosarcoma	Malignant fibrous histiocytoma

Adapted from Enneking WF. Staging of musculoskeletal tumors. In: Enneking WF, *Musculoskeletal Tumor Surgery*, vol. 1, New York: Churchill Livingstone; 1983:87–88

Fig. 4.3 Schematic drawing showing the various planes of resection for distal femoral osteosarcoma with an extraosseous component. This represents the planes of dissection for all anatomic sites

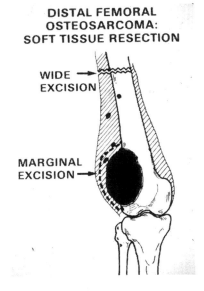

DISTAL FEMORAL OSTEOSARCOMA: SOFT TISSUE RESECTION

WIDE EXCISION

MARGINAL EXCISION

Figure 4.3 shows the planes of surgical resection for both malignant low-grade and high-grade bone lesions. Examples of bone and soft-tissue tumors in each of these categories are described within this chapter.

Mechanism of Tumor Spread

Unlike carcinomas, bone and soft-tissue sarcomas disseminate almost exclusively through the blood (i.e., to the lungs and other bones). About 5–10% of soft-tissue tumors spread through the lymphatic system to regional nodes. Hematogenous spread is manifested by pulmonary involvement in the early stages and by bony involvement in later stages. Bone metastasis occasionally is the first sign of dissemination.

The histologic hallmark of malignant sarcomas is their potential to break through the pseudocapsule to form satellite lesions called *skip metastases*. A skip metastasis is a tumor nodule that is located within the same bone as the main tumor but not contiguous to it. Transarticular skip metastases are located in the joint adjacent to the main tumor. Although relatively uncommon, skip metastases occur most frequently with high-grade sarcomas.

Sarcoma Tumor Staging

Selection and use of a prognostically significant staging system are fundamental both for the selection of appropriate treatment protocols and for the development of tumor registries necessary for basic research analysis. In 1980, the Musculoskeletal Tumor Society adopted a surgical staging system (SSS), proposed by Dr. William F. Enneking, for both bone and soft-tissue sarcomas [1]. This system is based upon the fact that mesenchymal sarcomas of bone and soft tissue behave alike, irrespective of histogenetic type. The SSS encompasses the "GTM" classification: grade (G), location (T), and lymph node involvement and metastases (M).

1. *Surgical grade*: The letter G incorporates both the histological grade of a lesion and as clinical factors related to aggressiveness, such as growth rate. A low-grade tumor is rated G1 while a high-grade tumor is rated G2. Low-grade lesions are malignancies with small potential to metastasize.
2. *Surgical site*: The letter T represents anatomic site, either intracompartmental (T1) or extracompartmental (T2). A compartment is defined as "an anatomic structure of space bounded by natural barriers of tumor extension." T1 lesions are easier to delineate clinically, surgically, and radiographically than T2 lesions and have a correspondingly higher chance of adequate removal without amputative procedures.
3. *Lymph nodes and metastases*: Local disease without evidence of metastasis is designated M0. When a bone or soft-tissue sarcoma has metastasized (M1), the prognosis is extremely poor. Lymphatic spread is a sign of extensive dissemination. Regional lymphatic involvement is equated with distal metastases.

The SSS developed for surgical planning and assessment of bone sarcomas is summarized as follows:

Stage IA	(GI, T1, M0) Low-grade intracompartmental lesion without metastasis.
Stage IB	(GI, T2P M0) Low-grade extracompartmental lesion without metastasis.
Stage IIA	(G2, TI, M0) High-grade intracompartmental lesion without metastasis.
Stage IIB	(G2, T2, M0) High-grade extracompartmental lesion without metastasis.
Stage IIIA	(GI or G2, M1) Intracompartmental lesion, any grade, with metastasis.
Stage IIIB	(GI or G2, T2, MI) Extracompartmental lesion, any grade, with metastasis.

Clinical and Radiographic Evaluation, Staging, and Biopsy

Staging of a bone or soft-tissue tumor mass means determining the local extension (anatomy) of the tumor and any possible sites of distal dissemination. If the clinical examination or plain radiographs suggest an aggressive or malignant tumor, staging studies should be performed before biopsy. All radiographic studies are influenced by surgical manipulation of the lesion, making interpretation more difficult. Bone scintigraphy, computed tomography or magnetic resonance imaging, and angiography are required to delineate local tumor extent, vascular displacement, and compartmental localization (Fig. 4.4). Recently, computed tomography angiography (CTA) has been proposed as a less invasive adjuvant modality for examining the vasculature associated with musculoskeletal tumors.

Radiographic Evaluation

X-Rays

Plain radiographs taken in perpendicular planes [anteroposterior (AP) and lateral] remain essential to the characterization and diagnosis of lesions involving the skeleton. Selection and interpretation of other imaging techniques is often guided by the radiographic properties of the lesion. Proper interpretation of a lesion seen on a radiograph can be summarized by answering "four questions" as proposed by Dr. William F. Enneking:

1. What are the anatomic location and extent of the lesion?
2. What is the lesion doing to the bone?
3. What is the bone doing to the lesion?
4. Are there any radiographic peculiarities of the lesion that give a hint as to its tissue type?

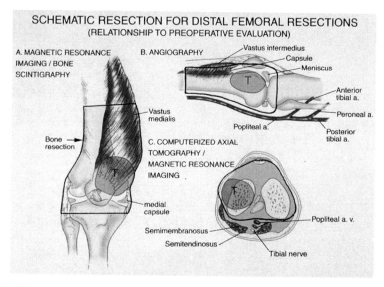

Fig. 4.4 Schematic illustration demonstrating the relationship and evaluation of the various imaging modalities to the various components of bone sarcoma. Plain radiographs assess bone and cortical breakthrough as well as overall pattern of biological growth. CT determines the exact extent of bone destruction and MRI determines the intramedullary and extraosseous components of the tumor. Bone scan most importantly determines the presence or absence of bony metastases. Angiography shows the anatomic relation of the tumor to the major blood vessels as well as the vascularity of the tumor and subsequent response to induction chemotherapy. (From Malawer MM, Link MP, Donaldson SS. Sarcomas of bone. In: DeVita VT, Hellman S, Rosenberg SA, eds. *Cancer: Principles and Practice of Oncology.* 5th ed. Philadephia, PA: Lippincott, Williams & Wilkins;1997:1789–1852. Reprinted with permission)

Distinction between benign, aggressive, and frankly malignant lesions can be made on the basis of this analysis. In general, the plain radiograph is the single most important study in determining the type of bone tumor.

Computed Tomography

CT allows accurate determination of intra- and extraosseous extension of skeletal neoplasms. CT accurately depicts the transverse anatomic relationship of a tumor to the surrounding structures. By varying window settings, one can study cortical bone, intramedullary space, adjacent muscles, and extraosseous soft-tissue extension. The anatomic compartmental involvement by soft-tissue sarcomas is easily determined. High-resolution CT scans (1 mm cuts) and two-dimensional or three-dimensional reconstruction can be extremely valuable in preoperative planning, particularly in the pelvis or spine. CT evaluation must be individualized to obtain the maximum benefit of image reconstruction. Close interaction between the surgeon and the radiologist facilitates accurate and effective imaging. CT is most useful for bony lesions.

Magnetic Resonance Imaging

MRI provides valuable imaging of both bone and soft tissues in multiple planes. Excellent visualization of anatomic compartments, neurovascular bundles, and areas of reactive tissue allow for detailed preoperative planning. Although signal

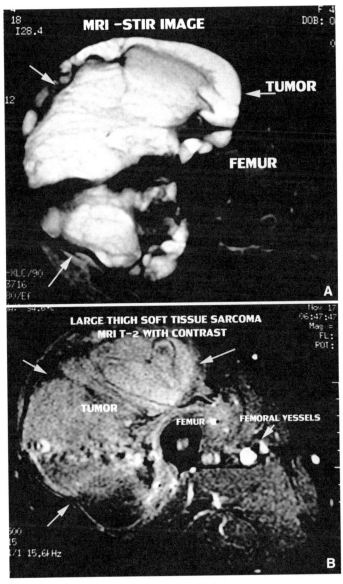

Fig. 4.5 (**a, b**) Stir MRI and T2-weighted MRI with contrast demonstrating a very large soft-tissue sarcoma of the thigh. Arrows delineate the extension of tumor. MRI scans are extremely accurate

characteristics of any given mass on the traditional T1- or T2-weighted images (or on the more recent fat-suppressed and gradient-echo images) can be diagnostic, distinction between benign or low-grade malignant lesions (such as lipomas versus well-differentiated liposarcomas) cannot be reliably made on the basis of MRI images alone (Fig. 4.5).

Bone Scans

Bone scintigraphy is useful for evaluation of both bony and soft-tissue tumors. Bone scans determine whether other bones are involved by tumor. They assist in determining metastatic disease, polyostotic involvement, intraosseous extension of tumor, and the relation of the underlying bone to a primary soft-tissue sarcoma. Malignant bone tumors may present with skeletal metastasis (1.6%). The initial flow phase correlates to the vascularity of the tumor. Recent studies using quantitative techniques and the isotope thallium-201 have shown that the histologic tumor response

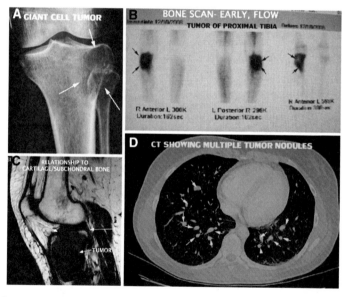

Fig. 4.6 Common imaging studies for bone and soft-tissue sarcomas. (**a**) Plain radiograph showing a typical giant cell tumor of the proximal tibia. (**b**) Bone scan showing marked uptake during the early flow phases of the corresponding bone scan. (**c**) MRI scan of the same patient showing a tumor of the proximal tibia (*dark area*), T_1-weighted image sequence. The arrows indicate a very thin bony cortex. (**d**) CT scan of the chest demonstrating several metastases to the lungs. Pulmonary metastases are the most common site of sarcoma spread. (**e**) Computerized tomography angiography (CTA) demonstrating in three dimensions a parosteal osteosarcoma arising from the distal femur. The popliteal artery is markedly displaced by the tumor, but remains patent. CTA has mostly replaced traditional angiography for staging of bony sarcomas. It shows the surgeon the true anatomic location of the displaced vessels, which greatly helps in the planning of a surgical procedure

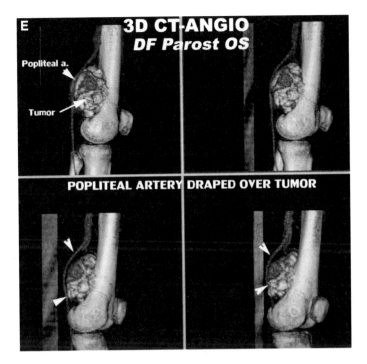

Fig. 4.6 (continued)

to chemotherapy can be predicted based upon comparison of pre- and posttreatment studies (Fig. 4.6).

Angiography

The arteriographic technique for bone and soft-tissue lesions differ from that used for arterial disease. A minimum of two views (biplane) is necessary to determine the relation of the major vessels to the tumor. Extraosseous tumor extension is easily demonstrated by angiography. As experience with limb-sparing procedures has increased, surgeons have become more aware of the need to determine the individual vascular patterns prior to resection. This is especially crucial for tumors of the proximal tibia, where vascular anomalies are common, and in metastatic lesions such as renal cell carcinoma which are known to be quite vascular. The increasing preoperative use of intraarterial chemotherapy also has increased the need for accurate angiography. Reduction of vascularity following chemotherapy can be correlated to overall histologic response of the tumor. Preoperative embolization of highly vascular tumors prior to surgical resection can significantly reduce blood loss and intraoperative morbidity (Fig. 4.6).

Computed Tomography Angiography

A less invasive but relatively equally sensitive modality has been explored to determine the vasculature associated with musculoskeletal tumors. CT angiograms are beginning to be utilized in this oncology subspecialty. Utilizing a very fast computed tomography machine and injectable contrast, the affected limb's vasculature can be examined. The main purposes of CT angiography include identification of the major arteries and veins, revealing the local anatomy with respect to the tumor to determine if any vascular anomalies occur, and identifying the presence of tumor thrombi within a vein to determine patency. Each of these pieces of information proves quite important for surgical planning and determining if a limb-sparing procedure can be performed.

The combination of plain radiographs, bone scintigraphy, cross-sectional anatomic imaging (via CT or MRI), and longitudinal imaging of vascular supply (via angiography) allows the surgeon to develop a three-dimensional construct of the local tumor area prior to resection and to formulate a detailed surgical approach for limb salvage (Fig. 4.6d).

Positron Emission Tomography

Positron emission tomography (PET) is a relatively newer diagnostic imaging technique that provides very different information from that obtainable with other imaging modalities. The purpose of this scan assess active metabolism in the body. The most widely used radiotracer is F-18 fluoro-2-deoxy-D-glucose (FDG), which is an analog of glucose. The FDG uptake in cells is directly proportional to traditional glucose metabolism, which is increased many times in malignant cells. FDG-PET, in addition to other imaging modalities, is now the standard of care in initial staging, monitoring the response to therapy and management of various cancers (e.g., breast cancer, lung cancer, and lymphoma). The introduction of combined PET-CT scanners, which provide s functional and structural information, leading to a detection of very small (<1 cm) lesions, make this technique useful in the early detection of the disease process and decreased false-positive lesions. The FDG uptake is measured in standardized uptake value (SUV) units, which quantifies uptake and thereby differentiates malignant disease from other possible causes (i.e., inflamatory or infectious processes) (Fig. 4.7).

Classification of Surgical Procedures by the Biological Margins Obtained for Bone and Soft-Tissue Tumors

Surgical removal – including curettage, resection, and amputation – is the traditional method of managing skeletal neoplasms. The advent of advanced imaging techniques, improved understanding of the biologic behavior of sarcomas, and adoption of effective adjuvant therapy has led to widespread acceptance of limb-sparing techniques. Retrospective analyses of disease-free survival and overall survival have

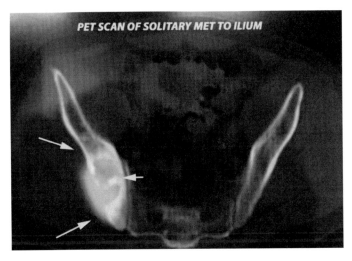

Fig. 4.7 Positron emission tomography (PET) scan showing metabolic activity in the right ilium caused by a solitary bony metastatic lesion. PET scans are accurate for both bony and soft-tissue sarcomas

shown no difference between limb salvage and amputation for osteosarcoma (the most common bone sarcoma) of the distal femur.

A classification scheme of surgical procedures based on the surgical plane of dissection in relation to the tumor and the method of accomplishing the removal has recently been developed. This system, summarized below, permits meaningful comparisons of various operative procedures and gives surgeons a common language.

1. *Intralesional.* An intralesional procedure passes through the pseudocapsule and directly into the lesion. Macroscopic tumor is left and the entire operative field is potentially contaminated. Biopsies are by definition intralesional.
2. *Marginal.* A marginal procedure is one in which the entire lesion is removed in one piece. The plane of dissection passes through the pseudocapsule, or reactive zone, around the lesion. When performed for a sarcoma, it leaves macroscopic disease because of tumor involvement of the pseudocapsule.
3. *Wide (intracompartmental).* This is commonly termed en bloc resection. A wide excision includes the entire tumor, the reactive zone, and a marginal cuff of normal tissue. The entire structure of origin of the tumor is not removed. In patients with high-grade sarcomas, this procedure may leave skip nodules (see Fig. 4.3).
4. *Radical (extracompartmental).* The entire tumor and the structure of origin of the lesion are removed. The plane of dissection is beyond the limiting fascial or bony borders (see Fig. 4.3).

5. It is important to note that any of these procedures may be accomplished *either* by local (i.e., limb-sparing) surgery or by amputation. An amputation may entail a marginal, wide, or radical excision, depending upon the plane through which it passes in relationship to the tumor.

Therefore, an amputation is not automatically an adequate cancer operation; careful consideration to the desired final margin is required prior to selection of the amputation level. The local anatomy dictates how a specific margin can be obtained surgically, and proper preoperative staging (as discussed above) is necessary to assess both local tumor extent and relevant local anatomy. In general, benign bone tumors can be adequately treated with either an intralesional procedure (curettage) or a marginal excision. Malignant tumors require a minimum of wide (intracompartmental) excision or radical (extracompartmental) resection. This can be accomplished by amputation or by an en bloc procedure (limb salvage). Similarly, benign soft-tissue tumors are treated by marginal excision, aggressive tumors by wide excision, and malignant tumors by wide or radical resection.

Overview of Indications and Surgical Procedures

Biopsy Techniques

Biopsy Considerations and Importance

The planning and technique of a biopsy is extremely important. A biopsy should be performed after the staging studies are obtained. If a resection is to be performed, it is crucial that the location of the biopsy be in line with the anticipated incision for the definitive procedure. Extreme care should be taken not to contaminate potential tissue planes or flaps that will compromise the management of the lesion. Improper biopsy technique often eliminates the opportunity for limb salvage. Mankin documented that 60% of referred patients had a major error in diagnosis and 18% had less-than-optimal treatment secondary to problems related to the biopsy (Fig. 4.8).

Core Needle Biopsy

To minimize contamination and reduce patient morbidity, needle biopsy of soft-tissue masses or of extraosseous components should be attempted prior to an incisional biopsy whenever possible. Needle or core biopsy of bone tumors often provides adequate specimen for diagnosis. Cooperation between the radiologist and pathologist is vital to ensuring that adequate tissue is obtained to provide a diagnosis. Radiographs should be obtained to document the position of the trocar. Core biopsy is preferable if a limb-sparing option exists, since it entails less local contamination than open biopsy does.

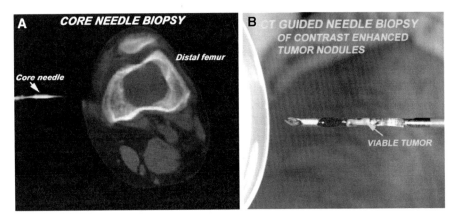

Fig. 4.8 (**a**) CT scan demonstrating a core needle biopsy of a distal femoral bone tumor. (**b**) Gross specimen of needle biopsy of a soft-tissue tumor. Core or needle biopsies are preferred to open, incisional biopsy for most tumors. They are less likely to cause local contamination

Open Incisional Biopsy

Proper techniques for open biopsies are necessary to minimize contamination. A tourniquet is used if feasible to facilitate visualization of the tumor. Transverse incisions are to be avoided at all cost, and consideration of subsequent surgery for limb salvage should guide positioning of the biopsy incision. Since sarcomas are characteristically surrounded by the most immature cells, biopsy of the lesion's peripheral tissue is recommended. If a soft-tissue component is present, there is no need to biopsy the underlying bone. If it is necessary to biopsy the underlying bone, a small, rounded cortical window should be used. This is especially true for a tumor that requires primary radiotherapy. Large segments do not reossify, leading to fracture and subsequent amputation.

When a patient presents with a bone or soft-tissue tumor, it is the initial surgical intervention, combined with neo- and adjuvant therapy, that affords the individual the best opportunity for cure. Therefore, it is imperative to have a good preoperative plan for the extent of surgery required. Frequently, radiographic studies can help recreate a three-dimensional approximation of the tumor and affected tissues. Knowing the tumor size and extension, in combination with clinical findings during the physical examination, will enable the surgeon to determine what surgical intervention is most appropriate. The three most common procedure types performed by orthopedic oncologists are curettage, resection, and amputation.

Curettage of Bone Tumors

Curettage and the most common surgical procedure for most benign and aggressive but benign bone tumors: unicameral bone cysts, aneurysmal bone cysts, chondroblastomas, fibrous lesions, and giant cell tumors. Once a defect is created, it is necessary to reconstruct the surgical defect by various techniques, e.g., bone graft, cementation with PMMA, and/or biologic fillers.

Curettage is the technique of creating a window by removing the overlying bone and "scooping" the underlying (intramedullary) tumor with small, sharp, scoop-shaped instruments (curettes) under direct visualization. Frequently following mechanical curettage, a high-speed burr drill is utilized to ablate the curetted bone defect. The benefit of this type of resection is that minimal collateral bone loss occurs, and the resulting defect can be reconstructed with bone cement, internal fixation, bone graft, or a combination of the three (Fig. 4.9). In specific tumors, especially giant cell tumor of bone, enchondroma, and even occasionally metastatic

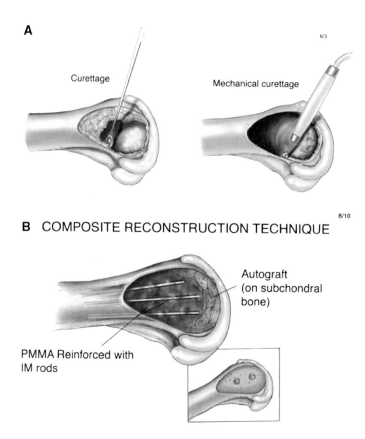

Fig. 4.9 Surgical illustrations demonstrating use of curettage (**a**) with both hand curettes and mechanical curettage (high speed burr), followed by (**b**) method of bone reconstruction involving intramedullary pins, PMMA, and bone graft. It is essential to reconstruct the bony defect following curettage and cryosurgery. This permits early weight bearing and avoids the risk of fracture through the reconstructed defect. (From Bickels J, Meller I, Shmookler BM, et al. The role and biology of cryosurgery in the treatment of bone tumors: a review. *Acta Orthop.* 1999; 70(3):308–315. Reprinted with permission from Taylor & Francis Group, http://www.informaworld.com)

carcinoma of bone, the use of liquid nitrogen (cryosurgery) accompanies curettage to kill any tumor cells that may remain in the bone cavity.

Cryosurgery (Adjuvant Following Curettage)

Cryosurgery has been used more successfully for giant cell tumors than for any other type of bone tumor. Cryosurgery is effective in eradicating the tumor while preserving joint motion and avoiding the need for resection or amputation. Liquid nitrogen is a very effective physical adjuvant and is recommended following curettage resection. Curettage alone is not recommended because of the associated high rate of local recurrence (Fig. 4.10).

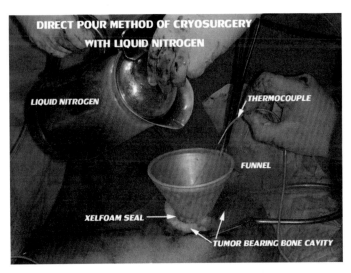

Fig. 4.10 Intraoperative photograph showing the direct pour method of cryosurgery following curettage of a benign-aggressive bone tumor. The decanter is filled with liquid nitrogen. The liquid nitrogen is poured into the funnel that is securely fitted inside the curetted bone defect. Gelfoam protects the skin and adjacent soft tissues from inadvertent freezing. The temperature probe is placed inside of the bone defect to ensure that an appropriate freezing temperature is obtained. A rapid freeze and slow thaw cycle is required to kill tumor cells; a total of two to three cycles are required

Resection of Bone and Soft-Tissue Tumors

Malignant Tumors

En bloc resection of bone sarcomas is the most commonly performed surgical procedure. This requires a large, carefully planned incision to allow adequate visualization of all structures critical to the affected limb. It is imperative that adequate healthy tissues be available following surgical resection in order to have a stable, functional, pain-free limb.

Wide (en bloc) excision entails removal of the tumor, its pseudocapsule, and a cuff of normal tissue surrounding the tumor in all directions. This is the desired resection margin for sarcoma; however, the adequate thickness of the normal tissue cuff is a matter of some controversy. For both soft-tissue and bone sarcomas, it is generally believed to be between 0.5 and 2 cm.

Radical excision or resection involves removal of the tumor and the entire anatomical compartment within which it arises. It does not define the component of the tumor that is left behind. In other words, a radical excision can achieve a marginal or a wide margin, depending on how close the tumor is to the border of the compartment. However, radical excision excludes the possibility of skip metastases.

Amputation

Amputations are radical surgical treatments for those patients in whom surgical resection is not feasible. Only approximately 5–10% of patients with bone and soft-tissue tumors require amputation due to successful adjuvant modalities such as chemotherapy and radiation. The most common cause for a patient requiring amputation is contamination of soft tissue during the initial biopsy. Additional reasons for amputation include involvement of the vascular plexus, infection, skeletal immaturity, especially in very young children, and non-healing pathological fractures.

When the decision to perform an amputation has been made, the surgeon must take into account the age, expected oncological outcome, and functional outcome of the individual. Typically, the more proximal the amputation occurs, the greater the functional loss.

An amputation involves the entire removal of bone and some soft tissues of the affected limb distal to the arising tumor. The affected hand or foot on the ipsilateral limb is always sacrificed. The decision of where the osteotomy is performed depends on the location of the tumor within the bone. The longer the bone remnant (stump), the greater the functional outcome for the patient tends to be. However, a curative procedure is absolutely superior to an improved functional outcome; therefore the amount of bone removed must be proportionate with the tumor extension and required tumor-free margins.

Common Types and Indications of Amputations Performed

> *Hemipelvectomy (H/P)*: An amputation of the ipsilateral ilium, ischium pubic ramus, and distal thigh and leg structures. This radical amputation is performed for unresectable primary tumors of the upper thigh, hip, or pelvis (Fig. 4.11).

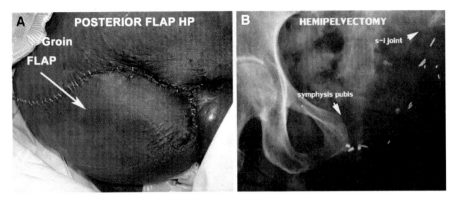

Fig. 4.11 (**a**) Operative photograph following posterior flap hemipelvectomy. Following rehabilitation, some patients choose to be fitted with an external prosthesis for cosmetic purposes. (**b**) Postoperative radiograph demonstrating the resultant bony pelvis. The amputation is through the sacro-iliac (S-I) joint and the symphysis pubis. Hemipelvectomy is often required for large, high-grade bone and/or soft-tissue sarcomas of the pelvis, proximal thigh, and/or groin. Today, this procedure is only occasionally required

Hip disarticulation: An amputation through the hip joint capsule. The purpose is to remove the entire lower extremity while maintaining the integrity of the resultant acetabulum and pelvis. This procedure is not frequently necessary due to success with chemotherapy and limb-sparing resections.

Above knee amputation (AKA): An amputation most frequently performed for advanced soft-tissue sarcomas of the distal thigh and leg or for high-grade bone sarcomas of the distal femur or proximal tibia. The levels of osteotomy can be performed in the supercondylar area of the femur (distally), the diaphyseal femur, or just below the lesser trochanter (high above knee). This amputation is typically reserved for those tissues involving the neurovascular structures or with significant contamination of the soft tissues (Fig. 4.12).

Below-knee amputation (BKA): An amputation performed for extensive high-grade soft-tissue sarcomas of the lower leg, ankle, or foot. Patients undergoing this procedure have resultant good function and frequently less complications than those attempting a limb-sparing surgery (Fig. 4.13).

Lisfranc amputation: Extensive tumors involving the first and second interspace in adjacent metatarsals or multiple metatarsals are treated with this type of amputation. A midfoot incision with long planar flaps allow for disarticulation of the Lisfranc joint.

Chopart amputation: Tumors extending to the tarsometatarsal joint with soft-tissue extension require this amputation which is performed through a transverse incision dorsal or distal to the talonavicular joint. Most of the cuboid and the distal structures are removed (Fig. 4.14a).

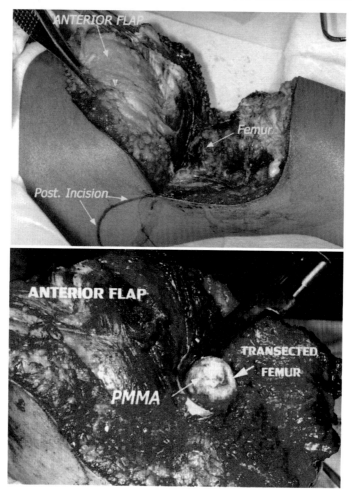

Fig. 4.12 Series of intraoperative photographs demonstrating the incisions and flaps utilized for an above-knee amputation. The distal portion of the transected femur is packed with bone cement prior to stump reconstruction to avoid postoperative bleeding and hematoma formation

Transmetatarsal amputation: An amputation performed for tumors distal to the metatarsophalangeal joint. These can be treated by amputation through the metatarsophalangeal joint with minimal disruption to function. The only exception is the first ray, which typically bears 50% of the weight with toe-off during each gait cycle. Therefore, preservation of as much proximal phalanx as possible is important to optimize this important structure (Fig. 4.14b).

Ray resection of foot: The indications for ray resections include tumors involving the toe or metatarsal bone. Benign tumors make up the majority of these

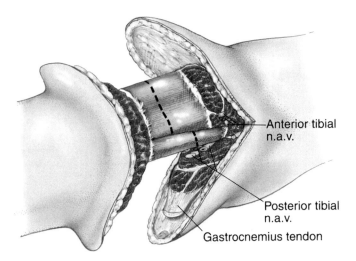

Anterior tibial
n.a.v.

Posterior tibial
n.a.v.

Gastrocnemius tendon

Fig. 4.13 Surgical illustration showing the levels of osteotomy (*dashed lines on the tibia and fibula*) and relationship to ligated vessels and structures for a below-knee amputation. The distal end of the fibula is transected about 2 cm proximal to the distal tibia osteotomy. (Originally published in Malawer M, Bickels J, Sugarbaker PH. Below-knee amputation. In: Malawer MM, Sugarbaker PH, eds. *Musculoskeletal Cancer Surgery: Treatment of Sarcomas and Allied Diseases.* Dordrecht, The Netherlands: Kluwer; 2001:363–369, [5])

lesions. An osteotomy of the metatarsal occurs, or the metatarsal is disarticulated at the tarsometatarsal joint. The resection then is performed from proximal to distal. The flexor tendon is identified and transected. The entire metatarsal is then excised along with the adjacent soft tissue.

Forequarter amputation: Entails surgical removal of the entire upper extremity including the scapula and clavicle. It is used in the treatment of unresectable sarcomas of the shoulder girdle, particularly osteosarcomas or high-grade soft-tissue sarcomas of the axilla, brachial plexus, and suprascapular area, or those tumors which tend to extend out of the anatomical compartment of the shoulder, cause fungation of the skin, or involve the neurovascular structures (Fig. 4.15).

Above elbow amputation: This amputation is indicated for advanced bone and soft-tissue sarcomas of the forearm. A longer length of the resultant humeral stump is proportional increased functionality for the patient fitted with a prosthetic device. Typically, the osteotomy is performed in the metaphyseal (high), diaphyseal, or supercondylar regions.

Below elbow amputation: This amputation is performed for uncontrolled tumors of the forearm and hand. As with all amputation, the greater the length of the preserved limb stump, the better the functional outcome with respect to prosthesis use.

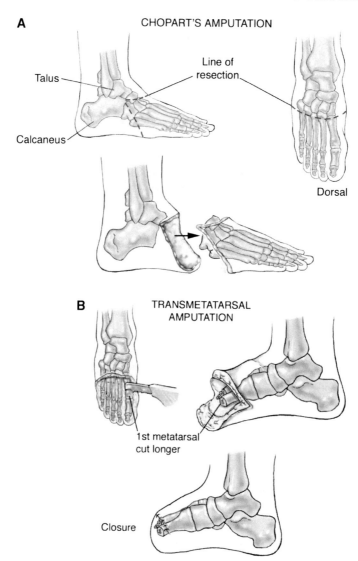

Fig. 4.14 Surgical illustrations depicting the lines of resection for Chopart's amputation (**a**) and transmetatarsal amputation (**b**)

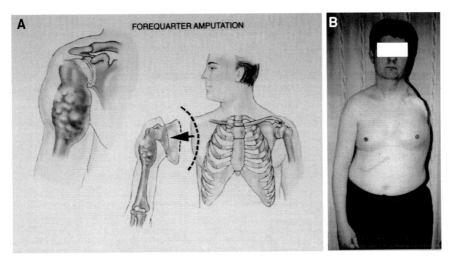

Fig. 4.15 (**a**) A schematic diagram of forequarter amputation, also known as an interscapu-lothoracic amputation. (From Bickels J, Malawer MM. Forequarter amputation. In: Wiesel S, ed. *Operative Techniques in Orthopedic Surgery*. Philadelphia, PA: Lippincott, Williams & Wilkins. In press.) (**b**) Clinical photograph of patient following forequarter amputation

Principles and Technique of Limb-Sparing Surgery for Bone and Soft-Tissue Tumors

Malignant Bone Sarcomas

Successful limb-sparing surgery consists of three phases:

1. *Resection of tumor.* Resection strictly follows the principles of oncologic surgery. Avoiding local recurrence is the criterion of success and the main determinant of the amount of bone and soft tissue to be removed.
2. *Skeletal reconstruction.* The average skeletal defect following adequate bone tumor resection measures 15–20 cm. Techniques of reconstruction (prosthetic replacement arthrodesis, allograft, or combination) vary and are independent of the resection, although the degree of resection may favor one technique over the other.
3. *Soft-tissue and muscle transfers.* Muscle transfers are performed to cover and close the resection site and to restore lost motor power. Adequate skin and muscle coverage is mandatory to decrease postoperative morbidity.

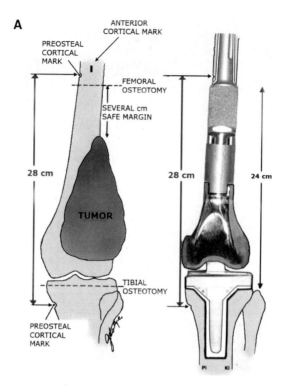

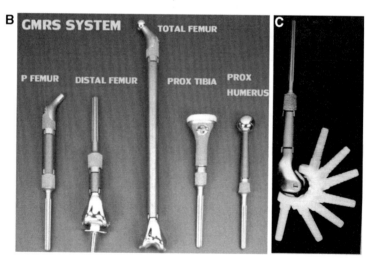

Fig. 4.16 (a) Schematic replacement of the distal femur with a modular endoprosthesis. (From Eckardt J, Malawer MM, Bickels J, Kiatisevi P. Distal femoral sections with endoprosthetic replacement.In: Wiesel S, ed. *Operative Techniques in Orthopedic Surgery*. Philadelphia, PA: Lippincott, Williams & Wilkins. In press.) (**b**) Clinical (MRS) for the distal femur manufactured

Guidelines for Surgical Resection

The surgical guidelines and technique of limb-sparing surgery used by the authors and by surgeons at most cancer centers in the United States are summarized as follows:

1. The major neurovascular bundle must be free of tumor.
2. Wide resection of the affected bone with a normal muscle cuff in all directions should be done.
3. All previous biopsy sites and all potentially contaminated tissues should be removed en bloc.
4. Bone should be resected 3–4 cm beyond abnormal uptake as determined by bone scan. (This is a safe margin to avoid intraosseous tumor extension.)
5. The adjacent joint and joint capsule should be resected.
6. Adequate motor reconstruction must be accomplished by regional muscle transfers.
7. Adequate soft-tissue coverage is needed to decrease the risk of skin flap necrosis and secondary infection.

Prostheses for Skeletal Reconstruction

Appropriate candidates for prosthetic reconstruction meet the above-mentioned guidelines for surgical resection. It is imperative that critical neurovascular structures and soft tissues remain following surgical resection in order to achieve a stable, well-functioning limb. Titanium alloy prostheses are available for reconstruction of each of the major joints: proximal humerus, scapula, distal humerus and elbow, proximal femur, total femur, distal femur, proximal tibia, and calcaneus. Due to their modularity, multiple systems can be utilized if a patient requires an extensive resection (Fig. 4.16). Additionally, the modular endoprosthetic systems allow for great flexibility during the surgical procedure in that trial-sized components can be utilized in order to achieve the best fit (Figs. 4.17 and 4.18).

Endoprosthetic reconstruction is a highly successful and durable method for reconstruction of the affected joint and accompanying bone. It allows for immediate fixation which in turn facilitates early mobilization or ambulation and rehabilitation. The metallic implants generally allow good to excellent function of the resected limb and allow patients to return to normal activities of daily living.

Fig. 4.16 (continued) by Stryker Orthopaedics (Mahwah, New Jersey). This is the most common type of endoprosthesis for limb-sparing surgery of the distal femur. The knee component is a rotating hinge mechanism. (c) Note the range of motion achieved by this kinematic knee. (Originally published in Henshaw RM, Malawer MM. Review of endoprosthetic reconstruction in limb-sparing surgery. In: Malawer MM, Sugarbaker PH, eds. *Musculoskeletal Cancer Surgery: Treatment of Sarcomas and Allied Diseases*. Dordrecht, The Netherlands: Kluwer; 2001: 383–403)

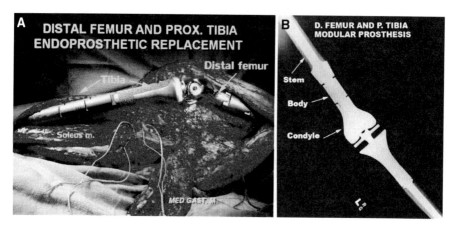

Fig. 4.17 (**a**) Operative photograph of the modular replacement system (MRS) used to replace an osteosarcoma of the proximal tibia as well as the distal femur (Stryker Orthopaedics, Mahwah, New Jersey). The medial gastrocnemius muscle will be rotated and serve as the soft-tissue coverage for the proximal tibial prosthesis and a technique for extensor mechanism reconstruction. A medial gastrocnemius flap is required, due to the lack of inherent soft tissues in this anatomic region following resection. This procedure has allowed for fewer complications (infection, wound necrosis, etc.) for proximal tibial prostheses. (**b**) Radiograph of implanted distal femur and proximal tibial modular prostheses (MRS) for a large tumor of the knee. Both the distal femur and proximal tibia have to be resected due to a "skip" metastasis. This demonstrates the usefulness of the modularity of this type of prosthesis

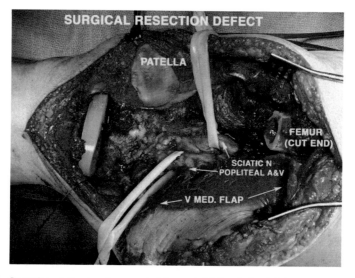

Fig. 4.18 Operative photo showing resected femur (*right*) and the tibial poly component (*left*). The sciatic nerve and popliteal vessels are identified and protected with Penrose drains. The large vastus medialis flap will provide soft-tissue coverage for the implanted prosthesis

While endoprosthetic reconstruction is normally limited to those patients who are or are nearing skeletal maturity (because of concerns in achieving proper oncologic margins), expandable prosthetic types, such as the Phenix growing prosthesis system (Phenix Medical, Paris, France), are being utilized in an attempt to avoid primary amputation in young children.

Soft-Tissue Sarcomas (STS) – Wide Excision (Resection)

General Surgical Technique and Considerations

The general surgical and oncological principles are as follows (Figs. 4.19–4.21):

1. All tissue at risk for gross tumor or micrometastatic cell involvement should be removed with a wide, en bloc excision that includes the tumor, a cuff of normal tissue, and all potentially contaminated tissues. The entire muscle group need not be removed. The biopsy site should be removed with 3 cm of normal skin and subcutaneous tissue en bloc with tumor.
2. The tumor or pseudocapsule should never be visualized during the procedure. Contamination of the wound with tumor greatly increases the risk of local recurrence.
3. Distant flaps should not be developed at the time of resection. This may contaminate a noninvolved area.

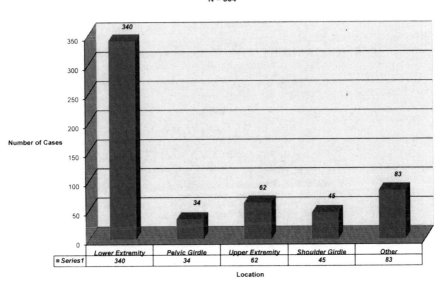

Fig. 4.19 Distribution of soft-tissue sarcoma resections by anatomic location

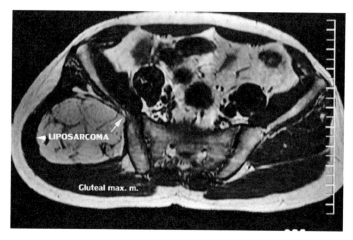

Fig. 4.20 MRI scan of a large soft-tissue sarcoma (liposarcoma) of the right buttock. It appears to have grown to the edge of the bony pelvis and to have compressed the soft tissues laterally

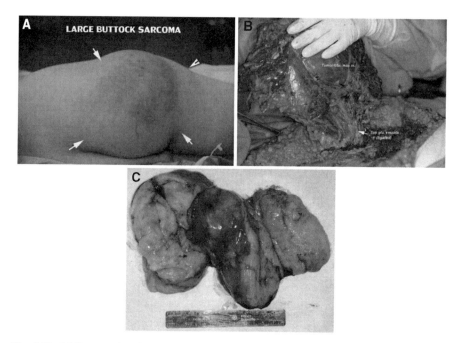

Fig. 4.21 (a) Preoperative photograph of patient in Figure 4.20. Arrows depict the tumor extension. (b) Intraoperative photograph of tumor reflected out of the surgical field. Note that the gluteal vessels have been ligated. (c) Gross photograph of the buttock liposarcoma

4. The margin surrounding the surgical wound should be marked with metallic staples. This helps the radiotherapist determine the high-risk area, should radiation treatment be needed later.
5. Reconstruction of the defect should include local muscle transfers to protect exposed neurovascular bundles and bone cortex.
6. All dead space should be closed, and there should be adequate drainage to prevent hematoma.

Perioperative antibiotics should be given. These procedures have a low but significant rate of postoperative infection. The risk of infection following preoperative adjuvant therapy is particularly high.

Surgical Treatment of Pathological Fractures

A pathological fracture is a fracture through a site of metastatic cancer or multiple myeloma of the bone. The bone is weakened and often partially destroyed by the tumor. Minimal trauma is required for a fracture to occur. The treatment of a pathological fracture differs significantly from a primary sarcoma of the bone. There is no need or attempt to remove the affected bone as is the purpose for primary malignant tumors. The aim is to reconstruct and to stabilize the fracture and to mobilize the patient quickly. The most common techniques are as follows:

1. *Curettage and internal fixation* of the tumor and immediate fixation with an intramedullary nail supplemented with bone cement (PMMA). Occasionally, a plate and screw fixation is preferred in some anatomic sites.
2. *Endoprosthetic replacement*: This technique is most commonly used for tumors around the hip. Immediate fixation is obtained with bone cement. Occasionally, comminuted fractures of the elbow and the distal femur are similarly treated with an endoprosthesis and bone cement.

Malignant Bone Tumors

Primary malignancies of bone arise from mesenchymal cells (sarcoma) and bone marrow cells (myeloma and lymphoma). Bone is also a common site of metastasis from a variety of carcinomas. Osteosarcoma and Ewing's sarcoma, the most common malignant mesenchymal bone tumors, usually occur during childhood and adolescence. Other mesenchymal tumors [malignant fibrous histiocytoma (MFH), fibrosarcoma, chondrosarcoma], while occasionally seen in childhood, are more common in adults (Table 4.2). Multiple myeloma and metastatic carcinoma

Table 4.2 General classification of musculoskeletal tumors

Histologic type	Benign	Malignant
Hematopoietic (41.4%)		Myeloma
		Reticulum cell sarcoma
Chondrogenic (20.9%)	Osteochondroma	Primary chondrosarcoma
	Chondroma	Secondary
	Chondroblastoma	chondrosarcoma
	Chondromyxoid	Dedifferentiated
	fibroma	chondrosarcoma
		Mesenchymal
		chondrosarcoma
Osteogenic (19.3%)	Osteoid osteomas	Osteosarcoma
	Benign osteoblastoma	Parosteal osteosarcoma
Unknown origin (9.8%)	Giant cell tumor	Ewing's sarcoma
		Malignant giant cell tumor
		Adamantinoma
Fibrogenic (3.8%)	Fibrous histiocytoma	Malignant fibrous
	Fibroma	histiocytoma
	Desmoplastic fibroma	Fibrosarcoma
Notochordal (3.1%)		Chordoma
Vascular (1.6%)	Hemangioma	Hemangioendothelioma
		Hemangiopericytoma
Lipogenic (0.5%)	Lipoma	Liposarcoma
Neurogenic (0.5%)	Neurilemmoma	

Source: From Sim FH, Bowman W, Chao E. Limb salvage surgery and reconstructive techniques. In: Sim FH, ed. *Diagnosis and Treatment of Bone Tumors: A Team Approach. A Mayo Clinic Monograph*. Thorofare, NJ: Slack; 1983

typically increase in frequency with increasing patient age and is usually seen in patients over 40 years of age. This section describes the clinical, radiographic, and pathological characteristics and treatment of the primary bone sarcomas.

Osteosarcoma provides the model on which treatment of all other sarcomas is based. The effectiveness of multiagent chemotherapy regimens has been proved by increasing overall survival rates from the bleak, 15–20% with surgery alone in the 1970s to 55–80% by the 1980s. In parallel with improved survival, dramatic advances in reconstructive surgery have made it possible for limb salvage to supplanting amputation as the standard method of treatment.

Classic Osteosarcoma

Osteosarcoma (OS) is a high-grade malignant spindle cell tumor arising within a bone. Its distinguishing characteristic is the production of "tumor" osteoid, or immature bone, directly from a malignant spindle cell stroma.

Clinical Characteristics and Physical Examination

OS typically occurs during childhood and adolescence. In patients over the age of 40, it is usually associated with a preexistent disease such as Paget's disease, irradiated bones, multiple hereditary exostosis, or polyostotic fibrous dysplasia. The most common sites are bones of knee joint (50%) and the proximal humerus (25%). Between 80 and 90% of OS occur in the long tubular bones; the axial skeleton is rarely affected. With the exception of the level of serum alkaline phosphatase, which is elevated in 45–50% of patients, laboratory findings are usually not helpful. Furthermore, an elevated alkaline phosphatase level per se is not diagnostic since it is also found in association with other skeletal diseases such as hyperparathyroidism, (brown tumor), fibrous dysplasia, and Paget's disease. Pain is the most common complaint on presentation, with a firm, soft-tissue mass fixed to the underlying bone found on physical examination. Systemic symptoms are rare. Incidence of pathologic fracture is less than 1%.

Radiographic Characteristics

Typical radiographic findings include increased intramedullary sclerosis (due to tumor bone or calcified cartilage), an area of radiolucency (due to nonossified tumor), a pattern of permeative destruction with poorly defined borders, cortical destruction, periosteal elevation, and extraosseous extension with soft-tissue ossification. This combination of characteristics is not seen with any other lesion. There are three broad categories: sclerotic OS (32%), osteolytic OS (22%), and mixed (46%) (Fig. 4.22). Although there is no statistically significant difference among overall survival rates of these types, it is important to recognize the patterns. The sclerotic and mixed types offer few diagnostic problems. Errors of diagnosis most often occur with pure osteolytic tumors. The differential diagnosis of osteolytic OS includes giant cell tumor, aneurysmal bone cyst, fibrosarcoma, and MFH.

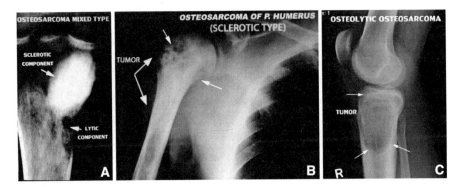

Fig. 4.22 Plain radiographs indicating three radiographic variants of an osteosarcoma. The most common observation is mixed variety (**a**), which has both sclerotic and lytic pattern components. (**b**) A mainly sclerotic lesion of the proximal humerus; and (**c**) a lytic proximal tibia osteosarcoma

Microscopic Characteristics

The diagnosis of OS is based on the identification of a malignant stroma that produces unequivocal osteoid matrix. The stroma consists of a haphazard arrangement of highly atypical cells. The pleomorphic cells contain hyperchromatic, irregular nuclei. Mitotic figures, often atypical, are usually easy to identify. Between these cells is a delicate, lacelike eosinophilic matrix, assumed to be malignant osteoid. The term osteoblastic osteosarcoma is used for those tumors in which the production of malignant osteoid prevails. Calcification of the matrix is variable. Some tumors reveal a predominance of malignant cartilage production, hence the term chondroblastic osteosarcoma. Even though the malignant cartilaginous elements may be overwhelming, the presence of a malignant osteoid matrix warrants the diagnosis of OS. Yet another variant is characterized by large areas of proliferating fibroblasts, arranged in intersecting fascicles. Such areas are indistinguishable from fibrosarcoma, and thorough sampling may be necessary to identify the malignant osteoid component (Figs. 4.23 and 4.24).

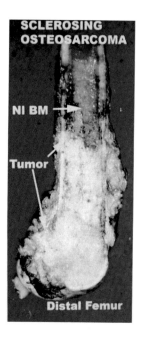

Fig. 4.23 Gross specimen (sagittal section) of a "sclerotic" type of osteosarcoma. Tumor and abnormal bone (*arrows*) are clearly visible

Natural History, Prognosis, and Chemotherapy

Prior to the development of adjuvant chemotherapy, effective treatment was limited to radical margin amputation. Metastasis to the lungs and other bones generally occurred within 24 months. Overall survival rates 2 years after surgery ranged from 5 to 20%. No significant correlation between overall survival and histologic

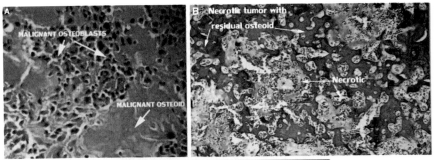

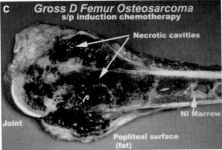

Fig. 4.24 Pathology slides demonstrating microscopic evaluation of osteosarcoma. (**a**) Classic osteosarcoma prior to induction chemotherapy. (**b**) Microscopic appearance of osteosarcoma following chemotherapy. (**c**) Gross specimen following induction chemotherapy. Significant tumor necrosis following chemotherapy is a positive prognostic indicator for osteosarcoma patients. (From Malawer MM, Helman LJ, O'Sullivan B. Sarcomas of bone. In: DeVita VT Jr, Lawrence TS, Rosenberg SA, eds. *Cancer: Principles and Practice of Oncology.* 8th ed. Philadelphia, PA: Lippincott, Williams & Wilkins; 2007:1794–1833. Reprinted with permission)

subtypes, tumor size, patient age, or degree of malignancy was seen. The most significant clinical variable was anatomic site: pelvic and axial lesions had a lower survival rate than extremity tumors, while tibial lesions had a better survival rate than femoral lesions.

The dismal outcome associated with osteosarcoma has been dramatically altered by adjuvant chemotherapy as well as by aggressive thoracotomy for pulmonary disease. A recent update of 227 patients showed that 48% remained alive at an average 11 years after surgery. Of critical importance was that no difference in local recurrence or overall survival was seen between patients undergoing amputation versus limb-sparing surgery. Chemotherapy protocols have typically included various combinations and dosage schedules of high-dose methotrexate (HDMTX), doxorubicin hydrochloride (Adriamycin), and cisplatin. Ifosfamide, which is as effective as adriamycin in single-agent studies, recently has supplanted methotrexate in many ongoing protocols. Multiagent chemotherapy, using various dosing schedules, is now considered standard treatment for osteosarcoma. Success with adjuvant chemotherapy led to investigation of treatment in the neoadjuvant (preoperative) setting. When used in that setting, tumor response results in shrinkage of the soft-tissue components, facilitating surgical excision and subsequent limb salvage.

Limb-Sparing Resection

Limb-salvage surgery is a safe operation for approximately 85–90% of individuals. This technique may be used for all spindle cell sarcomas, regardless of histogenesis. The majority of OS can be treated safely by a limb-sparing resection combined with effective adjuvant treatments. The successful management of localized OS and other sarcomas requires careful coordination and timing of staging studies, biopsy, surgery, and preoperative and postoperative chemotherapy, and/or radiation therapy. The site of the lesion is evaluated as previously described (Fig. 4.25; also see Fig. 4.18). Preoperative studies allow the surgeon to conceptualize the local anatomy and the volume of tissue to be resected and reconstructed.

Overall Treatment Strategy

The patient with a primary tumor of the extremity without evidence of metastases requires surgery to control the primary tumor and chemotherapy to control micrometastatic disease. Eighty to ninety percent of all patients with osteosarcoma fall into this category.

Surgery alone results in a 15–20% cure rate at best. The choice between amputation and limb-sparing resection must be made by an experienced orthopedic oncologist taking into account tumor location, size or extramedullary extent, the presence or absence of distant metastatic disease, and patient factors such as age, skeletal development, and lifestyle preference that might dictate the suitability of limb salvage or amputation. Routine amputations are no longer performed; all patients should be evaluated for limb-sparing options. Intensive, multiagent chemotherapeutic regimens have provided the best results to date. Patients who are judged unsuitable for limb-sparing options may be candidates for presurgical chemotherapy; those with a good response may then become suitable candidates for limb-sparing operations. The management of these patients mandates close cooperation between chemotherapist and surgeon.

Variants of Osteosarcoma

There are 11 recognizable variants of the classic OS. OS arising in the jaw bones is the most common of all variants. Parosteal and periosteal OS are the most common variants of the classic OS occurring in the extremities. In contrast to classic OS, which arises within a bone (intramedullary), parosteal and periosteal OS arises on the surface (juxtacortical) of the bone. Parosteal osteosarcoma is the most common of the unusual variants, representing about 4% of all osteosarcomas.

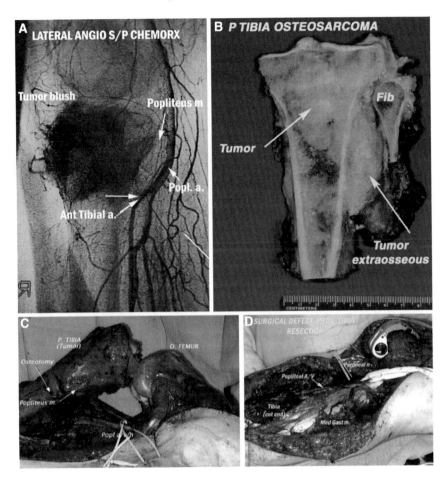

Fig. 4.25 (**a**) Angiogram of vascular bone tumor arising from the proximal tibia. The tumor blush is demonstrated as a proliferation of small vessels which "feed" the growing tumor. (**b**) Gross specimen of proximal tibia, tibio-fibular joint, and proximal fibula following resection. The specimen has been transected lengthwise to reveal the tumor extension. (From Malawer MM, Helman LJ, O'Sullivan B. Sarcomas of bone. In: DeVita VT Jr, Lawrence TS, Rosenberg SA, eds. *Cancer: Principles and Practice of Oncology*. 8th ed. Philadelphia, PA: Lippincott, Williams & Wilkins; 2007:1794–1833. Reprinted with permission.) (**c**) Intraoperative photograph of proximal tibial tumor in situ. (**d**) Surgical field following specimen resection and prior to proximal tibial modular replacement system (MRS) placement. Note that a distal femur articulating surface has been placed. (**e**) The medial gastrocnemius muscle will be rotated over the prosthesis to provide soft-tissue coverage. (**f**) Schematic diagram of soft tissue and extensor mechanism reconstruction following a proximal tibia replacement and reconstruction with a modular endoprosthesis (MRS). Coverage of the prosthesis with the medial gastrocnemius decreases the likelihood of local complications and permits a reliable reconstruction of the extensor mechanism. (Originally published in Malawer MM, Bickels J. Proximal tibial resections with endoprosthetic reconstruction. In: Malawer MM, Sugarbaker PH, eds. *Musculoskeletal Cancer Surgery: Treatment of Sarcomas and Allied Diseases*. Dordrecht, The Netherlands: Kluwer; 2001:485–505.) (**g**) Angiogram of an osteosarcoma arising from the left scapula. (**h**) The scapula and glenohumeral joint is removed and replaced with a snap fit endoprosthesis. Gore-Tex® graft (W.L. Gore & Associates, Inc., Newark, Delaware) is used to create an artificial capsule of the joint. (**i**) Plain radiograph demonstrating the implanted scapula and proximal humeral prostheses

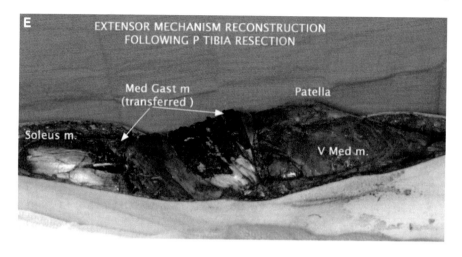

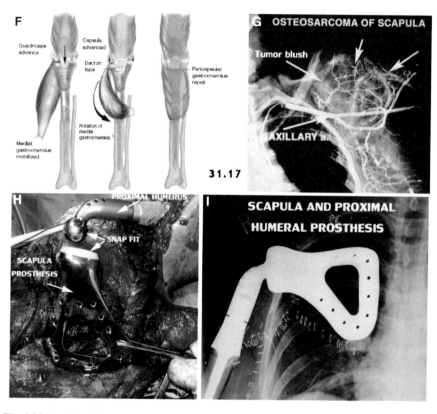

Fig. 4.25 (continued)

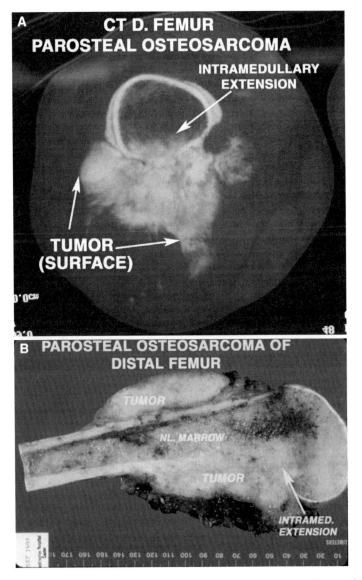

Fig. 4.26 (a) Parosteal osteosarcoma of the distal femur. This CT scan shows a large surface tumor with extension into the medullary space. (From Malawer MM, Helman LJ, O'Sullivan B. Sarcomas of bone. In: DeVita VT Jr, Lawrence TS, Rosenberg SA, eds. *Cancer: Principles & Practice of Oncology.* 8th ed. Philadelphia, PA: Lippincott, Williams & Wilkins; 2007:1794–1833. Reprinted with permission.) (**b**) Gross specimen of the same resected tumor. The CT scan accurately depicted the medullary involvement. Parosteal osteosarcomas represent about 4% of all osteosarcomas

Parosteal Osteosarcoma

Parosteal osteosarcoma (POS) is a distinct variant of conventional osteosarcoma, accounting for 4% of all OS. It arises from the cortex of a bone and generally occurs in older individuals. It has a better prognosis than classical osteosarcoma (Fig. 4.26).

Radiographic Findings

X-rays characteristically show a large, dense, lobulated mass broadly attached to the underlying bone without involvement of the medullary canal. If old enough, the tumor may encircle the bone. The periphery of the lesion is characteristically less mature than the base.

Periosteal Osteosarcoma

Periosteal osteosarcoma is a rare, less aggressive tumor than conventional osteosarcoma. It is a relatively well-differentiated chondroblastic osteosarcoma occurring on the surface of the long bones of the extremities (Fig. 4.27).

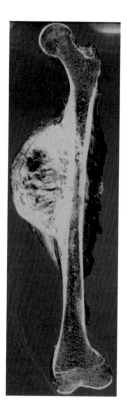

Fig. 4.27 Coronal section of a total femur resected for a large surface periosteal osteosarcoma. Periosteal osteosarcoma represents about 1% of all osteosarcomas and is one of the rarest variants

Radiographically, it is a small radiolucent lesion with some bone spiculation. The cortex remains intact with a scooped out Codman's triangle appearance.

Chondrosarcoma

Chondrosarcoma, the second most common primary malignant spindle cell tumor of bone, is a heterogeneous group of tumors whose basic neoplastic tissue is cartilaginous without evidence of direct osteoid formation. Bone formation occasionally results from differentiation of cartilage. If there is evidence of direct osteoid or bone production, the lesion is classified as an OS. There are five types of chondrosarcoma: central, peripheral, mesenchymal, differentiated, and clear cell. The classic chondrosarcomas are central (arising within a bone) or peripheral (arising from the surface of a bone). The other three are variants and have distinct histological and clinical characteristics.

Both central and peripheral chondrosarcomas can arise as a primary tumor or secondary to underlying neoplasm. Seventy-six percent of primary chondrosarcomas arise centrally. Secondary chondrosarcomas most often arise from benign cartilage tumors. The multiple forms of the benign osteochondromas or enchondromas have a higher rate of malignant transformation than do the corresponding solitary lesions.

Central and Peripheral Chondrosarcomas

Clinical Characteristics and Physical Examination

Half of all chondrosarcomas occur in persons above the age of 40. The most common sites are the pelvis, femur, and shoulder girdle (Fig. 4.28). The clinical presentation varies. Peripheral chondrosarcomas may become quite large without causing pain, and local symptoms develop only because of mechanical irritation. Pelvic chondrosarcomas are often large and present with referred pain to the back or thigh, sciatica secondary to sacral plexus irritation, urinary symptoms from bladder neck involvement, unilateral edema due to iliac vein obstruction, or as a painless abdominal mass. Conversely, central chondrosarcomas present with dull pain. A mass is rarely present. Pain, which indicates active growth, is an ominous sign of a central cartilage lesion. This cannot be overemphasized. An adult with a plain radiograph suggestive of a "benign" cartilage tumor but who is experiencing pain most likely has a chondrosarcoma.

Radiographic Findings

Central chondrosarcomas have two distinct radiological patterns. One is a small, well-defined lytic lesion with a narrow zone of transition and surrounding sclerosis with faint calcification. This is the most common malignant bone tumor that may

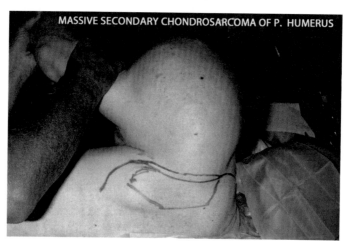

Fig. 4.28 Preoperative photograph of a patient with a massive chondrosarcoma of the proximal humerus secondary to an osteochondroma. This photo illustrates the extremely large size low-grade chondrosarcomas may obtain, especially of the shoulder girdle and the pelvis. This patient did not have metastatic disease and was able to undergo a limb-sparing procedure despite the large size of the tumor

appear radiographically benign. The second type has no sclerotic border and is difficult to localize. The key sign of malignancy is end steal scalloping. This type is difficult to diagnose on plain radiographs and may go undetected for a long period of time. In contrast, peripheral chondrosarcoma is easily recognized as a large mass of characteristic calcification protruding from a bone. Correlation of the clinical, radiographic, and histological data is essential for accurate diagnosis and evaluation of the aggressiveness of cartilage tumor. In general, proximal or axial location, skeletal maturity, and pain point toward malignancy, even though the cartilage may appear benign (Fig. 4.29).

Grading and Prognosis

Chondrosarcomas are graded I, II, and III; the majority are either grade I or grade II. The metastatic rate of moderate grade versus high grade is 15–40% versus 75% [2]. Grade III lesions have the same metastatic potential as osteosarcomas.

In general, peripheral chondrosarcomas are a lower grade than central lesions. Ten-year survival rates among those with peripheral lesions are 77% compared with 32% among those with central lesions. Secondary chondrosarcomas arising from osteochondromas also have a low malignant potential; 85% are grade 1. The multiple forms of benign osteochondromas or enchondromas have a higher rate of malignant transformation than the corresponding solitary lesions.

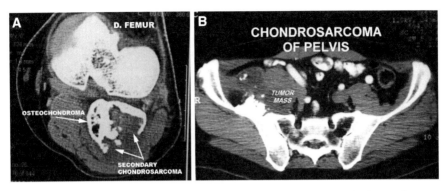

Fig. 4.29 (a) CT scan of the distal femur demonstrating an osteochondroma (benign) and an area of chondrosarcoma arising from the cartilaginous cap. This is termed a secondary chondrosarcoma; most are low grade with a high survival rate. (b) MRI scan showing a large chondrosarcoma of the right ilium. The pelvis is the most common site for chondrosarcomas. Almost all cartilage tumors of the pelvis are malignant

Microscopic Characteristics

The histological spectrum of this neoplasm varies tremendously: High-grade examples can be easily identified, whereas certain low-grade tumors (Fig. 4.30) are exceedingly difficult to distinguish from chondromas. Correlation of the histological features with both the clinical setting and the radiographic changes is therefore

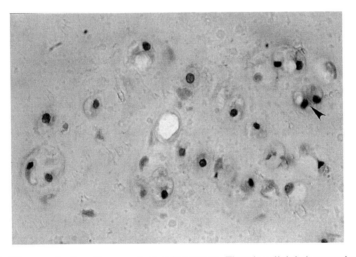

Fig. 4.30 Microscopic view of low-grade chondrosarcoma. There is a slightly increased amount of cellularity. The arrow indicates a binucleated cell. The nuclei of these cells are atypical. (Originally published in Shmookler B, Bickels J, Jelinek JS, et al. Bone and soft tissue sarcomas: epidemiology, radiology, pathology and fundamentals of surgical treatment. In: Malawer MM, Sugarbaker PH, eds. *Musculoskeletal Cancer Surgery: Treatment of Sarcomas and Allied Diseases.* Dordrecht, The Netherlands: Kluwer; 2001:3–35)

of utmost importance in avoiding serious diagnostic error. The grade of malignant cartilaginous tumors correlates with clinical behavior. Grade I tumors are characterized by an increased number of chondrocytes set in a matrix that is chondroid to focally myxoid.

Areas of increased cellularity with more marked variation in cell size, significant nuclear atypia, and frequent pleomorphic forms define a grade II lesion. Binuclear forms are more common in this group.

Grade III chondrosarcomas, which are relatively uncommon, show even greater cellularity, often with spindle cell areas, and reveal prominent mitotic activity. Chondrocytes may contain large, bizarre nuclei. Areas of myxoid changes to the chondroid matrix are common.

Treatment

The treatment of chondrosarcoma is surgical removal. Guidelines for resection for high-grade chondrosarcomas are similar to those for OS. The sites of origin and the fact that chondrosarcomas tend to be low-grade make them amenable to limb-sparing procedures. The four most common sites are the pelvis, proximal femur, shoulder girdle, and diaphyseal portions of long bones.

Variants of Chondrosarcoma

There are three less-common variants of classic chondrosarcoma. Each is briefly described below.

Clear Cell Chondrosarcoma

Clear cell chondrosarcoma, the rarest form of chondrosarcoma, is a slow-growing, locally recurrent tumor resembling a chondroblastoma but with some malignant potential that typically occurs in adults. The most difficult clinical problem is early recognition; it is often confused with chondroblastoma. Metastases occur only after multiple local recurrences. Primary treatment is wide excision. Systemic therapy is not required.

Mesenchymal Chondrosarcoma

Mesenchymal chondrosarcoma is a rare, aggressive variant of chondrosarcoma characterized by a biphasic histological pattern, i.e., small, compact cells intermixed with islands of cartilaginous matrix. This tumor has a predilection for flat bones; long tubular bones are rarely affected. It tends to occur in the younger age group and has a high metastatic potential. The 10-year survival rate is 28%. This entity responds favorably to radiotherapy.

Dedifferentiated Chondrosarcoma

Approximately 10% of chondrosarcomas may dedifferentiate into either a fibrosarcoma or an OS [2, 3]. They occur in older individuals and are often fatal. Surgical treatment is similar to that described for other high-grade sarcomas. Adjuvant therapy is warranted.

Giant Cell Tumor of Bone

Giant cell tumor of bone (GCT) is an aggressive, locally recurrent tumor with a low metastatic potential (4–8%). Giant cell sarcoma of bone refers to a de novo, malignant GCT, not to the tumor that arises from the transformation of a GCT previously thought to be benign. These two lesions are separate clinical entities.

Clinical Characteristics and Physical Examination

GCTs occur slightly more often in females than in males. Eighty percent of GCTs in the long bones occur after skeletal maturity; 75% of these develop around the knee joint (Fig. 4.31). A joint effusion or pathologic fracture, uncommon with other sarcomas, is common with GCTs. GCTs occasionally occur in the vertebrae (2–5%) and the sacrum (10%) [2].

Natural History and Potential Malignancy

Although GCTs are rarely malignant de novo (2–8%), they may undergo transformation and demonstrate malignant potential histologically and clinically after multiple local recurrences. Between 8 and 22% of known GCTs become malignant following local recurrence [2]. This rate decreases to less than 10% if patients who have undergone radiotherapy are excluded. Approximately 40% of malignant GCTs become malignant at the first recurrence. The remainders typically become malignant by the second or third recurrence; thus, each recurrence increases the risk of malignant transformation. A recurrence after 5 years is extremely suspicious for a malignancy. Primary malignant GCT generally has a better prognosis than secondary malignant transformation of typical GCT does, especially if the transformation occurs after radiation therapy. Local recurrence of a GCT is determined by the adequacy of surgical removal rather than by histologic grade.

Radiographic and Clinical Evaluation

GCTs are eccentric lytic lesions without matrix production occurring at the end of long bones. About 10% are axial. They have poorly defined borders with a wide area of transition. They are juxtaepiphyseal with a metaphyseal component. Although the cortex is expanded and appears destroyed, at surgery it is usually found to be attenuated but intact. Periosteal elevation is rare; soft-tissue extension is common.

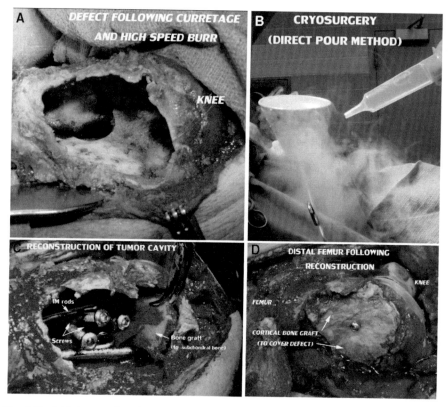

Fig. 4.31 (**a**) Intraoperative photograph following curettage and high speed burr of a giant cell tumor of the distal femur. A large cavity typically remains following this procedure. Although all gross tumor has been removed, it is important to use a local "adjuvant" to decrease the local recurrence rate. (**b**) The use of cryosurgery as an adjuvant modality prevents and kills residual tumor cells. (**c**) Reconstruction of the defect is required to prevent fracture and to permit early mobilization. Bone cement, screws, intramedullary nails, and (**d**) autograft bone (along the subchondral surface) is routinely used for reconstruction

In the skeletally immature patient, aneurysmal bone cyst must be differentiated, although both lesions are closely related. GCTs are classified as Type I, II, or III (Enneking staging system).

Microscopic Characteristics

Two basic cell types constitute the typical GCT. The stroma is characterized by polygonal-to-somewhat spindled cells containing central round nuclei. Scattered diffusely throughout the stroma are benign, multinucleated giant cells. Small foci of osteoid matrix, produced by the benign stroma cells, can be observed; however, chondroid matrix never occurs (Fig. 4.32).

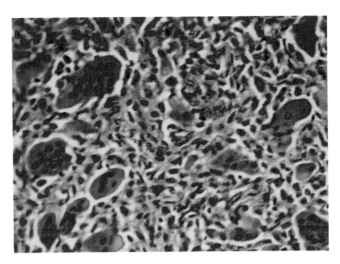

Fig. 4.32 Microscopic appearance of giant cell tumor of bone. There is a normal distribution of orthoclastic giant cells in this image. The stromal cells appear similar to the nuclei of the giant cells and in fact coalesce to form new giant cells. (Originally published in Shmookler B, Bickels J, Jelinek JS, et al. Bone and soft tissue sarcomas: epidemiology, radiology, pathology and fundamentals of surgical treatment. In: Malawer MM, Sugarbaker PH, eds. *Musculoskeletal Cancer Surgery: Treatment of Sarcomas and Allied Diseases.* Dordrecht, The Netherlands: Kluwer; 2001:3–35)

Treatment

Treatment of GCT of bone is surgical removal. In general, curettage of the bony cavity with "cleaning" of the walls with a high-speed burr drill and the use of a physical adjuvant will kill any cells remaining within the cavity wall. The author prefers the combined use of cryosurgery (either liquid nitrogen or a closed system of argon/helium) to obtain temperatures of –40°C. The cavity is then reconstructed with bone graft, PMMA, and internal fixation devices, which permit early mobilization.

Malignant Fibrous Histiocytoma

Clinical Characteristics

Malignant fibrous histiocytoma (MFH) is a high-grade bone tumor histologically similar to its soft-tissue counterpart. Osteoid production is absent. It is a disease of adulthood. The most common sites are the metaphyseal ends of long bones, especially around the knee. Alkaline phosphatase values are normal, helping rule out an osteosarcoma or fibrosarcoma. Pathologic fracture is common. MFH disseminates rapidly. Lymphatic involvement, although rare for other bone sarcomas, has been reported.

Radiographic Characteristics

MFH is an osteolytic lesion associated with marked cortical disruption, minimal cortical or periosteal reaction, and no evidence of matrix formation. The extent of the tumor routinely exceeds plain radiographic signs. MFH may be multicentric (10%) and associated with bone infarcts (10%).

Treatment

Treatment is similar to that of other high-grade sarcomas. Adjuvant chemotherapy has similar results to that seen in the treatment of osteosarcoma.

Fibrosarcoma of Bone

Clinical Characteristics

Fibrosarcoma of bone is a rare entity, accounting for only 1% of bone tumors. It is characterized by interlacing bundles of collagen fibers (herringbone pattern) without any evidence of tumor bone or osteoid formation. Fibrosarcoma occurs in middle age. The long bones are most affected. Fibrosarcomas occasionally arise secondarily in conjunction with an underlying disease such as fibrous dysplasia, Paget's disease, bone infarcts, osteomyelitis, postirradiation bone, and GCT. Fibrosarcoma may be either central or cortical (termed *periosteal*). The histological grade is a good prognosticator of metastatic potential. Overall, survival rate is 27 and 52% for central and peripheral lesions, respectively. Late metastases do occur, and 10- and 15-year survival rates vary. In general, periosteal tumors have a better prognosis than central lesions do.

Radiographic Features

Fibrosarcoma is a radiolucent lesion that shows minimal periosteal and cortical reaction. The radiographic appearance closely correlates with the histological grade of the tumor. Low-grade tumors are well defined, whereas high-grade lesions demonstrate indistinct margins and bone destruction similar to those of osteolytic OS. Plain radiographs often underestimate the extent of the lesion. Pathologic fracture is common (30%) because of the lack of matrix formation. Differential diagnosis includes GCT, aneurysmal bone cyst, MFH, and osteolytic OS.

Ewing's Sarcoma and Other Small Round Cell Sarcomas of Bone

Round cell sarcomas of bone behave differently and require different therapeutic management than do spindle cell sarcomas. Round cell sarcomas of bone consist of poorly differentiated small cells without matrix production. They present radiographically as osteolytic lesions. These lesions are best treated with radiation and chemotherapy; surgery is reserved for special situations. Non-Hodgkin's lymphoma and Ewing's sarcoma are the most common small cell sarcomas. The differential diagnosis of round cell sarcomas includes metastatic neuroblastoma, metastatic undifferentiated carcinoma, histiocytosis, small cell OS, osteomyelitis, and multiple myeloma.

Ewing's Sarcoma

Ewing's sarcoma is the second most common bone sarcoma of childhood; it is approximately one-half as frequent as OS. The lesion is characterized by poorly differentiated, small, round cells with marked homogeneity. The exact cell of origin is unknown. The clinical and biological behavior is significantly different from that of spindle cell sarcomas. Within the past two decades, the prognosis of patients with Ewing's sarcomas has dramatically been improved by the combination of adjuvant chemotherapy, improved radiotherapy techniques, and the select use of limited surgical resection.

Clinical Characteristics and Physical Examination

Ewing's sarcomas tend to occur in young children, though rarely in those below the age of 5 years. Characteristically the flat and axial bones (50–60%) are involved. When a long (tubular) bone is involved, it is most often the proximal or diaphyseal area. In contrast, OSs occur in adolescence (average age 15), most often around the knees, and involve the metaphysis of long bones. Another unique finding with Ewing's sarcomas is systemic signs, i.e., fever, anorexia, weight loss, leukocytosis, and anemia [2]. All may be a presenting sign of the disease (20–30%); this is in contrast to the distinct absence of systemic signs with OS until late in the disease process. The most common complaint is pain and/or a mass. Localized tenderness is often present with associated erythema and induration. These findings, in combination with systemic signs of fever and leukocytosis, closely mimic those of osteomyelitis.

Radiographic Findings

Ewing's sarcoma is a highly destructive radiolucent lesion without evidence of bone formation. The typical pattern consists of a permeative or moth-eaten destruction associated with periosteal elevation. Characteristically there is multilaminated periosteal elevation or a sunburst appearance. When Ewing's sarcoma occurs in flat bones, however, these findings are usually absent. Tumors of flat bones appear as a destructive lesion with a large soft-tissue component (Fig. 4.33). The ribs and pelvis are most often involved. Pathologic fractures occur secondary to extensive bony destruction and the absence of tumor matrix. The differential diagnosis is osteomyelitis, osteolytic OS, metastatic neuroblastoma, and histiocytosis.

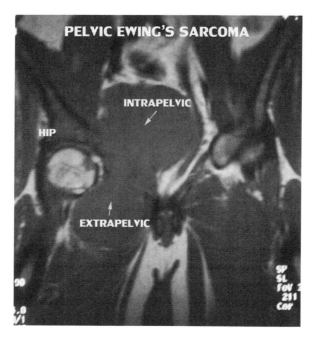

Fig. 4.33 This scan demonstrates a huge pelvic Ewing's sarcoma with both intra- and extrapelvic extension. Almost all Ewing's sarcomas are accompanied by a soft-tissue component, as they readily break through the originating bone cortex. Ewing's sarcomas arise mostly from flat bones in contrast to osteosarcomas that most often arise from the metaphyseal ends of long bones. Ewing's sarcomas have approximately one-half the incidence of osteosarcomas and tend to occur in younger children

Natural History

Ewing's sarcoma is highly lethal and rapidly disseminates. Historically, fewer than 10–15% of patients remained disease free at 2 years [2]. Many patients present with metastatic disease. The most common sites are the lungs and other bones. Ewing's sarcoma was once thought to be a multicentric disease because of the high incidence of multiple bone involvement. Unlike other bone sarcomas, Ewing's sarcoma is associated with visceral, lymphatic, and meningeal involvement, and these must be searched for.

Radiographic Evaluation and Staging

There is no general staging system for Ewing's sarcoma. The musculoskeletal staging system does not apply to the round cell sarcomas of the bone. Because these lesions have a propensity to spread to other bones, bone marrow, the lymphatic system, and the viscera, evaluation is more extensive than that for spindle cell sarcomas. It must include a careful clinical examination of regional and distal lymph nodes and radiographic evaluation for visceral involvement. Liver–spleen scans and bone marrow aspirates are required, in addition to CT of the lungs and the primary site. Angiography is required only if a primary resection is planned.

Biopsy Considerations

Because of the frequent difficulty of accurate pathological interpretation and potential problems with bone heating, the following are guidelines for the biopsy of suspected round cell tumors:

1. Adequate material must be obtained for histological evaluation and electron microscopy.
2. Routine cultures should be made to aid in the differentiation from an osteomyelitis.
3. Biopsy of the bony component is not necessary. The soft-tissue component generally provides adequate material. Bone biopsy should be through a *small* hole on the compressive side of the bone. Pathologic fracture through an irradiated bone often does not heal.

Microscopic Characteristics

Large nests and sheets of relatively uniform round cells are typical. The sheets are often compartmentalized by intersecting collagenous trabeculae. The cells contain round nuclei with a distinct nuclear envelope. Nucleoli are uncommon, and mitotic activity is minimal. There may be occasional rosette-like structures, although neuroectodermal origin has never been confirmed. In the vicinity of necrotic tumor, small pyknotic cells may be observed. Vessels in these necrotic regions often are encircled by viable tumor cells. The cells often contain cytoplasmic glycogen. This neoplasm belongs to the category of small blue round cell tumors, a designation that also includes neuroblastoma, lymphoma, metastatic OS, and, occasionally, osteomyelitis and histiocytosis. When confronted with this differential diagnosis, the pathologist may turn to electron microscopy or immunohistochemistry for additional information.

Combined Multimodality Treatment

Ewing's sarcomas are generally considered radiosensitive. Radiation therapy to the primary site has been the traditional mode of local control. Within the past decade, surgical resection of selected lesions has become increasingly popular. Though detailed management is beyond the scope of this chapter, the following sections summarize some common aspects of the multimodality approach.

Chemotherapy

Doxorubicin, actinomycin D, cyclophosphamide, and vincristine are the most effective agents. There are a variety of different combinations and schedules. All patients require intensive chemotherapy to prevent dissemination. Overall survival in patients with lesions of the extremities now ranges between 40 and 75%.

Radiation Therapy

Radiation to the entire bone at risk is required. The usual dose ranges between 4,500 and 6,000 cGy delivered in 6–8 weeks. In order to reduce the morbidity of radiation, it is recommended that between 4,000 and 5,000 cGy be delivered to the whole bone, with an additional 1,000–1,500 cGy to the tumor site.

Surgical Treatment

The role of surgery in the treatment of Ewing's sarcoma is currently undergoing change. The Intergroup Ewing's Study recommends surgical removal of expendable bones such as the ribs, clavicle, and scapula. In general, surgery is reserved for tumors located in high-risk areas, e.g., the ribs, ilium, and proximal femur. *Risk* is defined as an increased incidence of local recurrence and metastases. In general, surgery is considered an adjunct to the other treatment modalities.

Recently there has been increased interest in primary resection of Ewing's sarcoma following induction (neoadjuvant) chemotherapy, similar to the treatment of OS. When this is performed, radiation therapy is not given if the surgical margins are negative (wide resection). The goal of this approach is to increase local control as well as minimize the complications and functional losses that are associated with high-dose radiotherapy.

Multiple Myeloma/Plasmocytoma

Clinical and Physical Examination

Multiple myeloma is often referred to as the most common primary malignancy of bone, with an incidence between 2 and 3 cases per 100,000. It is a disease of older adults and frequently presents with signs and symptoms related to bone marrow suppression, hypercalcemia, and renal failure. Bone pain and spontaneous vertebral fractures are often present. The radiographic hallmark of this disease is multiple osteolytic (punched-out) lesions involving both the axial and appendicular skeleton. Bone scans are typically less sensitive than plain radiographs because osteoclast activity predominates in the lytic process. Myeloma should be suspected when routine laboratory studies reveal anemia, increased serum creatinine, elevated calcium, and elevated serum protein. Confirmation can be readily made by demonstrating a monoclonal spike on a serum protein electrophoresis (SPEP). Infection and renal failure are the most common causes of death, and the presence of either is a poor prognostic indicator.

Metastatic Bone Disease and Pathologic Fracture Overview

Approximately 100,000 patients a year in the United States develop metastatic bony disease. The orthopedic surgeon is commonly asked to manage patients with skeletal metastases. The operative and nonoperative treatment of metastatic disease is continuously evolving. Approximately 85% of all patients dying of cancer will have skeletal involvement, although only 5% will sustain a pathological fracture.

Diagnosis

Clinical Characteristics and Physical Examination

Metastatic carcinoma is the most common bone tumor in patients over 40 years of age. Despite the wide variety of carcinomas, the hallmark of skeletal involvement is pain. A patient with a known cancer who develops skeletal pain must be assumed to have a bony metastasis until proved otherwise. Approximately 10% of cancer patients present with bony metastasis as the first sign of the disease. Plain radiographs may appear normal for weeks or months after the onset of pain. Thus, clinical suspicion is the key to accurate diagnosis. The most common primary sources of skeletal metastases are the lungs, breast, prostate, pancreas, and stomach (Figs. 4.34–4.36).

Patterns of Metastases and Batson's Plexus

Bone scans are highly accurate and demonstrate increased uptake of contrast medium. The most common sites of involvement are spine (thoracic, then lumbar), pelvis, femur, and ribs. This distribution reflects the pattern of hematogenous spread. Vertebral lesions are thought to be secondary to seeding via Batson's plexus, i.e., perivertebral via the valveless venous plexus that permits retrograde flow. The hip and femur are the most common sites of pathologic fracture. Spinal involvement presents with back pain or neurological deficit secondary to epidural compression. Laboratory data may show hypercalcemia, reflecting accelerated bone resorption. An elevated alkaline phosphatase level is less common and is due to a secondary osteoblastic attempt to repair the destructive lesion. An elevated acid phosphatase level is pathognomonic of metastatic prostate cancer.

Staging Studies

Staging studies are similar to those used in the evaluation of primary sarcomas. The information obtained is useful in local evaluation and in therapy.

Radiographic Findings

Most metastatic carcinomas tend to be irregularly osteolytic with some osteoblastic response. Characteristically, osteoblastic metastases occur in the breast, prostate, lung, or bladder. In general, most endocrine tumors tend to be osteoblastic, whereas nonendocrine tumors tend to be radiolucent or osteolytic. Between 75 and 90% of

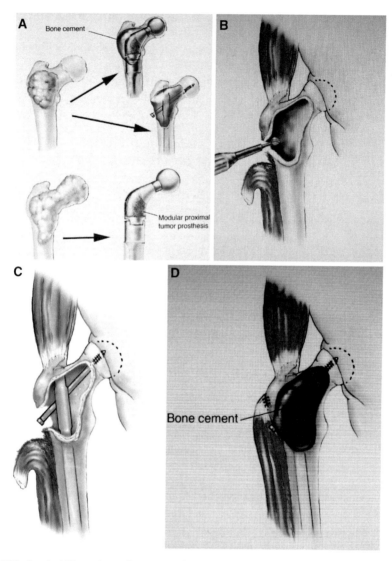

Fig. 4.34 Surgical illustrations of treatment of metastatic bone disease. The proximal femur (hip) is one of the most common sites and often requires surgical reconstruction due to the presence or risk of fracture (termed a "pathological" fracture). (**a**) Femoral head and neck reconstruction by internal fixation with a nail and screw and bone cement or modular femoral endoprosthetic replacement. (From Bickels J, Malawer MM. Surgical management of metastatic bone disease, general considerations. In: Wiesel S, ed. *Operative Techniques in Orthopedic Surgery*. Philadelphia, PA: Lippincott, Williams & Wilkins. In press.) (**b**) Intraoperative illustration of curettage of a metastatic lesion with its resultant cavity. (**c**) Fixation with an intramedullary rod and nail followed by (**d**) polymethylmethacrylate (PMMA) cementation. (From Bickels J, Malawer MM. Surgical management of metastatic bone disease, femoral lesions. In: Wiesel S, ed. *Operative Techniques in Orthopedic Surgery*. Philadelphia, PA: Lippincott, Williams, & Wilkins. In press)

Fig. 4.35 Plain radiograph showing an impending pathological fracture of the proximal femur due to several areas of metastatic disease

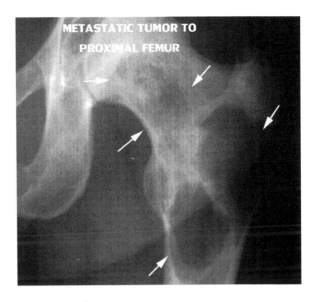

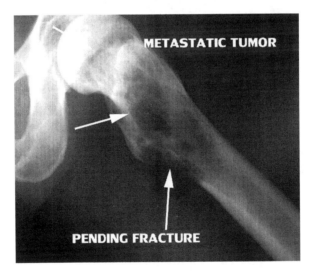

Fig. 4.36 Lateral radiograph of a pending pathological fracture through a large metastatic lesion of the femoral head. The hip (i.e., proximal femur) is the most common site of pathological fractures. The large majority requires either prosthetic replacement or reconstruction with a combined internal fixation with an intramedullary device and supplemented by polymethylmethacrylate (PMMA) for immediate fixation. Early immobilization is the main goal in the surgical treatment of hip metastases

patients with metastatic disease have multiple lesions at initial presentation. Soft-tissue extension is rare for metastatic disease. Periosteal elevation is rare except with prostate cancer. Radiographic diagnosis of metastatic disease tends to be simple (Figs. 4.35 and 4.36). Factors favoring metastasis are irregular osteolytic and/or mixed osteoblastic lesion, multiple lesions, and age above 40 years. A few metastatic lesions may mimic a primary sarcoma. Specifically, a metastatic prostate (osteoblastic) lesion may appear as a primary osteosarcoma and a solitary hypernephroma as an osteolytic sarcoma, e.g., MFH of bone.

Bone Scans

Bone scintigraphy is the most helpful study in evaluating metastatic disease. Presence of multiple lesions favors the diagnosis of metastatic carcinoma and often suggests that there is involvement of other anatomic areas not suspected from clinical examination. Intraosseous extension beyond the area indicated by the plain radiographs is not unusual; this is due to the propensity of carcinoma cells to permeate between the bony trabeculae.

Computed Tomography/Magnetic Resonance Imaging

Axial studies of the body are not only helpful in the definition of localized skeletal disease but are of great importance in diagnosing the site of primary disease in patients initially presenting with a bone lesion. CT scans of the chest and contrast-enhanced CT scans of the abdomen and pelvis allow for accurate screening for solid tumors of the major organ systems. Despite this, however, approximately 10% of all patients will never have an identifiable site of primary disease. MRI has become increasingly useful in patients with spinal, pelvic, and hip lesions. Thus, both CT and MRI are useful in evaluation of patients with metastatic disease.

Biopsy

The principles and techniques of biopsy are similar to those described for primary bone tumors. If a metastatic lesion is strongly suspected, a needle biopsy is often sufficient (90%) for a correct diagnosis. Needle biopsies are most useful for confirming metastatic carcinoma in a patient with a known cancer.

Microscopic Characteristics

The primary site determines, to a large degree, the histological appearance of the metastatic focus. Unequivocal epithelial features such as acinar formation, papillae with epithelial lining, or keratin pearl formation indicate that the lesion is not primary in bone; furthermore, based on both the pattern and certain histochemical properties, a likely primary site can be suggested. For example, the presence of epithelial mucins within tumor cell vacuoles suggests lung, gastrointestinal tract, or pancreas, among others, as possible primary sites. The Fontana stain confirms the presence of melanin pigment, as would be expected in malignant melanoma. Immunohistochemical studies, as for thyroglobulin or prostate-specific acid phosphatase, offer an additional means of tumor identification.

Treatment

Treatment considerations for patients with metastatic skeletal disease differ from those for patients with primary bone neoplasms. In general, overall survival is less than 1 year. The main goals of treatment are relief of bone pain, prevention of fracture, continued ambulation, and avoidance of cord compression from metastatic vertebral disease. The treatment for each patient must be highly individualized, but there are certain guidelines:

1. Bone pain can be relieved by analgesics and radiation therapy. Lesions of the lower extremity often require prophylactic fixation to avoid fracture. Closed intramedullary rodding reduces the local morbidity of diaphyseal lesions.
2. If multiple sites are involved, the lower extremity (especially the hips) should be treated early to permit ambulation.
3. Early spinal cord compression should be treated aggressively with radiotherapy. If symptoms persist, early decompression is required. Increasing back pain is an early sign of cord compression.
4. Intramedullary fixation is preferred over screw-and-plate fixation. Endoprosthetic replacement is preferred for the hip in lieu of nail or plate fixation (Fig. 4.34).
5. Polymethylmethacrylate is required to permit immediate stable fixation and to prevent loosening.
6. Perioperative antibiotics are required because of the increased risk of infection.
7. Hematologic parameters should be carefully evaluated before, during, and after surgery because of the increased risk of bleeding in cancer patients (coagulopathy). The platelet count, prothrombin time (PT), and partial prothrombin time (PTT) are routinely obtained.

Common Operative Procedures for Metastatic Tumors Involving Common Anatomic Site-Guidelines

Curettage and cementation: Curettage and cementation combined with internal fixation for diaphyseal fractures (femur, humerus, tibia). Alternatively in some particular sites (e.g., elbow, shoulder), cementation and fixation is accomplished by a cortical plate and screw combination

Endoprosthetic replacement (hip): The hip is the most common area of bony metastases after the pelvis and spine (vertebral bodies).

Pelvis: Usually treated with radiation therapy only except for large tumors of the periacetabular areas. These are often treated by curettage and cementation or possible total hip replacement.

Benign Bone Tumors

Benign bone tumors are more common than malignant bone tumors and usually occur during childhood or adolescence. Some can be treated successfully by simple curettage (intralesional procedure), while others require extensive resection (marginal or wide). Treatment is based upon the natural history of the specific entity. Treatment must be individualized; preservation of function is important. The important clinical aspects of these tumors are emphasized in this section. In general, the preoperative staging studies are extremely accurate, and the plain radiographs often suggest the correct diagnosis.

Solitary and Multiple Osteochondromas (Exostosis)

Osteochondromas are the most common benign bone tumor. They are characteristically sessile or pedunculated, arising from the cortex of a long tubular bone adjacent to the epiphyseal plate. Osteochondromas are usually solitary except in patients with multiple hereditary exostosis. Plain radiographs are usually diagnostic and no further tests are required. Sessile osteochondromas present difficulty in diagnosis, especially when found in unusual sites such as the distal posterior femur, in which case they must be differentiated from a parosteal OS. Bone scintigraphy and CT are helpful in distinguishing between these two entities (Fig. 4.37).

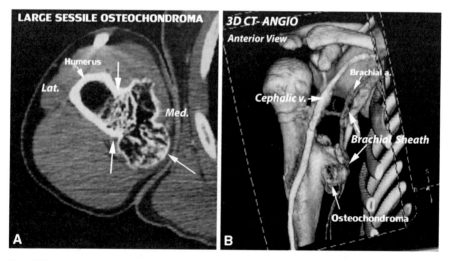

Fig. 4.37 (a) CT scan showing a large sessile osteochondroma of the humerus. (b) Three-dimensional CT angiography showing osteochondroma displacing the neurovascular structures

Osteochondromas grow along with the individual until skeletal maturity is reached; growth of an osteochondroma during adolescence therefore does not signify malignancy. Pain is not a sign of malignancy in children or adolescents, although in an adult it is a significant warning sign. Pain in a child may be due to local bursitis, mechanical irritation of adjacent muscles, or pathologic fracture.

Between 1 and 2% of solitary osteochondromas undergo malignant transformation; patients with multiple hereditary exostosis are at a higher (5–25%) risk. Malignant tumors arising from a benign osteochondroma are usually low-grade chondrosarcomas. Proximal osteochondromas are at a higher risk to undergo malignant transformation than are distal lesions. In general, surgical removal is recommended only for symptomatic osteochondromas or for those arising along the axial skeleton and pelvic and shoulder girdle.

Enchondromas

Enchondromas may be solitary or multiple (Ollier's disease). They have been reported in most bones. These lesions are often difficult to diagnose radiographically and histologically. The biological potential is often overestimated or underestimated. Malignant transformations do occur, but the rate is difficult to determine. In general, lesions of the pelvis, femur, and ribs are at higher risk than are more distal sites.

Enchondromas are rarely painful unless a pathologic fracture exists. Otherwise, pain is a sign of local aggressiveness and possible malignancy. Enchondromas of the hands and feet, irrespective of pathological findings, are benign, whereas cartilage tumors of the pelvic or shoulder girdle are often malignant, despite a benign-appearing histological appearance. Plain radiographs may be helpful in this differentiation. Radiographic scalloping is a sign of local aggressiveness. Bone scintigraphy is not helpful in differentiating a low-grade chondrosarcoma from an active enchondroma. Age is an important indicator of possible malignancy; enchondromas rarely undergo malignant transformation prior to skeletal maturity. Painful, benign-appearing, proximal enchondromas in an adult are often malignant, despite the histological findings. The correlation of symptoms, plain radiographs, and histological findings is crucial in assessing an individual cartilage tumor.

Curettage of enchondromas, with or without bone graft, in a child is usually curative. Pathologic fracture may require internal fixation in addition to curettage. In an adult, curettage has a significant rate of local recurrence; resection or curettage combined with cryosurgery has a high success rate.

Microscopic Characteristics

When chondroid lesions are under evaluation, histological features must be correlated with both radiographic changes and the clinical setting. There may be variable cellularity, but the chondrocytes tend to remain small and uniform. Nuclear atypia is minimal, and occasional binucleate forms are not inconsistent with the diagnosis of a benign lesion. As a rule, the chondrocytes are situated in individual lacunae. Correlating with the gross findings, foci of calcification and endochondral ossification can be observed. Features such as marked nuclear atypia, mitotic activity, myxoid degeneration of matrix, and multiple cells in individual lacunae should raise a strong suspicion of chondrosarcoma.

Chondroblastoma, Osteoblastoma, and Osteoid Osteoma

Chondroblastoma and osteoblastoma are characterized by immature but benign chondroid and osteoid production, respectively. Both may undergo malignant transformation in rare cases, and osteoblastoma can metastasize. Osteoid osteomas are small (less than 1 cm), painful, bone-forming tumors that are always benign. Chondroblastomas typically occur in the epiphysis of a skeletally immature child. Although osteoblastomas may be found in any bone, the spine and skull account for 50% of all reported cases. The differential diagnosis of chondroblastoma includes GCT, aneurysmal bone cyst, and clear cell chondrosarcoma. Osteoblastoma must be differentiated from osteosarcoma and osteoid osteoma. Clinical correlation of age, site, and histological findings often points to the correct diagnosis.

Chondroblastomas and osteoblastomas are aggressive benign lesions with a high recurrence rate following simple curettage. Local control can be obtained by primary resection; however, routine resection cannot be recommended for tumors adjacent to a joint. Cryosurgery has avoided the need for resection and extensive reconstruction in select patients.

Osteoid Osteoma

Clinical Characteristics and Physical Examination

This lesion has classic symptoms and radiographic appearance in 80% of patients. Osteoid osteomas are extremely painful (equivalent to a severe toothache) and well localized. Pain is often worse at night. The pain is relieved by salicylates; narcotics often are not helpful. The response to salicylates is dramatic, occurring in 20–30 min with a minimal dose of one or two tablets of regular-strength aspirin. This pain pattern may exist for 6–9 months before the appropriate diagnosis is considered. Occasionally, the pain precedes the appearance of radiographic abnormalities and therefore leads to multiple incorrect diagnoses, including neuroses. The most common anatomic sites are the femur and tibia, although any bone, including the skull, spine, and small bones of the hands and feet, may be involved. When the lesion is located near a joint, symptoms may mimic those of monoarticular arthritis.

Osteoid osteomas of the spine often present as a painful scoliosis mimicking a vertebral osteomyelitis, spinal cord tumor, or abdominal disease. There is an interfacing network of irregular partially calcified bony trabeculae that resembles that seen in osteoblastoma.

Radiographic Appearance and Evaluation

The tumor can be found in any portion of a bone. The position relative to the cortex, periosteum, and spongiosa determines the radiographic appearance (Fig. 4.38). The most common site is intracortical. Plain radiographs may show the nidus (lesion), which is radiolucent but often obscured by a large amount of dense, white, reactive bone that is stimulated in response to the tumor. When the lesion is intramedullary, there is less sclerotic response. Detection and localization of the lesion are difficult. Bone scintigraphy is the most useful staging study and demonstrates markedly increased uptake of contrast medium.

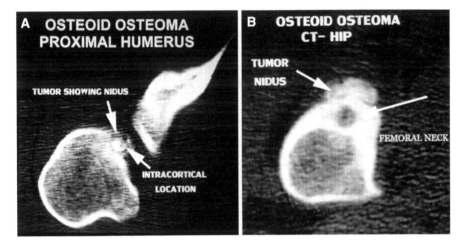

Fig. 4.38 (**a, b**) CT scans demonstrating osteoid osteomas of the proximal humerus and the hip, respectively. These small tumors produce prostaglandins and are extremely painful. Relief of symptoms following treatment with aspirin can be of diagnostic significance for these tumors. Today, most osteoid osteomas are treated by radiofrequency ablation (RFA) in lieu of surgical excision

Treatment

Surgical removal of the nidus is required; the sclerotic, reactive bone need not be removed. Pain is dramatically resolved if the nidus has been excised. Incomplete removal routinely results in a clinical recurrence. Recently, nonsurgical removal by CT-guided radiofrequency ablation has been recommended.

Aneurysmal Bone Cysts

Aneurysmal bone cysts (ABCs) are benign tumors of childhood, occurring typically before skeletal maturity. They never become malignant. They often involve
the metaphyseal regions of the long bones or the vertebrae. Radiographically,
ABCs are eccentric, lytic, and expansile, characterized by cortical destruction
and periosteal elevation. They can grow rapidly and appear extremely aggressive,
and distinguishing them from a primary malignancy may be difficult. Differential
diagnosis includes GCT and telangiectatic osteosarcoma. ABCs contain some
osteoid; however, careful examination reveals this to be reactive and not neoplastic.
Approximately one-third arise in conjunction with another bony neoplasm.

Unicameral (Simple) Bone Cysts

Unicameral bone cysts (UBCs) are benign lesions that occur during growth. They
involve the metaphysis and/or the diaphysis of a long bone. They are not believed to
be true neoplasms.

The most common sites are the proximal humerus (67%) and proximal femur
(15%). UBCs are usually asymptomatic until a fracture occurs. Radiographically,
UBCs are radiolucent and slightly expansile, with well-defined margins. UBCs
are rarely confused with other benign or malignant tumors. Plain radiograph is
the primary imaging study utilized for diagnosis when these tumors arise in common locations. Other preoperative staging studies usually are not required. Bone
scintigraphy is the most useful study when the diagnosis is in doubt. The bone scan
typically shows a photon-deficient area corresponding to detail on the plain radiograph. A small area of increased uptake of contrast reflects a typical hairline crack
that initiates pain and radiographic investigation.

Treatment

The traditional treatment has been curettage. Recently, aspiration, flushing, and
injection with methylprednisolone acetate have successfully treated UBCs.

UBCs are treated by aspiration, high-pressure Renografin injection (diatrizoate meglumine and diatrizoate sodium), and intracavitary methylprednisolone.
Pathologic fractures should be allowed to heal *before* injection is performed. If the
diagnosis is in doubt, a Craig needle procedure or small incisional biopsy should be
performed. There may be radiographic recurrence; this can be successfully treated
with repeat injections. UBCs should not be left untreated in the hope that they will
spontaneously regress. Less than 1% of UBCs do so; the remainders often become
large before the appropriate treatment is undertaken, making definitive treatment
more difficult. Alternatively, UBCs are treated by curettage and bone grafting.

Eosinophilic Granuloma (Histiocytosis X)

Langerhans' cell histiocytosis is a more descriptive and recently accepted term to describe the disease commonly referred to as histiocytosis X. Eosinophilic granuloma (EG) is a solitary destructive lesion arising presumably from the reticuloendothelial system during the first decade of life. There is slight male predominance. Any bone may be involved, but the most common sites are the long bones and commonly the periacetabular region. The skull, mandible, ribs, and vertebrae are frequent sites. Multiple bony involvement is common; between 10 and 20% of patients develop multiple lesions. Plain radiographs characteristically show a lytic, punched-out lesion with some evidence of cortical destruction. Approximately 50% of patients have periosteal elevation. The differential diagnosis includes osteomyelitis, Ewing's sarcoma, and lymphoma. The diaphysis and the metaphysis are equally affected. Primary epiphyseal involvement or extension is rare:

Good results have been achieved with the use of steroids to treat localized bony EG. The natural history of EG of bone is to spontaneously heal. Curettage or intralesional steroid is recommended for documented lesions, especially in a weight-bearing bone.

Tumors Originating from the Joint

Specific Diagnoses

Pigmented Villonodular Synovitis (Aggressive Synovitis)

Pigmented villonodular synovitis (PVNS) is a rare primary disease of the synovium characterized by exuberant proliferation with the formation of villi and nodules. It presents with localized pain, joint swelling, a thickened synovium, and an effusion which on aspiration shows either a brownish or a serosanguineous discoloration. PVNS commonly occurs between the second and the fifth decades of life. The knee is most commonly involved (75–90%), followed by the hip and ankle joints. Treatment is often delayed because PVNS is not considered in the differential diagnosis. Clinical suspicion is the key to early diagnosis. PVNS should be considered in the differential diagnosis of a monoarticular arthritis of the knee or hip joint. Simple aspiration is often suggestive, and synovial biopsy is definitive. Plain radiographs demonstrate juxtacortical erosions of both sides of an affected joint and may show marked joint or bone destruction if the disease has been present for a long time. Arthrography and arthroscopy are helpful in establishing the correct diagnosis. Arthrography shows diffuse nodular masses, while arthroscopy shows a brownish, discolored synovium with large, flattened nodules and villous proliferation. Rarely, PVNS may present as a primary bony or soft-tissue tumor due to marked proliferation of the synovium with destruction of the adjacent joint or a soft-tissue mass. The histological findings in this situation may incorrectly suggest an MFH.

PVNS is treated by surgical excision. Localized lesions require simple excision, while extensive involvement requires a synovectomy. If the anterior or posterior compartments of the knee may be extensively involved, a staged approach is required (Fig. 4.39). The anterior joint is treated through a standard midline incision and arthrotomy. The posterior knee is best approached by a popliteal incision with complete exposure of the posterior capsule. The author's preference is to begin by performing an anterior synovectomy, which should enable the patient to regain knee motion, and then perform a posterior synovectomy. Recurrent disease should be treated by surgical excision. If there is extensive bony destruction, arthrodesis or prosthetic replacement, combined with an extraarticular joint resection, is required. Low-dose radiation treatment may be beneficial in improving local control, particularly in high-risk patients.

Fig. 4.39 Lateral view of MRI showing pigmented villonodular synovitis (PVNS) of the knee. Arrows delineate the anterior and posterior tumor extension. PVNS is often difficult to cure and require extensive anterior and posterior synovectomies, sometimes followed by radiation therapy

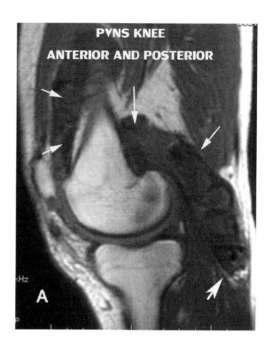

Microscopic Characteristics

The typical lesion consists of heterogeneous population of cells. The villi are lined by several layers of plump synovial cells. Beneath the synovium are sheets of histiocytes, xanthoma cells, hemosiderin-laden macrophages, and multinucleated giant cells, all in variable proportions. Occasionally, slitlike spaces are present within the more cellular areas.

Ganglia

Ganglia are among the most common soft-tissue lesions. The wrist is the most common location; other sites include the metatarsophalangeal joints and the ankle and knee joints. When the lesions are located in unusual sites, the diagnosis is often less obvious. Ganglia represent benign myxoid degeneration. It must be emphasized that all masses are not ganglia and should be critically evaluated. All too often, a sarcoma of the hand or ankle is assumed to be a ganglion. Excision is undertaken, and the correct diagnosis is made only after extensive soft-tissue contamination has occurred. This unfortunate circumstance leads to many lost limbs. Treatment of ganglia is simple excision or aspiration.

Soft-Tissue Sarcomas

Soft-tissue sarcomas (STSs) are malignant tumors arising from or within the soft tissues of the extremities or the shoulder and/or the pelvic girdle. These heterogeneous groups of tumors arise specifically from the supporting extraskeletal mesenchymal tissues of the body, i.e., muscle, fascia, connective tissues, fibrous tissues, and fat. They are rare lesions, constituting less than 1% of all cancers. There are wide morphological differences among these tumors, probably resulting from the different cells of origin; however, all STSs, like bone sarcomas, share certain biological and behavioral characteristics.

The clinical, radiographic, and surgical management of most STSs is identical, regardless of histogenesis. The surgical grading system developed by the Musculoskeletal Tumor Society applies to both bone sarcomas and soft-tissue sarcomas.

Clinical Findings and Physical Examination

Soft-tissue sarcomas are a disease of adulthood, occurring in persons between 30 and 60 years of age. The sole exception is rhabdomyosarcoma, which occurs in young children. Approximately one-half of STSs are found in the extremities; the remainders arise in the head/neck and trunk. The lower extremity is the most common anatomic site; 40% of all STSs occur in this location. The anterior thigh (quadriceps) is the most common compartment, followed by the adductors and hamstrings.

Most STSs present as a painless mass. Systemic signs such as fever, weight loss, or anemia are rare. There are no useful laboratory screening examinations. Clinical suspicion is therefore crucial to diagnosis. Any adult presenting with an extremity mass must be presumed to have a sarcoma until proved otherwise and should be further evaluated. History of coincident trauma often can be especially misleading. Unfortunately, a presumptive diagnosis of lipoma, ganglion, hematoma, or muscle tear is often made, thereby delaying definitive evaluation and treatment. Local examination reveals a well-localized, nontender mass that may be movable. The lesion may be firm or, rarely, cystic.

Biological Behavior and Natural History

The pattern of growth, metastasis, and recurrence of STSs is similar to that of spindle cell sarcomas arising in bone. The major distinctions are the tendency of STSs to remain intracompartmental and a significant incidence of lymphatic involvement in a few of the less-common entities, such as the epithelioid, synovial, and alveolar soft-part sarcomas. The prognosis of an STS is most closely related to its histological grade and the presence or absence of metastases. Historically, high-grade STSs have an overall survival rate of 40–60%. In half of all cases, wide local excision is followed by local recurrence within 12–24 months, followed by pulmonary metastases resulting from hematogenous dissemination to the lungs. Visceral involvement and lymphatic involvement are rare. Pulmonary recurrence and local recurrence are the most common sites of relapse. Aggressive surgical resection of local recurrences should be considered. If distant metastasis has not occurred, a 5-year salvage rate of 50–80% can be achieved.

Pathology and Staging

STSs are classified on the basis of histologic cell of origin. Individual grading is often difficult; in general, however, the extent of pleomorphism, atypia, mitosis, and necrosis correlates with the degree of malignancy. Notable exceptions are synovial sarcomas, which tend to behave like high-grade lesions even in the absence of these findings. The exact histogenesis of some soft-tissue sarcomas often cannot be accurately defined, although grading can still be adequately performed. The surgical stage is determined by grade, location, and the presence or absence of pulmonary or lymphatic metastases similar to other malignancies. Staging studies must be done prior to treatment.

Radiographic Evaluation

Magnetic Resonance Imaging

Because of better visual contrast and the ability to image in coronal and sagittal planes, MRI has surpassed CT as the most useful study for evaluating STSs of the extremities. CT remains valuable for retroperitoneal tumors and for assessment of lung metastases. Either imaging method can delineate the cross-sectional anatomic extent and compartmentalization of the lesion. Unique features of modern MRI, including use of gadolinium contrast, mixed spin-echo images and fat-suppression images, appear to facilitate visualization of tumor extent and may prove crucial to longitudinal study of postoperative patients to allow for early detection of local recurrences.

Angiography

Biplane angiography remains the standard technique for demonstrating the position of the major vessels. Although MRI and contrast-enhanced CT often show the vessels, angiography is helpful in planning an operative approach, especially if displacement is noted on the CT scan (Fig. 4.40).

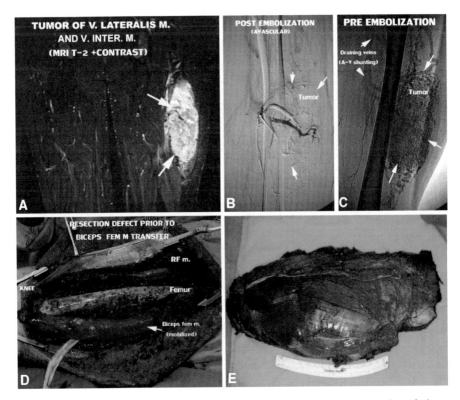

Fig. 4.40 Large soft-tissue sarcoma of the thigh. (**a**) MRI showing a large, vascular soft-tissue sarcoma of the vastus lateralis and intermedius muscles. The thigh is the most common site of soft-tissue sarcomas. (**b**) There is very significant vascularity prior to embolization. (**c**) The tumor blush is virtually non-existent following embolization, making tumor resection safer. (**d**) Surgical defect following resection of the vastus lateralis and medialis. The biceps femoris muscle has been mobilized to reconstruct the defect. (**e**) Gross specimen. Note the tumor is not seen; it is covered in all dimensions by normal muscle

Bone Scans

Bone scintigraphy is used to determine the relation of adjacent bony structures to the tumor. Increased contrast-medium uptake by a bone in close proximity to an STS usually indicates a reactive rim of tumor near the periosteum, rather than direct intraosseous tumor extension.

Treatment

The treatment of high-grade STS has undergone fundamental changes within the past decade. Treatment of these patients requires a multimodality approach and successful management requires cooperation of the surgeon, chemotherapist, and radiation oncologist. The appropriate role of each modality is continuously changing, but can be described in general as follows.

Chemotherapy

Combination chemotherapy has been shown to be more effective in preventing pulmonary dissemination from high-grade sarcomas than single-agent therapy. The most effective drugs in use today are doxorubicin hydrochloride (Adriamycin) and ifosfamide. Dacarazine (DTIC), methotrexate, and cisplatin also have activity and are included in many current protocols. The various combinations are traditionally given in an adjuvant (postoperative) setting and are presumed effective against clinically undetectable micrometastases. Neoadjuvant (preoperative) chemotherapy is being evaluated in several institutions. Early results have indicated that significant reduction in tumor size can occur, thereby facilitating attempts at limb salvage.

Radiation Therapy

Radiation typically consists of 5,000–6,500 cGy over many fractions. This modality is effective in an adjuvant setting in decreasing local recurrence following nonablative resection. The degree to which the initial surgical volume should be decreased in these circumstances is controversial, although the local recurrence following a wide excision and postoperative radiotherapy is 5–10%. The technique of radiation therapy includes irradiating all the tissues at risk, shrinking fields, preserving a strip of unirradiated skin, and using filters and radiosensitizers. Local morbidity has been greatly decreased within the past decade. Preoperative radiation is effective in reducing tumor volume but is associated with increased morbidity resulting from significant wound-healing complications.

Surgery and Chemotherapy as a Multimodality Approach

Removal of the tumor is necessary to achieve local control. This may be accomplished either by a nonablative resection (limb salvage) or by an amputation. The procedure chosen depends on results of the preoperative staging studies.

A prospective randomized National Cancer Institute (NCI) trial established that a multimodality approach employing limb-salvage surgery combined with adjuvant radiation and chemotherapy offered local control and survival rates comparable to those of amputation plus chemotherapy, while simultaneously preserving a functional extremity.

The use of adjuvant therapy (chemotherapy or radiation) permits limb-sparing procedures for the majority of extremity soft-tissue sarcomas. Enneking has shown that a radical resection for an STS has about a 5% local recurrence rate with surgery alone [1, 4]. Wide excision (without adjuvant radiation or chemotherapy) has a 50% rate of local failure. Results from the NCI showed that the rate of local recurrence decreased to 5% following local excision (either a marginal or a wide excision) when combined with postoperative radiation therapy and chemotherapy. Others have reported similar good results from preoperative radiation, with or without pre-operative chemotherapy. Contraindications to limb-sparing surgery are similar to those for the bony sarcomas. In general, nerve or major vascular involvement is a contraindication.

Studies of referred patients show that approximately half of all patients with soft-tissue sarcomas treated with attempted excisional biopsy by the referring surgeon will have microscopic or gross tumor remaining. As a result, referred patients undergo routine re-resection of the surgical site to ensure adequate local control prior to administration of adjuvant treatment.

Specific Soft-Tissue Sarcomas

The five most common soft-tissue sarcomas are briefly described below.

Malignant Fibrous Histiocytoma

Malignant fibrous histiocytoma (MFH), first described as a specific entity in 1963, is the most common STS in older adults. MFH occurs in primarily in adults and is most prevalent in the lower extremity, followed in frequency by the upper extremity and retroperitoneum. The histological grade (usually intermediate to high grade) is a good prognosticator of metastatic potential. The myxoid variant, particularly when located in the superficial soft tissues, tends to have a more favorable prognosis than the other subtypes. In fact, the pure myxoid tumors with bland spindle cells are considered to be low-grade neoplasms with minimal metastatic potential. It has been suggested that high-grade pleomorphic MFHs are a heterogeneous collection of poorly differentiated sarcomas, many of which can be specifically classified with the application of immunohistochemical and electron microscopic techniques.

Liposarcoma

Liposarcoma is the second most common STS. It has a wide range of malignant potential dependent upon the grade of the individual tumor. Determination

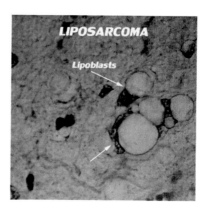

Fig. 4.41 Microscopic examination of a low-grade liposarcoma. This is a well-differentiated specimen with a few lipoblasts. (Originally published in Shmookler B, Bickels J, Jelinek JS, et al. Bone and soft tissue sarcomas: epidemiology, radiology, pathology and fundamentals of surgical treatment. In: Malawer MM, Sugarbaker PH, eds. *Musculoskeletal Cancer Surgery: Treatment of Sarcomas and Allied Diseases.* Dordrecht, The Netherlands: Kluwer; 2001:3–35)

of subtype and grade is essential to appropriate management. Well-differentiated (grade I) liposarcomas rarely metastasize (Fig. 4.41). Unlike other sarcomas, liposarcomas may be multiple and may occur in unusual sites within the same individual. Careful evaluation of other masses in a patient with a liposarcoma is mandatory. Occasionally, these lesions occur in children. Liposarcomas very rarely arise from preexisting benign lipomas.

Fibrosarcoma

Fibrosarcoma used to be considered the most common STS. Following the identification of MFH as a distinct entity and the establishment of reproducible criteria for the recognition of other definitive spindle cell sarcomas, fibrosarcoma is less commonly diagnosed. Clinical and histological difficulties occasionally arise in differentiating low-grade fibrosarcoma from fibromatosis and its variants. The anatomic site, age, and histological findings must be carefully evaluated. This is a neoplasm of midadulthood and most commonly affects the lower extremity.

Synovial Sarcoma

Synovial sarcomas are the fourth most common STS. They characteristically have a biphasic pattern that gives the impression of glandular formation, which was originally thought to be indicative of synovial origin. These tumors, however, rarely arise within a joint, but rather have a distribution similar to those of other STSs. Uncommon primary sites include the retropharynx, orofacial area, and retroperitoneum. Synovial sarcomas occur in a younger age group than other sarcomas; 72%

of patients in one large study were below the age of 40 years. There is a propensity for the distal portions of extremities: hand (5%), ankle (9%), or foot (13%). The plain radiograph often shows small calcifications within a soft-tissue mass; this should alert the physician to the diagnosis. Lymphatic spread occurs occasionally (5–7%). Virtually all synovial sarcomas are high grade.

Epithelioid Sarcoma

Epithelioid sarcoma was first described in 1970. It is an unusually small tumor that is often misdiagnosed as a benign lesion. Half of these lesions occur in the forearm and wrist, and it is the most common sarcoma of the hand. This lesion has a propensity for eventual lymph node involvement. Rarely, it presents as a metastasis to the epitrochlear lymph node. Unlike other sarcomas, it occurs predominantly in adolescents and young adults (average age 26 years). When it arises in the dermis, in which case it presents as a nodular or ulcerative process, it often clinically simulates benign cutaneous diseases, such as granulomatous dermatitis.

Benign Soft-Tissue Tumors

All mesenchymal tissue can give rise to benign lesions. They may occasionally be confused with malignant lesions, or they may become symptomatic because of their size, anatomic location, or both. Although these tumors are benign, local recurrence or difficult anatomic location can cause significant morbidity. Some, such as lipomas, are easily cured by simple removal, while others, most notably fibromatoses, require extensive resection. Thus, it is important to differentiate these lesions from their malignant counterparts, establish a correct diagnosis, and remove them surgically.

There are a large number of benign lesions. The more common lesions and their unique characteristics are described.

Benign Adipose Tumors

Simple Lipoma

Lipomas, the most common mesenchymal neoplasms, arise from normal fat and appear during adulthood. They may be single or multiple; the latter occur in only 5% of all patients. They are found either subcutaneously or deeply embedded. Eighty percent of all lipomas are of the simple type. The shoulder girdle and proximal thigh are the two most common sites. Simple surgical excision is curative.

Microscopic Characteristics

Both types of lipomas consist of monotonous sheets of mature fat cells that are ovoid to round and usually contain a single fat droplet that compresses the nucleus along the cell membrane. Capillary-like vessels occasionally appear between the fat lobules. Areas of myxoid change or dense fibrous trabeculae are sometimes seen.

Episacral Lipomas

Although these are not true lipomas, they are encountered by orthopedic surgeons and general practitioners. These are lumbar fat herniations that occur most commonly in women and cause significant pain in the SI joint or hip region. They palpate similar to small lipomas in that they are small, firm nodules; however, they are composed entirely of subfascial fat that has herniated through the overlying fascial layer. MRI, ultrasound, and other imaging studies are of little diagnostic value. These herniations do occur in predictable regions adjacent to the sacrospinalis muscle proximal to the iliac crest. Surgical repair of the fascia and removal of the herniated fat pad is the definitive treatment.

Spindle Cell Lipoma

This is a variant of lipoma consisting of benign spindle cells in addition to mature fat. The tumor has a predilection for males (90%) and most commonly occurs in the neck and shoulder. Spindle cell lipomas are encapsulated and are easily removed by simple excision. It is essential to distinguish this lesion clinically from a well-differentiated liposarcoma.

   Pleomorphic lipomas also consist of mature fat cells, but they are more variable in size. They contain both pleomorphic and distinctive multinucleated giant cells instead of spindle cells. These giant cells contain multiple overlapping nuclei at their peripheries. Occasionally, lipoblast-like cells occur.

Intramuscular and Intermuscular Lipomas

Lipomas occurring within (intramuscular) and between (intermuscular) muscle groups often become large, produce few symptoms, and present as a mass mimicking an STS. Clinical evaluation and staging are similar to those of any suspected sarcoma. The pathologist must be aware of the clinical setting, and an adequate sample must be obtained in order to differentiate a low-grade liposarcoma from a true benign lipoma. Unlike superficial lipomas, these lesions often do not have a capsule and tend to infiltrate the surrounding muscle. A marginal or wide resection is required to obtain local control. These lesions never become malignant.

Benign Tumors of Peripheral Nerves

The two most common nerve tumors are neurilemmoma and neurofibroma.

Neurilemmoma (Schwannoma)

These benign growths arise within a nerve and are surrounded by a true capsule composed of the epineurium. They are composed of Antoni A (cellular) and Antoni B (loose myxoid) components. These lesions generally are not associated with von Recklinghausen's disease (multiple neurofibromatosis). Surgical treatment entails opening the capsule and enucleating the growth from the nerve. "Ancient" neurilemmoma is cystic degeneration of a neurilemmoma. These lesions clinically present as a large mass with some cellular atypia. They must be differentiated from malignant lesions. Simple excision, done for diagnostic purposes or if the lesion is symptomatic, is curative.

Neurofibroma

Neurofibromas may be solitary or multiple. Unlike neurilemmomas, they are not encapsulated. They often enlarge the nerves and may undergo malignant degeneration. Histologically, they consist of Schwann cells associated with collagen fibrils and myxoid material. Multiple neurofibromas are found in patients with von Recklinghausen's disease. These lesions cannot be surgically detached from the underlying nerve. Surgery is indicated only if malignant degeneration is suspected. Between 20 and 65% of patients with neurofibromatosis ultimately develop a sarcoma.

Benign Fibrous Tumors

There are a large variety of benign fibrous tumors. Most are treated by simple excision. Aggressive fibromatosis is a benign but locally aggressive lesion deserving special consideration.

Aggressive Fibromatosis

This tumor, which appears bland microscopically, is the most serious of all the benign soft-tissue tumors. It does not have a capsule and tends to infiltrate far beyond its clinically recognized boundaries. This lesion does not respect fascial borders and thus can attain a large size and involve multiple anatomic compartments if left untreated. The most common locations are the neck, shoulder, and pelvic girdle. Death results from intrathoracic or retroperitoneal extension. The clinical history often reveals multiple recurrences despite supposedly adequate surgical removal. The appropriate surgical procedure is wide excision. Local recurrence uniformly follows excision with positive margins. Surgical staging studies should be performed prior to resection. Amputation is occasionally required. Radiation and chemotherapy have recently been used for unresectable fibromatosis.

Benign Vascular Tumors

Hemangioma

Benign tumors of the blood vessels consist of a variety of hemangiomas. It is not certain whether these are true neoplasms, hamartomas, or vascular malformations. There are two types of hemangiomas: generalized and localized; the latter are more common. Hemangiomas are classified on the basis of their pathological appearance – capillary, cavernous, venous, or arteriovenous. Capillary hemangiomas are the most common type. Most hemangiomas occur during childhood. Venous hemangiomas occur during adulthood and are often deeply situated. Intramuscular hemangiomas are rare and are occasionally difficult to differentiate from angiosarcomas. Evaluation requires angiography and venography. Surgery is indicated if symptoms develop. Hemangiomas rarely become malignant.

Angiomatosis is a benign condition characterized by involvement of multiple types of mesenchymal tissues. Large anatomic regions, even an entire limb, may be affected. These extensive vascular lesions, which are probably hamartomatous, can involve the skin, subcutaneous fat, skeletal muscle, fascia, and bone. Involvement of an entire extremity can cause hypertrophy of the limb.

References

1. Dahlin DC. *Bone Tumors: General Aspects and Data on 6,221 Cases.* 3rd ed. Springfield, IL: Charles C. Thomas; 1978.
2. Marcove RC. Chondrosarcoma: diagnosis and treatment. *Orthop Clin North Am.* 1977;8(4):811–820.
3. Enneking WF, Spanier SS, Malawer MM. The effect of the anatomic setting on the results of surgical procedures for soft parts sarcoma of the thigh. *Cancer.* 1981;47(5):1005–1022.
4. Enneking WF, Spanier SS, Goodman MA. A system for the surgical staging of musculoskeletal sarcoma. *Clin Orthop Relat Res.* 1980;153:106–120.
5. Malawer MM, Sugarbaker PH, eds. *Musculoskeletal Cancer Surgery: Treatment of Sarcomas and Allied Diseases.* Dordrecht, The Netherlands: Kluwer; 2001.

Suggested Reading

1. Dahlin DC. *Bone Tumors: General Aspects and Data on 6,221 Cases.* 3rd ed. Springfield, IL: Charles C. Thomas; 1978.
2. Edeiken J. Bone tumors and tumor-like conditions. In: Edeiken J, ed. *Roentgen Diagnosis of Diseases of Bone.* Baltimore, MD: Williams & Wilkins; 1981.
3. Enneking WF, Spanier SS, Goodman MA. A system for the surgical staging of musculoskeletal sarcoma. *Clin Orthop Relat Res.* 1980;153:106–120.
4. Enneking WF, Spanier SS, Malawer MM. The effect of the anatomic setting on the results of surgical procedures for soft parts sarcoma of the thigh. *Cancer.* 1981;47(5):1005–1022.
5. Malawer MM, Sugarbaker PH, eds. *Musculoskeletal Cancer Surgery: Treatment of Sarcomas and Allied Diseases.* Dordrecht, The Netherlands: Kluwer; 2001.

6. Mankin HJ, Lange TA, Spanier SS. The hazards of biopsy in patients with malignant primary bone and soft-tissue tumors. *J Bone Joint Surg Am.* 1982;64(8):1121–1127.

7. Marcove RC. Chondrosarcoma: diagnosis and treatment. *Orthop Clin North Am.* 1977;8(4):811–820.

8. Marcove RC, Miké V, Hajek JV, Levin AG, Hutter RV. Osteogenic sarcoma under the age of twenty-one. A review of one hundred and forty-five operative cases. *J Bone Joint Surg Am.* 1970;52(3):411–423.

9. Rougraff BT, Simon MA, Kneisl JS, Greenberg DB, Mankin HJ. Limb salvage compared with amputation for osteosarcoma of the distal end of the femur. A long-term oncological, functional, and quality-of-life study. *J Bone Joint Surg Am.* 1994;76(5):649–656.

10. Sim FH, Bowman W, Chao E. Limb salvage in primary malignant bone tumors. *Orthopedics* 1985:574–581.

Chapter 5
Children's Orthopedics

John N. Delahay and William C. Lauerman

Introduction

Children are different! This statement has been presented in many different ways; but it is critically important that this central fact be recognized, if one is to successfully diagnose and treat disease in this age group. Even within this rather broad range of ages there are dramatic differences among specific subsets: neonate, child, and adolescent.

These differences are not only biological, but psychological, social, and emotional. It is likewise inappropriate to focus only on one aspect of these differences. For example, it would be unwise to ignore a young child's activity level when treating a fracture – inadequate immobilization or cast removal too early will have disastrous end results.

Recognition of this special group actually gave orthopedics its name. The word means "straight child" and alludes to the interest and time spent correcting deformities in children. These deformities can result not only from injury but also from systemic and local disease states, both congenital and acquired. Because the child is *growing*, these diseases produce anatomic and physiologic effects not expected in the adult. Before discussing specific entities, it would, therefore, be appropriate to review some of the biological differences of the child's musculoskeletal system and the influences that act on the immature skeleton.

J.N. Delahay (✉)
Department of Orthopedic Surgery, Georgetown University Medical Center, 3800 Reservoir Road NW, Pasquerilla Healthcare Center (PHC), Ground Floor, Washington, DC 20007, USA
e-mail: delahayj@georgetown.edu

S.W. Wiesel, J.N. Delahay (eds.), *Essentials of Orthopedic Surgery*,
DOI 10.1007/978-1-4419-1389-0_5, © Springer Science+Business Media, LLC 2010

Biological Differences

Growth

As mentioned, the fact that the child's skeleton is growing, both longitudinally and latitudinally, positions it uniquely for damage due to the adverse effects of trauma and disease. The extent of this damage is a reflection of the rate of growth and the immaturity of the skeleton. Hence, an insult will have a greater impact, if applied at the time of more rapid growth (a growth spurt) or when the skeleton is very young (neonate).

Remodeling

The immature skeleton can remodel to a much greater degree than that of the adult. Due to the presence and activity of multiple cell populations, damage to the skeleton can be repaired more extensively than one should anticipate in the adult. The challenge for the physician is to be able to recognize the limitations of this remodeling process and work within the boundaries of this potential.

Specific Anatomic Structures

Bone

Although a child's bone is historically lamellar in pattern, there remains enough flexibility in the skeleton to permit what has been called "biological plasticity," a phenomena not nearly as extensive in adult bone. Essentially, this allows a bone to "bend without breaking"; in point of fact, it is responsible for some of the unique types of fractures seen in the pediatric age groups, specifically torus and greenstick fractures.

In addition, the mechanical properties of a child's bone vary from those of the adult. Such characteristics as modulus of elasticity, ultimate tensile strength, and yield point all reflect the elasticity and plasticity unique in this age group. However, the overall "strength" tends to be less than that of the adult in certain modes of loading, such as tension and shear.

Ligament

As a tissue, ligament is one of the most age-resistant tissues in the human body. The tensile strength in the child and the adult is virtually the same. Therefore, these structures remain as a constant in the musculoskeletal system. While the strength of bone, cartilage, and muscle tends to change, the ligamentous structures remain unchanged with growth and development.

Periosteum

The outer covering of the bone is a dense fibrous layer, which in the child is significantly thicker than that of the adult. The periosteum of the child actually has an outer fibrous layer and an inner cambial or osteogenic layer. Hence, the child's periosteum confers both mechanical strength and biologic activity. The effect of these biologic differences is far reaching when one discusses fractures in children. Due to this thickened periosteum, fractures do not tend to displace to the degree seen in adults, and the intact periosteum can be used as an aid in fracture reduction and maintenance. In addition, fractures will heal significantly faster than similar injuries in adults due to the fact that all the cellular precursors are already present. The osteogenic layer supplies active osteoblasts, ready to make bone for the fracture callus. The generation of these precursor elements in adults takes a period of time not required in the child.

Cartilage

As one will recall, the skeleton is developed embryologically within a cartilage model. At birth, large portions of any given bone remain largely cartilaginous. Unfortunately, cartilage is *not* seen on standard X-rays. The cartilage anlage is very labile and dramatically affected by external influences such as mechanical loading. It is important to realize that, in examining an X-ray, one should not be lulled into a false sense of security if all appears well; what you do not see (i.e., the cartilage) is more important than what you do! Aberrant cartilaginous growth will drastically affect the ultimate shape of bones and, more importantly, joints. The best example is the proximal femur where most of the upper end is cartilaginous. Adverse influences due to eccentric loading seen in developmental dysplasia of the hip can have far-reaching effects when applied to the immature cartilage of the neonatal hip.

The Growth Plate

By far and away, the most unique characteristic of the immature skeleton – indeed, what is the defining component of the immature skeleton – is the growth plate, or the "physis." The physis is a cartilage plate interposed between the epiphysis (the secondary ossification center) and the metaphysis (Fig. 5.1). It is essential for long-bone growth to occur. The downside is that this anatomic structure creates a "normal flaw" in the overall skeletal structure and thus a point of mechanical weakness. The physis historically has four zones (Fig. 5.2), each with its own physiologic role:

a. Resting zone: The top layer of flattened cells is germinal and metabolically stores materials for later use, since they will ultimately "move their way" down the plate

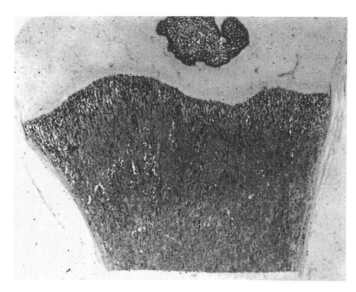

Fig. 5.1 Early secondary ossification center of mature fetus. The formation of the secondary ossification centers in the lower tibia and upper femur coincides with fetal maturity. The secondary center begins not in the center of the epiphysis, but nearer the growth plate. Expansion, therefore, is eccentric. (From Bogumill GP. Orthopaedic Pathology: A Synopsis with Clinical Radiographic Correlation. Philadelphia: Saunders, 1984. Reprinted with permission)

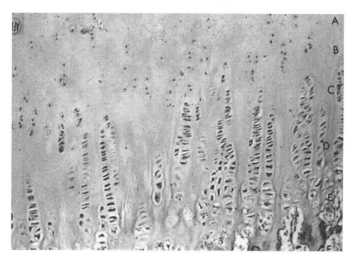

Fig. 5.2 Growth plate. Low-power view showing entire plate. (**a**) Resting zone has isolated cartilage cells in the upper portion together with empty lacunae. (**b**) Cell reproduction produces cloning of cells that "stack up" longitudinally. Successive generations occupy more space than each single progenitor cell and thus increase the length of the cartilage model. Secretion of new matrix at (**c**) is followed by dehydration with accompanying fibrillation of the territorial cartilage matrix between the "dinner plates" at (**d**). Hypertrophy of cartilage cells at (**e**) is due to imbibition of water. Calcification of matrix is followed by vascular invasion at (**f**). (From Bogumill GP. *Orthopaedic Pathology: A Synopsis with Clinical Radiographic Correlation.* Philadelphia, PA: WB Saunders Company; 1984. Reprinted with permission)

toward the metaphysis. The chondrocytes in this zone also are synthetic, as they fabricate the matrix within which they lie.

b. Proliferating zone: The cells in this region are actively replicating and extending the plate. Their appearance has been described as a "stack of plates." In this region, the cells use the materials that they have previously stored for their "trip to the metaphysis."

c. Hypertrophic zone: Having extended the plate in the former zone, the cells now tend to swell and switch over to a more catabolic state. They prepare the matrix for calcification and ultimately for conversion to bone. Due to large swollen cells and the disorganized matrix, this zone has been cited as being the weakest mechanically; hence, it is here that failure tends to occur. Most, however, would agree that crack propagation can be seen throughout all zones in the case of trauma.

d. Calcified zone: Metabolically, the matrix has been readied for the deposition of calcium salts, and the task of forming the osteoid is left for this lowest region of the plate. In the adjacent metaphysis, small vascular twigs can be seen arborizing toward the basal layers of the plate.

Peripheral Structures of the Plate

Two defined histologic regions have been identified with specific functional roles to play in skeletal development.

a. Zone of Ranvier: Around the circumference of the plate is an identifiable clustering of cells that are responsible for latitudinal growth of the plate.

b. Perichondral ring of Lacroix: As the periosteum is continuous around the margins of the plate, this fibrous structure is apparent. Its function arguably has been to serve as a "girdle" for the plate and give mechanical support against translational movement.

Factors Affecting the Skeletal Growth

Numerous factors, both intrinsic and extrinsic, affect the way in which the skeleton develops. Some examples are noteworthy, as indicated below.

Genetic Impact

Inborn errors of metabolism (renal rickets) as well as chromosomal alterations (Down's syndrome) can cause phenotypic variations in the development of the skeleton. Abnormal histology, aberrational growth, and variational development all will affect the ultimate shape and behavior of the skeleton.

Nutrition

Vitamins and proteins are required for normal skeletal development and without appropriate levels, abnormalities will be seen. Rickets, for example, will alter the shape of the metaphysis, in addition to disrupting normal physical development.

Endocrine

Hormonal influences play a significant trophic or permissive role in the development of the skeleton. Shortages or excesses, therefore, will disrupt the way in which the skeleton matures. Thyroid hormone is a good example. Disrupted epiphyseal development is a hallmark of cretinism.

Environmental Factor

Mechanical effects as well as environmental toxins and drugs can adversely affect the development of the skeleton. Fetal alcohol syndrome and the use of illicit narcotics by the mother are just two examples of the growing compendium of skeletal aberrations due to externally applied toxins.

Coexistent Disease

Neuromuscular diseases of children, such as cerebral palsy, polio, and muscular dystrophy, provide good examples of the secondary effects seen in the skeleton due to extrinsic disease. In these examples, the final common pathway in the pathophysiology of the deformities is muscle imbalance; hence, eccentric mechanical loading and aberrational mechanical loading of the immature skeleton produce changes such as joint dislocations and deformities (e.g., scoliosis).

Developmental Variations in Skeletal Growth

It seems axiomatic to say that children grow and develop at different rates and in different ways. Yet, one of the most common reasons that children are brought to a physician is to evaluate the position of their lower extremities, and the way in which they stand and walk. Toeing-in and toeing-out, as well as knock knees and bow legs, are a major preoccupation of parents and especially grandparents – and a major source of orthopedic referrals. The simple fact is that the vast majority of these children – well over 90% – are normal children who are simply reflecting variational growth and development. Dr. Mercer Rang, a preeminent pediatric orthopedist, has tried to emphasize this important fact by referring to these conditions as "non-disease."

Rang further goes on to suggest that the appropriate management for "non-disease" is "non-treatment." It is important to recognize the difference between doing nothing and "non-treatment." As the physician seeing the child, one must be able to recognize the variational patterns and differentiate them from pathologic states. Once that has been accomplished, the physician may embark on a program of aggressive "non-treatment" which might include such things as the following:

1. Careful examination of the normal child
2. Reassurance of parents and grandparents
3. Supply educational information to strengthen one's diagnosis and approach
4. Consider use of benign shoe adjustment (scaphoid pad) for the "terminally skeptical"
5. Offer the option of yearly follow-up "to be sure that the non-disease is getting better"

Torsional Variations

The newborn typically will reflect the intrauterine position and environment. Therefore, a certain amount of "molding" is to be anticipated. This usually, but not always, results in an internally rotated position of the lower extremities and the ultimate manifestation of this rotation is toeing-in when the child begins to walk. The two most typical variations leading to intoeing are as follows:

1. Internal tibial torsion: Axial rotation of the tibias can best be identified by examining the child supine with hips and knees flexed and evaluating the transmalleolar axis at the ankle for its relation to the knee axis. Normally, it should lie 10–30° externally rotated from that of the knee. Neonates typically have an internally rotated axis which causes intoeing with the initiation of walking and spontaneously corrects after about 1 year of walking. Tibial external rotation can occasionally be seen, but is far less common. Neither requires any specific treatment other than those recommended for "non-treatment" (Fig. 5.3).
2. Internal femoral torsion (femoral anteversion): The plane of the femoral head and neck in the normal adult lies 15° externally rotated from that of the transcondylar plane of the distal femur. In the newborn, this relationship is more extreme: the head/neck plane is about 45° external to that of the transcondylar plate, and it corrects spontaneously at a rate of about 2° per year (Fig. 5.4). Persistence of this infantile pattern beyond the age of walking will cause intoeing as the leg internally rotates at the hip so that the femoral head sits properly in the acetabulum. The rate of correction varies widely and "non-treatment" is usually all that is required. Additionally, two other recommendations might be made: first, the child should be discouraged from sitting in the so-called W or TV position, since it seems to delay spontaneous correction; and second, lightweight footwear should be encouraged, since the child will toe-in less due to weight of shoes.

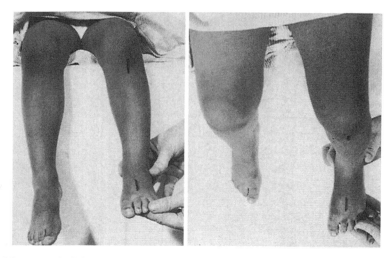

Fig. 5.3 Practical clinical method of measuring tibial torsion (see text for explanation). (From Tachdjian MO. *Pediatric Orthopedics*, 2nd ed, vol 1. Philadelphia, PA: Saunders; 1990. Reprinted with permission)

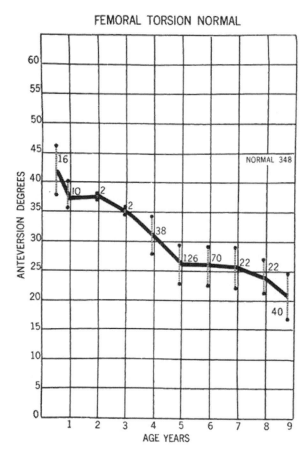

Fig. 5.4 The degree of normal femoral torsion in relation to age. The *solid lines* represent the mean; the *vertical lines* represent standard deviation. (From Tachdjian MO. *Pediatric Orthopedics*, 2nd ed, vol 1. Philadelphia, PA: Saunders; 1990. Reprinted with permission)

External femoral torsion is described, but most believe this actually represents the persistence of an infantile external rotational contracture of the soft tissues posterior to the hip; despite its etiology, spontaneous correction of this variation can similarly be anticipated.

When examining the child for femoral rotational patterns, it is best accomplished with the child prone, hips extended, and knees flexed 90° (Fig. 5.5). Internal and external rotation of the hips can then be easily estimated using the leg as an angle guide.

Fig. 5.5 Range of rotation of the hip in excessive femoral antetorsion. (**a**) Lateral rotation of the hip in extension is exaggerated. (**b**) Medial rotation of the hip in extension is limited to neutral. (From Tachdjian MO. *Pediatric Orthopedics*, 2nd ed, vol 1. Philadelphia, PA: Saunders; 1990. Reprinted with permission)

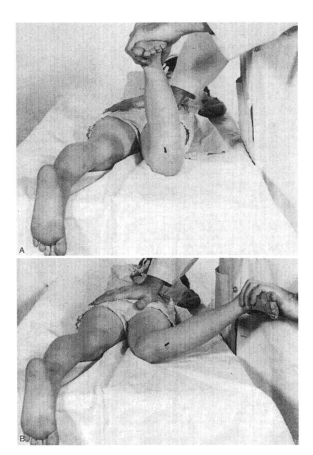

Angular Variations

Knock knees (genu valgum) and bow legs (genu varum) are another common source of physician referrals. Recognition of the normal allows relatively easy determination of pathologic states.

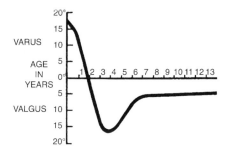

Fig. 5.6 Development of the tibiofemoral angle during growth. (From Tachdjian MO. Pediatric Orthopedics, 2nd ed, vol 1. Philadelphia, PA: Saunders; 1990. Reprinted with permission)

Salenius examined thousands of "normal" children and has provided us with standard expectations for this group (Fig. 5.6). Newborns demonstrate 4–10° of genu varus, which tends to spontaneously correct by 18 months of age. Thus, a child who presents with bow legs would be diagnosed as "physiologic genu varum." After 18 months of age, a child develops knock knees, which increases until about age 4 or 5 and then begins to improve. By age 7 or 8, most children have assumed more of an adult pattern: 5–7° of valgus in males and 7–9° of valgus in females.

It is best to record the degree of varus by measuring the number of finger breadths accommodated between the child's knees and the degree of valgus by recording the number of finger breadths accommodated between the medial malleoli.

Differential Diagnosis

Recognizing that the vast majority of children with angular patterns are normal and require "non-treatment," it is nonetheless important to realize that angular deformities can be a manifestation of pathologic states.

A. *Knock knees (genu valgum)* (Fig. 5.7)

1. Physiologic
2. Renal rickets
3. Skeletal dysplasias
4. Trauma

B. *Bow legs (genu varum)* (Fig. 5.8)

1. Physiologic
2. Blounts' disease
3. Rickets (nutritional)
4. Skeletal dysplasias (achondroplasia)
5. Trauma

As one can appreciate from these lists, symmetry is important. Physiologic angular deformity is virtually always symmetric; the finding of asymmetry should, therefore, suggest a pathologic state and trigger an appropriate workup.

Fig. 5.7 Bilateral genu valgum in an adolescent. (From Tachdjian MO. *Pediatric Orthopedics*, 2nd ed, vol 1. Philadelphia, PA: Saunders; 1990. Reprinted with permission)

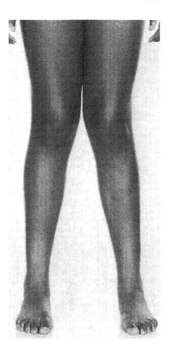

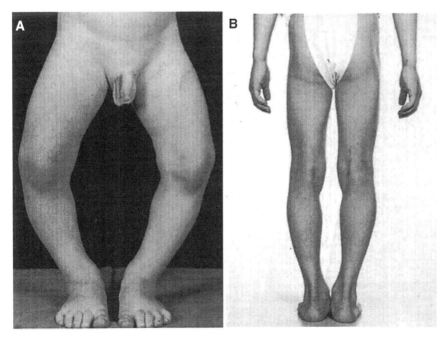

Fig. 5.8 Bilateral genu varum. (**a**) At age 1.5 years. (**b**) At 7 years, showing spontaneous correction without treatment. (From Tachdjian MO. *Pediatric Orthopedics*, 2nd ed, vol 1. Philadelphia, PA: Saunders; 1990. Reprinted with permission)

General Affectations of the Pediatric Skeleton

There are many diseases that have skeletal manifestations. This makes it impossible in one short chapter to fully discuss the vast array of pathologic states that have an impact on the musculoskeletal system. Rather, by being introduced to several specific examples in each disease category, one can appreciate some of the general ways in which the skeleton will react to various insults. Recalling the VITAMIN acronym introduced earlier in the text, this chapter will now focus on some of the vascular, infectious, arthritic, metabolic, and neurodevelopmental diseases that produce skeletal manifestations. An entire chapter of this book is devoted to a discussion of tumor and one to injury; therefore, these will only be mentioned insofar as their effects are unique to the growing skeleton.

Infection

Osteomyelitis

The pediatric skeleton is a prime location for bone and joint infections. In part, this is due to the many bacterial infections that small children seem to have – hence providing organisms capable of hematogenously spreading from skin, ear, and nasopharynx. In addition, the unique metaphyseal blood supply (Fig. 5.9) in the child establishes the battlefield for the host–organism interaction. Since the physis creates a barrier to the vessels, they must double back on themselves, thereby forming end-loop capillaries and creating an area of stasis in the bony metaphysis. This area of stasis "catches" bacteria as they are showered hematogenously from distant sites. Once entrenched, the bacteria establish a focus of infection, and the classic case of osteomyelitis develops. It is important to recognize that the changes are not simply the result of the damage the bacteria do to the bone, but also the reparative changes initiated by the bone in an effort to localize the infection.

The result of this activity is a mixture of bony destruction by the organisms and new bone formed to wall off the infection and shore up the areas of damage. The dead and dying bony fragments are referred to as "sequestra," and the new viable bone being formed is called "involucrum" (Fig. 5.10; see also Chapter 3).

Clinical Features

One should inquire about a past history of trauma, as well as infections elsewhere, that may have provided a source for the organism. Occasionally, no such history will be available and one is evaluating a child who presents with pain in a limb and fever. The combination of these two findings – pain in an extremity and fever – should be presumed to be osteomyelitis until proven otherwise.

In children under 1 year of age, the findings may be more nonspecific and poorly localized – e.g., irritability, changes in feeding habits, and few signs of sepsis. Pseudoparalysis (failure to use the limb) may be the only localized finding.

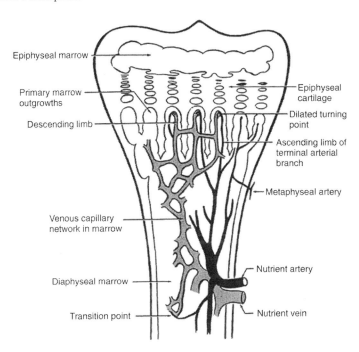

Epiphyseal marrow

Primary marrow
outgrowths

Descending limb

Epiphyseal
cartilage

Dilated turning
point

Ascending limb of
terminal arterial
branch

Metaphyseal artery

Venous capillary
network in marrow

Diaphyseal marrow

Transition point

Nutrient artery

Nutrient vein

Fig. 5.9 Localization of osteomyelitis due to structure of metaphyseal sinusoids. Diagram of blood supply of long bones in children showing the structure of metaphyseal sinusoids to be the cause for localization of pathogenic bacteria in the metaphysis. (From Tachdjian MO. *Pediatric Orthopedics*, 2nd ed, vol 1. Philadelphia, PA: Saunders; 1990. Reprinted with permission)

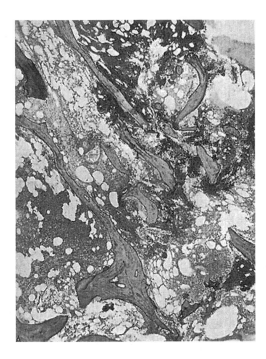

Fig. 5.10 Histologic findings in acute osteomyelitis. Necrotic trabeculae of bone surrounded by inflammatory cells (×25). (From Tachdjian MO. Pediatric Orthopedics, 2nd ed, vol 1. Philadelphia, PA: Saunders; 1990. Reprinted with permission)

Localized physical findings such as swelling, heat, localized tenderness, erythema, and signs of systemic sepsis are frequently seen in the older child.

Diagnosis

Standard laboratory studies will usually show an elevated white blood cell (WBC) count and sedimentation rate (ESR). The C-reactive protein (CRP) is similarly elevated. The ESR and CRP are both acute phase reactants; however, the latter responds more rapidly to the presence of infection and, therefore, tends to be a more sensitive measure of skeletal involvement. X-rays initially may be negative, since it takes 10 days for the pathology to become demonstrable radiographically. Bone resorption and new periosteal bone formation are the characteristic changes. However, neither of these may be seen initially. A standard total body bone scan is often quite helpful in the evaluation of these children. The bone scan is particularly useful in the localization of pathology (Fig. 5.11).

Appropriate cultures are essential. Blood cultures are reportedly positive in approximately 50% of cases of acute hematogenous osteomyelitis. Source cultures

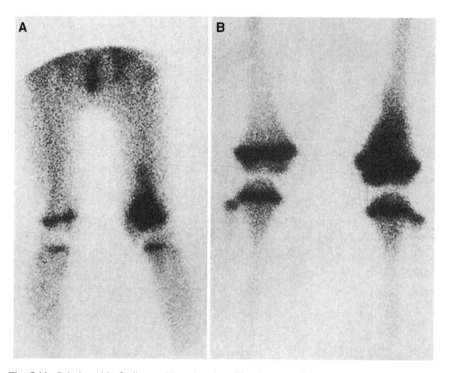

Fig. 5.11 Scintigraphic findings with technetium-99m in acute diphosphonate of the left distal femoral metaphysis. Note the increased localized uptake. (**a**) Early vascular flush. (**b**) Two hours later. (From Tachdjian MO. *Pediatric Orthopedics*, 2nd ed, vol 1. Philadelphia, PA: Saunders; 1990. Reprinted with permission)

from the throat, ear, skin, etc., should also be obtained. Bony aspiration is essential in the complete evaluation of these children. It is axiomatic that to diagnose a bone infection one must culture the bone. To that end, and using a large-bore needle, one should aspirate at the point of maximal tenderness in an effort to retrieve organisms. Reportedly, aspiration will be positive in approximately 60% of cases. The organisms vary slightly with age, but ordinarily either *Staphylococcus aureus* or *Streptococcus* species should be anticipated. In neonates, one needs to consider the possibility of gram-negative organisms.

Treatment

Diagnosis is critical prior to initiating antimicrobial treatment. All too often broad-spectrum antibiotics are given before a bacteriologic diagnosis is made. The result is a "partially treated osteomyelitis." These children present a challenging problem since the classical physical findings tend to be damped or eradicated completely. The problem, however, is that the organisms are frequently not killed – they only await antibiotic withdrawal before initiating a new wave of bony destruction. The principles of management have been established for many years and are best summarized as follows: (1) complete bacteriologic diagnosis, (2) appropriate antibiotic selection, (3) antibiotic delivery by the appropriate route and for the appropriate duration, (4) immobilization to decrease the risk of pathologic fracture, and (5) surgical drainage of abscesses. For many years, the tradition of intravenous (IV) antibiotic delivery has been accepted as essential. Although some would argue that the oral route is adequate, the IV route is still considered by most to be the standard mode of delivery despite the inconvenience caused to child, family, and physician. The traditional duration of 6 weeks has been altered in some protocols to 3 weeks intravenous and 3 weeks oral, based on clinical response.

The indication for surgical drainage is the presence of loculated pus. Typically, this will be seen within the metaphysis and/or under the periosteum (Fig. 5.12). These subperiosteal abscesses typically follow breakthrough of the thin cortical bone in the metaphyseal region. As these subperiosteal collections strip the periosteum from the underlying cortex, the cortex is devascularized and segments become avascular. In severe cases of acute hematogenous osteomyelitis, it is not uncommon to see sequestration of the entire bony diaphysis.

Septic Arthritis

Infection of a child's joint typically results from one of three pathologic mechanisms:

1. Hematogenous spread: Just as in osteomyelitis, organisms can localize in the joint finding the highly vascular synovium a favorable location for replication.

2. Breakthrough from a metaphyseal osteomyelitis: This occurs in specific joints where a portion of the metaphysis is intraarticular. Anatomically, the synovial reflection extends below the physis and includes a portion of metaphyseal cortical bone. The transverse Volkmann's canals provide a conduit for pus in the metaphysis to access the joint. In doing so, a secondary septic arthritis results. This phenomena of breakthrough is most typical in the hip (Fig. 5.13), but can also occur in the elbow, where the radial head is intraarticular, the shoulder, and the ankle.
3. Penetrating trauma: This results in joint sepsis when organisms are directly injected into the joint.

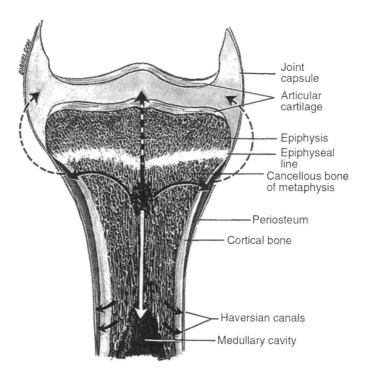

Fig. 5.12 Diagram showing spread of acute hematogenous osteomyelitis. The *interrupted lines* are rare routes. (From Tachdjian MO. *Pediatric Orthopedics*, 2nd ed, vol 1. Philadelphia, PA: Saunders; 1990. Reprinted with permission)

Clinical Features

Joint swelling and redness are the typical physical findings that one would expect. Systemic signs of sepsis are also usually readily apparent. In contradistinction to acute hematogenous osteomyelitis, children affected with septic arthritis tend to be

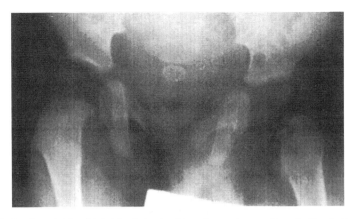

Fig. 5.13 Septic arthritis of left hip. Lateral subluxation and area of rarefaction in the femoral neck are evident. (From Tachdjian MO. *Pediatric Orthopedics*, 2nd ed, vol 1. Philadelphia, PA: Saunders; 1990. Reprinted with permission)

more toxic, exhibiting high fevers, listlessness, and poor feeding. In addition, these children will resist any attempt to move the involved joint.

Diagnosis

A workup similar to that for osteomyelitis should be carried out and at the risk of appearing repetitious, one cannot seriously consider this diagnosis in the differential without having made an attempt to retrieve organisms from the joint. It is important to be sure that the joint is, indeed, being aspirated and this frequently will require fluoroscopic control, especially if the joint in question is the hip. The pediatric hip is often difficult to enter under the best of circumstances and radiographic control using an arthrogram is recommended.

Microbiologically, the most common organism retrieved in the child is *S. aureus*. As is the case with osteomyelitis, neonates should be suspected of having unusual organisms, including gram negatives. In the adolescent patient, one must never forget the most common cause of septic arthritis: *Neisseria gonorrhoeae*.

Treatment

Septic arthritis, unlike acute hematogenous osteomyelitis, is a surgical emergency. It is imperative that the pus be removed from the joint as soon as possible. The articular cartilage is extremely vulnerable and easily damaged by enzymes – both those produced by the microorganisms and those produced by the white cells. It is, therefore, NOT enough to simply kill the organisms in the joint. The joint must be rid of all WBCs, bacterial byproducts, and enzymes. In most young children, this requires an arthrotomy. Occasionally, in the older child, arthroscopy is an appropriate technique for cleaning out a more accessible joint, such as the knee. Repeated needle aspirations are rarely effective in cleaning the inflamed joint. In addition, repetitive aspiration in the child is yet another example of "man's inhumanity to man."

Antibiotic management is similar to that for osteomyelitis. The choice of antibiotic and the route of delivery are usually identical. The duration of administration, however, is frequently shortened. The prognosis for septic arthritis in a child depends on early diagnosis, aggressive drainage, and appropriate antibiotic management. Delay in diagnosis or delay in adequate surgical drainage can have disastrous long-term effects on the joint, typically producing irreversible changes.

Complications of Bone and Joint Infections

Long-term sequelae can result from bacterial damage to these relatively vulnerable tissues (Fig. 5.14). In addition to the bone and articular cartilage, the child has a physis, which is likewise exposed to the insult.

Septic Joint Destruction

Loss of articular cartilage and arthrofibrosis ultimately result in joint contracture, deformity, and occasionally bony ankylosis (fusion). Salvage of the irreparably damaged articulations is difficult at best and frequently impossible.

Physeal Damage

Injury to the plate can have long-term effects, especially when it occurs in a very young child with significant growth remaining. Complete arrest and subsequent limb-length inequality or partial arrest and the resultant angular deformity are the two standard patterns of postinjury deformity.

Pathologic Fracture

Although infected bone will frequently look more dense (i.e., sclerotic) on X-ray, it should not be assumed that it is mechanically stronger. In point of fact, the dense bone is disorganized, its lamellar pattern disrupted, and, therefore, it is mechanically less sound. Pathologic fracture can occur even in the immobilized limb, although the risk is less.

Chronic Infection

Despite aggressive treatment, some infections are not completely eradicated, and a "stalemate" is established between the host and the organism. Occasionally, at times of psychological or environmental stress, the infection will reactivate and produce additional damage (see Chapter 3).

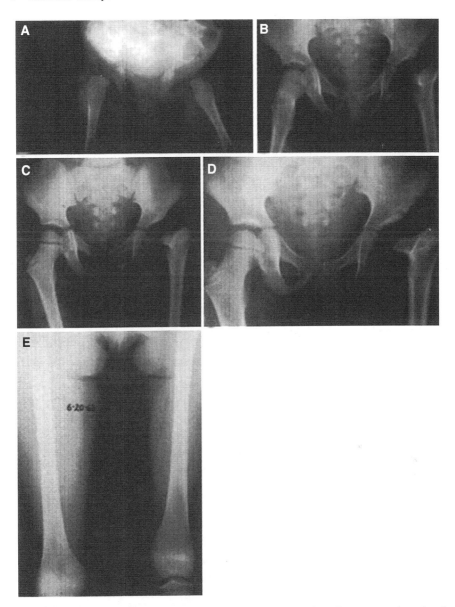

Fig. 5.14 Suppurative arthritis of the left hip in a 3-month-old infant. Onset was at 4 weeks of age. Erroneous diagnosis of fibrocystic disease and thrombophlebitis resulted in a 2-month delay in diagnosis. (**a**) Radiograms of hips show marked effusion of left hip with lateral subluxation. (**b–d**) Serial radiograms of hips show failure of ossification of the femoral head (due to avascular necrosis) and the development of coax vara. (**e**) Teleoradiograms taken 9.5 years after onset of sepsis in left hip. There is a 3.9 cm shortening of left femur. A subtrochanteric abduction osteotomy was performed 4 years earlier. The left hip has functional range of motion. Skeletal growth of lower limbs is being followed, and the plan is to perform distal femoral epiphyseodesis on the right at the appropriate age. (From Tachdjian MO. Pediatric Orthopedics, 2nd ed, vol 1. Philadelphia: Saunders, 1990. Reprinted with permission)

Arthritis in Childhood

Juvenile Rheumatoid Disease

Frequently referred to as Still's disease, juvenile rheumatoid disease (JRA) is the most common connective tissue disease in children. In fact, George Still specifically described the systemic form of the illness. Children have systemic symptoms – fever, rash, hepatosplenomegaly – and develop a polyarticular arthritis. This is the most destructive form of the disease and leaves multiple destroyed joints in its wake.

The other two forms of the disease are definitely less virulent. Polyarticular disease, as the name implies, takes its toll on the joints, but is not associated with systemic findings. Pauciarticular JRA is the most common and the most benign form of the disease. Typically, it is a monarticular arthritis, with the knee, elbow, and ankle being the joints most commonly involved. Frequently, children suffering from the pauciarticular form of the disease present with an isolated chronically swollen joint. This finding should trigger a diagnostic workup. Diagnostic blood studies are usually negative (rheumatoid factor is positive in only 10% of cases). X-rays usually only show juxtaarticular osteopenia, and frequently a synovial biopsy may be needed (Fig. 5.15). The histology of the synovium is similar to that of the adult disease – namely, hyperplasia and villous hypertrophy of the synovium. It is imperative to recognize JRA is the leading cause of blindness in children due to the

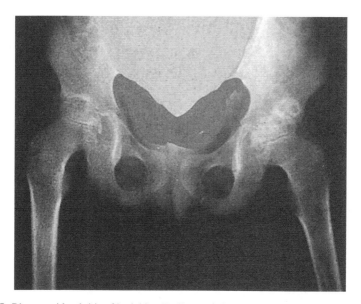

Fig. 5.15 Rheumatoid arthritis of both hips. Radiogram of hips taken 3 years later. The child was allowed to be ambulatory without protection of the hips. Note the destructive changes with fibrous ankylosis on the right and bony ankylosis on the left. (From Tachdjian MO. Pediatric Orthopedics, 2nd ed, vol 1. Philadelphia: Saunders, 1990. Reprinted with permission)

destructive iridocyclitis that can accompany the joint disease. All children with JRA should be under the care of an ophthalmologist since eye involvement does NOT parallel the degree of joint involvement; those with minimal joint disease can have the most severe eye changes.

Treatment should be directed toward control of the synovitis with medications, physical therapy to maintain joint motion, psychologic support for those chronically impaired children, and ultimately arthroplasties or fusions for those joints most severely involved.

Hemophilia

Children with bleeding dyscrasias frequently have repeated hemarthroses. Initially, the blood in the joint simply distends the capsular structures and causes a mild synovitis. With repeated bleeds, the synovium becomes hyperplastic and ultimately pannus formation is seen. At this point, the joint changes appear very similar to those seen in rheumatoid disease – e.g., osteopenia, enzymatic cartilage degradation, bony erosions, and lysis (Fig. 5.16).

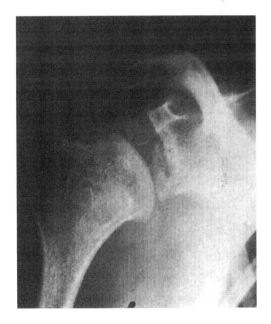

Fig. 5.16 Hemophilic arthropathy of shoulder. (From Tachdjian MO. Pediatric Orthopedics, 2nd ed, vol 1. Philadelphia: Saunders, 1990. Reprinted with permission)

Lyme Disease

In the endemic regions of the Northeast and Middle Atlantic states, the child who presents with a swollen knee needs to be considered as a potential victim of Lyme disease. This infectious arthritis is due to a specific spirochete, *Borrelia burgdorferi*.

The organism is transmitted to the human host by the bite of a deer tick. These ticks are significantly smaller than the common wood tick, and they are barely visible with the naked eye. Unfortunately, a history of a bite is rare and usually the diagnosis is reached by a high index of suspicion in a susceptible host. The combination of endemic region, erythematous annular skin lesions, and monarticular arthritis should lead the physician to order a Lyme titer.

Treatment is generally successful if begun early. Occasionally, despite adequate treatment, the arthritis can progress to chronic joint destruction mandating further care.

Metabolic Disease

Perhaps the classic metabolic disease to affect the pediatric skeleton is rickets. The etiologies of rickets are multiple (Table 5.1), but the important pathophysiologic step is a relative paucity of vitamin D. It will be remembered that vitamin D is essential for normal progression of physeal bone development, and without it provisional calcification will not occur in the deepest layer of the growth plate.

Table 5.1 Etiologies of rickets

1. Vitamin D dietary deficiency
2. Malabsorption states
3. Renal rickets
   a. Tubular defects (generally congenital)
   b. Glomerular disease (generally acquired)
4. Miscellaneous causes
   a. Associated with neurofibromatosis
   b. Complication of Dilantin (phenytoin) therapy

As a result, physeal disorganization (Fig. 5.17) can be anticipated with subsequent physeal widening, trumpeting of the metaphysis, and aberrant enchondral bone growth. The clinically apparent changes of knobby joints, beading of the costochondral joints, and genu varum are all phenotypic reflections of the underlying histologic disruption of bone formation (Fig. 5.18). Depending on the etiology of the rickets, the histologic pattern will vary slightly, but the overall skeletal changes remain relatively constant.

Vascular and Hematologic Disease

Vascular diseases of the pediatric skeleton are typified by osteochondroses such as Perthes' disease of the hip and Osgood-Schlatter's disease of the knee. These will be considered regionally, leaving the hematologic diseases to be discussed here.

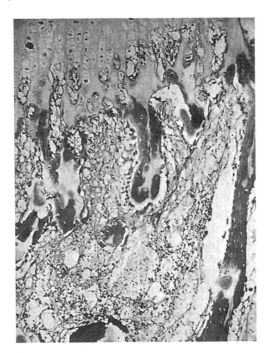

Fig. 5.17 Histologic appearance of rickets. Photomicrograph through the epiphyseal–metaphyseal junction. Note the uncalcified osteoid tissue, failure of deposition of calcium along the mature cartilage cell columns, and disorderly invasion of cartilage by blood vessels (× 25). (From Tachdjian MO. Pediatric Orthopedics, 2nd ed, vol 1. Philadelphia: Saunders, 1990. Reprinted with permission)

Sickle Cell Disease

The red cell deformation that occurs in sickle cell patients due to the abnormal hemoglobin is responsible for the skeletal changes. The abnormally shaped cells cause stasis and sludging in small arterioles and capillaries. The effect as expected is disrupted flow and bony necrosis. The bony infarcts seen in sickle cell disease can occur anywhere in the bone, but are more typical in the metaphysis (Fig. 5.19).

These children are also predisposed to osteomyelitis, probably due to the already sludged vessels in the metaphysis, making bacterial trapping even easier. Even though *Staphylococcus* is the most common organism retrieved, this patient population is also susceptible to infection with *Salmonella*. This organism gains access to the circulatory system through small infarcts in the intestinal wall and then enters the bone hematogenously. The incidence of *Salmonella* osteomyelitis is approaching that of *Staphylococcus* in this population.

The treatment for the infarcts is appropriate hematologic care – hydration, analgesics, etc. Antibiotic selection for osteomyelitis should take into consideration the incidence of salmonella.

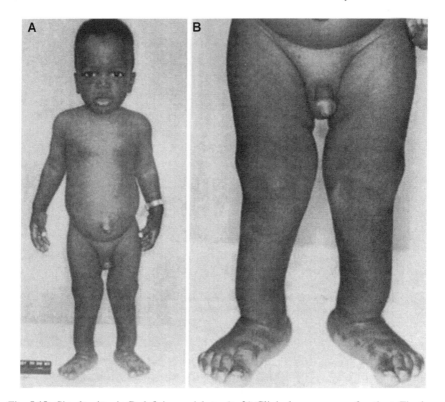

Fig. 5.18 Simple vitamin D deficiency rickets. (**a, b**) Clinical appearance of patient. The legs are bowed anterolaterally. Note the protuberant abdomen with the umbilical hernia. (From Tachdjian MO. Pediatric Orthopedics, 2nd ed, vol 1. Philadelphia: Saunders, 1990. Reprinted with permission)

Leukemia

This is the most common malignancy of childhood, and the skeleton is not spared its ravages. The bones by X-ray will show nondescript lytic changes most characteristically seen in the metaphyseal region and referred to as "metaphyseal banding" (Fig. 5.20). The areas of osteopenia parallel and are adjacent to the physis; although suggestive of leukemia, they are NOT pathognomonic of it.

Although usually the diagnosis has been made well before skeletal complications develop, occasionally a child will present for the evaluation of "growing pains" only to have a workup reveal this disease. Ordinarily "growing pains" occur in children 2–7 years of age, affect primarily the legs, are symmetric (although not simultaneous), occur in early evening or just after going to bed, and are NOT associated with any systemic complaints. Any variation from the usual pattern should suggest a basic workup to include X-rays and a white count with differential.

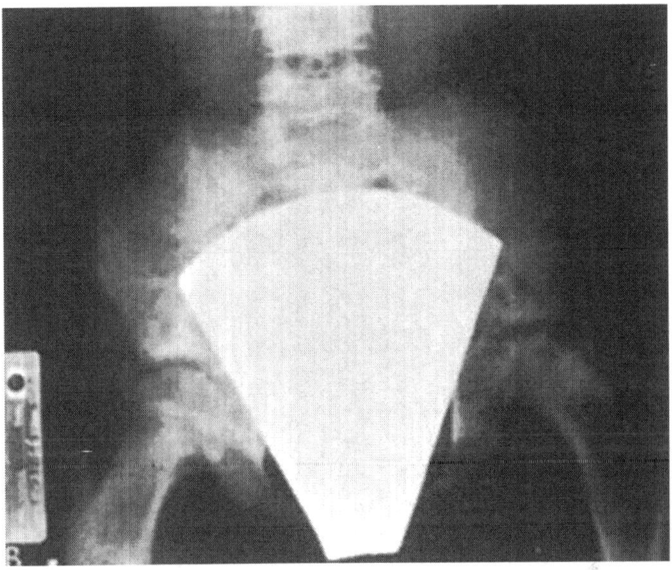

Fig. 5.19 Sickle cell disease in an 11-year-old girl. Anteroposterior radiogram of the hips. Note the avascular changes in the left femoral head. (From Tachdjian MO. Pediatric Orthopedics, 2nd ed, vol 1. Philadelphia: Saunders, 1990. Reprinted with permission)

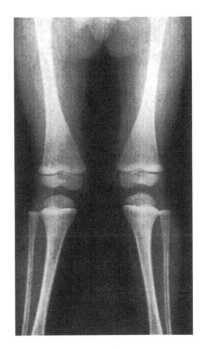

Fig. 5.20 Bone manifestations of acute leukemia. (From Tachdjian MO. Pediatric Orthopedics, 2nd ed, vol 1. Philadelphia: Saunders, 1990. Reprinted with permission)

Congenital and Neurodevelopmental

This is the largest and most nondescript "wastebasket" of pathologic states, many of which have severe impact on the pediatric skeleton. Included here are congenital birth defects of no known etiology, such as proximal femoral focal deficiency, as well as genetic diseases transmitted in classic Mendelian fashion (e.g., hemophilia) or due to chromosomal defects (e.g., Down's syndrome).

In addition, the neuromuscular diseases frequently have an immense impact on the skeleton, as aberrant and eccentric muscular forces are created. Unfortunately, it is difficult to find many common themes that make an appreciation of the skeletal impact easier to understand.

Osteogenesis Imperfecta

This disease is transmitted in a classic autosomal dominant pattern with only rare exception. The basic defect is one of abnormal collagen synthesis due to impotent osteoblasts. For this reason, it has been grouped with other "sick" cell syndromes. Certainly, the osteoblasts are normal in number, but incapable of normal synthetic activity. The collagenous product of their incompetence is poorly formed and poorly cross-linked, making it weak. The subsequent bone that is made is similarly architecturally thin and mechanically weak.

The severity of the disease is as expected – a function of the dose of abnormal genetic material. Some of the severe homozygotes are stillborn due to intracranial bleeds occurring in the perinatal period. As with most genetic diseases, penetrance varies such that some children have multiple fractures and severe shortening and others less involved have only the occasional fracture.

Typically, the bones are osteopenic (Fig. 5.21) with thinned cortices and decreased diameter. Multiple fractures with resulting deformities are the norm. These fractures respond to appropriate treatment, and healing is only slightly prolonged. Occasionally, it is necessary to correct long-bone deformities, and this is best accomplished operatively by performing multiple osteotomies in a single bone (Fig. 5.22) and lining the resultant fragments up on an intramedullary rod (Sofield "shish kabob").

Scoliosis can also complicate this disease, and its management can be very challenging, especially if surgical management is required to correct the deformity. It is very difficult to use spinal instrumentation in the face of this osteopenic, softened bone.

Down Syndrome

First described in England by Langdon Down in the 1800s, this syndrome has been shown to result from a trisomy of the number 21 chromosome. It is the most

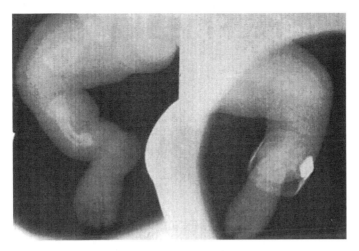

Fig. 5.21 Osteogenesis imperfecta congenita in a newborn. Radiogram of lower limbs, showing multiple fractures. (From Tachdjian MO. Pediatric Orthopedics, 2nd ed, vol 1. Philadelphia: Saunders, 1990. Reprinted with permission)

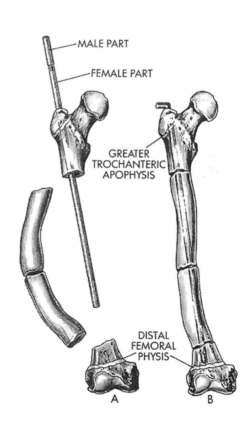

Fig. 5.22 Williams modification of Sofield–Millar intramedullary (**a, b**) rod fixation. (From Tachdjian MO. Pediatric Orthopedics, 2nd ed, vol 1. Philadelphia: Saunders, 1990. Reprinted with permission)

common chromosomal abnormality that is seen today and it occurs in approximately 1 in 500 live births. Because of its frequency, it is the prototype for the other chromosomal abnormalities and the orthopedic manifestations tend to be somewhat common to all.

Hypotonia and ligamentous laxity typify the group. The ligamentous laxity results from an inordinate number of elastic fibers relative to the number of collagen fibers in ligament and joint capsule. The joint changes typical of this disease and other chromosomal diseases can be traced directly to this ligamentous laxity. Specific manifestations include the following:

1. C1–C2 instability (Fig. 5.23): Due to laxity of the transverse ligament of the odontoid process, anterior translation of C1 on C2 occurs, frequently to alarming degrees. Routine lateral cervical spine radiographs in flexion and extension should be regularly obtained in these children to evaluate them for this problem.
2. Hip subluxation and dislocation can occur insidiously over time, again resulting from the capsular laxity about the joint.
3. Patellar subluxation is the cause of the typical gait seen in the older child with Down syndrome. These children often walk with a stiff-legged gait in an effort to preclude patellar subluxation.
4. Hypermobile flatfeet and bunions.

The management of these orthopedic problems is primarily directed at controlling the deformity, if possible, and minimizing the pain, which is rarely a significant problem. Despite fixed deformities, it is frequently surprising how well these children are able to compensate.

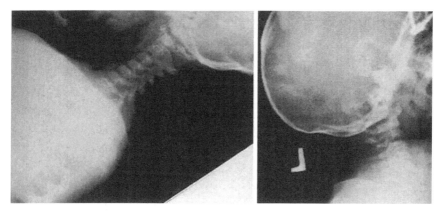

Fig. 5.23 Atlantoaxial instability in Down's syndrome. (From Tachdjian MO. Pediatric Orthopedics, 2nd ed, vol 1. Philadelphia: Saunders, 1990. Reprinted with permission)

Skeletal Dysplasias

There are several hundred recognized skeletal dysplasias, each with its own unique clinical characteristics and specific skeletal abnormalities. It is impossible to recall all of the features, which define a given dysplastic condition, especially in light of the fact that each is usually quite rare. At best, generalizations can be employed to assist in the diagnosis of a specific patient and thereby guide the appropriate workup and referral to an individual skilled in definitive diagnosis. The anticipated orthopedic problems, treatment, and prognosis will hinge on the diagnosis.

When presented with an individual displaying dysplastic findings, especially short stature, chromosomal evaluation and standard X-rays are good starting points once appropriate history (especially family history) and a careful physical examination have been carried out. The X-rays should include a lateral of the cervical and thoracolumbar spine, an anteroposterior view of the pelvis, and anteroposterior views of the wrists and the knees. These views will allow one to evaluate epiphyseal, physeal, metaphyseal, and diaphyseal growth and their aberrations.

Most of the dysplasias tend to affect a specific region of the bone; by assessing each region, clues can be gotten regarding the specific type of dysplasia. For example, spondyloepiphyseal dysplasia affects primarily epiphyseal growth as the name implies. One should expect to see deformities of the epiphyseal nuclei and disordered apophyseal growth. On the other hand, achondroplasia is a defect in physeal growth and will, therefore, produce significant dwarfing; in fact, it is the most common cause of pathologic short stature.

Most of the skeletal dysplasias are genetically transmitted, and a careful family history will define the pattern. Many, however, are spontaneous mutations or without a defined etiology. It is important to keep in mind that by definition a skeletal dysplasia is a GENERALIZED affectation of the skeleton with all bones showing some changes. Obviously, the end of the bone growing more rapidly will demonstrate the defect to a greater degree; thus, the knee and wrist films are more likely to show changes than the hip or elbow views.

Achondroplasia

As an example of how a dysplasia affects the skeleton, one should consider the most common, achondroplasia. Transmitted as an autosomal dominant in most cases, it is usually apparent at birth. The infant will be rhizomelically shortened; that is to say, the proximal segment of the limbs is relatively shorter than the middle or distal segments (Fig. 5.24). In addition, the child is disproportionately built since the limbs are preferentially involved and, therefore, very short relative to the spine and trunk.

These children follow the growth curve, but several standard deviations below normal, achieving a mature height between 3 and 4 ft. As with all of the true dysplasias, intelligence is not impaired and life expectancy is virtually normal.

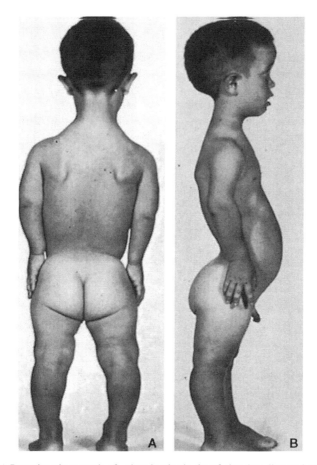

Fig. 5.24 (**a**) Posterior photograph of achondroplastic dwarf showing distorted growth of long bones. The proximal limb segments are proportionately shorter than the distal, with the hands reaching only to the hip region. The legs are bowed, and the scapulae and pelvis are smaller than normal. Scoliosis is uncommon. (**b**) Lateral photograph of child with achondroplasia. Note marked lumbar lordosis with prominent buttocks as a result of pelvic tilt. The lordosis is due in part to differential growth of vertebral body versus posterior elements. (From Bogumill GP. Orthopaedic Pathology: A Synopsis with Clinical Radiographic Correlation. Philadelphia: Saunders, 1984. Reprinted with permission)

Clinical Features

The child's head shows flattening of the nasal bridge and prominent frontal bones. Both findings are due to the disparity between the normal intramembranous calvarial growth and the retarded enchondral growth of the basilar portions of the skull.

The extremities are short, with each of the bones being short in length, but relatively normal in girth, since periosteal bone formation remains relatively unaffected. The spine and pelvis also show some decrease in height, but of greater significance is the decrease in the interpedicular distance which effectively creates a spinal stenotic syndrome. This, coupled with a hyperlordotic lumbar spine, creates many achondroplasts to develop disc symptoms at an early age.

The major problem of the older adolescent is obesity, which complicates many of the other abnormalities. As adults, problems with multiple tendonitises and bursitises are commonplace.

Neuromuscular Disease

Unlike the skeletal dysplasias which are intrinsic abnormalities of the skeleton, this group of diseases is extrinsic, but drastically alters the normal skeleton due primarily to the muscle imbalance they create.

Common themes can be seen that emphasize the fact that the problem is disparity in the agonist–antagonist relationship. Major joints tend to dislocate, with the hip being a prime example. The flexor pattern tends to become dominant, causing the femoral head to dislocate posteriorly. Scoliosis should be expected as asymmetry of spinal muscle action alters normal balance. If the neurologic defect is asymmetric, as in polio, then the growth plates in one leg will "feel" a different muscle pull than those of the other and a leg-length discrepancy can be anticipated.

Cerebral Palsy

This is a static neurologic disease of children due to an insult to the immature brain during the perinatal period. The defect is, therefore, central, damaging the normal inhibitory influences on the peripheral gamma efferent system. Without central damping, the peripheral reflex arc functions autonomously, and the result is increased tone or spasticity.

Cerebral palsy is classified in one of two ways:

1. Physiologic classification

   a. Spastic: Hypertonia, hyperflexia, and contractures are seen. This is the most common form of the syndrome.
   b. Athetoid: This is far less common today than it was in years past. Rh incompatibility and erythroblastosis fetalis was a common etiology of this form.
   c. Rigid
   d. Ballismic
   e. Mixed

2. Geographic classification

   a. Hemiplegia: The most common form, it is frequently associated with seizures.

b. Diplegia: Both lower extremities predominate the pattern.
c. Quadriplegia: The most severe cases involve children, many of whom are retarded and few of whom will ever walk.

Cerebral palsy is really a syndrome rather than a disease (Fig. 5.25), and no two children are really the same. This makes comparison of procedures and other treatments extremely difficult, if not impossible. The muscles all tend to be spastic; however, the muscle imbalance is created between spastic and more spastic muscles. Contractures, joint dislocations, limb deformities, and scoliosis should all be anticipated.

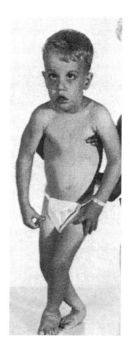

Fig. 5.25 Spastic quadriplegia with total body involvement. At 4 years of age. The marked scissoring of the hips and equinus deformity of the ankles provide a poor base upon which balance can develop. Note the pes valgus. (From Tachdjian MO. Pediatric Orthopedics, 2nd ed, vol 1. Philadelphia: Saunders, 1990. Reprinted with permission)

Polio

With the introduction of the Salk vaccine in 1954, this disease has become rare in the United States; however, it is certainly not eradicated in the Third World. Since immigrants are seen in our larger cities on an increasingly frequent basis with the sequelae of this disease some familiarity with it seems appropriate.

The polio virus has unique predilection for the anterior horn cells of the cord and the bulbar portion of the brain. In most cases, the involvement is spotty and the degree of paralysis is variable. The victim is left with a mix of normal muscle, weak muscle, and absent muscle – hence creating a broad spectrum of muscle imbalance, but in an asymmetric distribution. It is important to remember that the sensory fibers are NOT affected, which gives these children a clear and distinct benefit over the children with spina bifida.

Spina Bifida

Despite the improvement in antenatal testing, many children with myelodysplasia are still born in the United States each year. Due to open cord defects at a certain level (Fig. 5.26), these children are essentially congenital paraplegics. They are without motor and sensory modalities below the level of the defect. Needless to say, the higher their level of defect, the poorer their function and, hence, the prognosis (Fig. 5.27). For example, a child with a T12 level (the spinal roots that are the last to function are T12) has no motor power and no sensation below the waist. These children will be wheelchair-confined and have bowel and bladder compromise. On the other hand, children with an S1 level (the last functioning spinal level is S1) will have only minimal motor involvement and will usually walk without braces. Their major problems are the bowel and bladder malfunction.

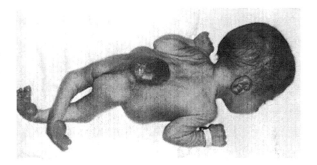

Fig. 5.26 Newborn infant with lumbosacral myelomeningocele. Note the severe equinovarus deformity of both feet. (From Tachdjian MO. Pediatric Orthopedics, 2nd ed, vol 1. Philadelphia: Saunders, 1990. Reprinted with permission)

The absence of sensation below the level of the lesion creates many additional problems for these children. Not unlike a diabetic patient with severe neuropathy, children with spina bifida are prone to foot ulceration, infection, and the development of neuropathic joints.

One recently identified problem in this group is latex allergy. Perhaps due to repeated catheterization with latex rubber catheters, these patients can become severely sensitized to all latex contact, to the point of anaphylaxis. Specific protocols are now used at the time of surgical procedures to avoid contact with any latex products, including gloves, catheters, and IV tubing.

Lastly, it is important to realize that these children, as well as many of those with cerebral palsy, are multiply handicapped. They have learning difficulties, perceptual problems, hearing and visual impairments, not to mention emotional issues – all of which require a coordinated effort by multiple specialists to provide optimal care.

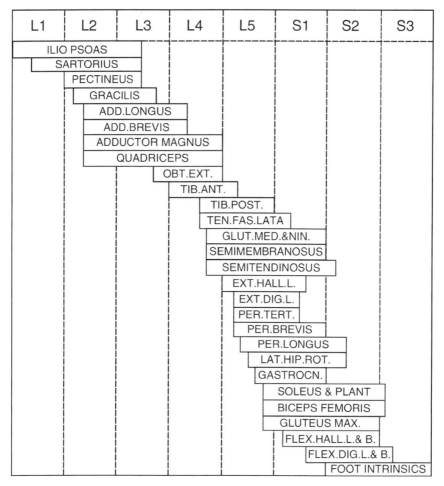

Fig. 5.27 Neurosegmental innervation of muscles of lower limb. (From Tachdjian MO. Pediatric Orthopedics, 2nd ed, vol 1. Philadelphia: Saunders, 1990. Reprinted with permission)

Regional Orthopedic Problems

The Pediatric Hip

Most of the showcase pediatric orthopedic maladies affect the hip. Developmental dysplasias, Perthes' disease, and slipped capital epiphysis have established the hip as the preeminent joint of a child's musculoskeletal system. Several unique anatomic features predispose this joint to long-term problems following septic, vascular, developmental, and traumatic insults.

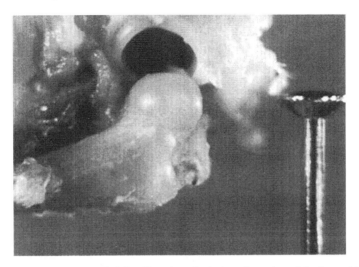

Fig. 5.28 Embryology of the hip joint. Note the spherical configuration of the femoral head and acetabulum. The limbus and transverse acetabular ligament are well-formed structures. (From Tachdjian MO. Pediatric Orthopedics, 2nd ed, vol 1. Philadelphia: Saunders, 1990. Reprinted with permission)

In the newborn, the upper end of the femur (Fig. 5.28) is entirely cartilaginous, representing the secondary ossification centers of both the greater trochanter and the femoral head (capital femoral epiphysis) as a composite chondroepiphysis. The two bony ossification centers will develop within this one cartilage mass and grow differentially to their ultimate adult size and shape. Implicit in this fact is that the growth of one is in part dependent on the growth of the other. Normally, the bony centrum of the capital femoral epiphysis should be radiographically visible by 3–6 months of age.

The growth of this epiphysis is dependent primarily on the blood supply of the upper end of the femur (Fig. 5.29). It is essential to recognize that up until 1 year of age there is communication between the metaphyseal and epiphyseal circulations. This protects the capital femoral epiphysis from isolation in the event of an insult to the epiphyseal side. Unfortunately, as the physis thickens and matures by 18 months of age, it becomes an impenetrable barrier between the two circulations, leaving the epiphysis of the head totally dependent on the epiphyseal vessels for its viability. Less than 10% of the femoral head is supplied by the branch of the obturator artery through the ligamentum teres. The epiphyseal vessels are supplied by the medial and lateral circumflex branches of the femoral artery. This vascular isolation of the upper end of the femur is largely responsible for the disastrous complications of developmental dislocation of the hip (DDH), Perthes' disease, and slipped capital femoral epiphysis (SCFE).

The acetabulum develops from two cartilage segments. The first is the triradiate cartilage, which a bilaminar physis forms at the junction of the ilium, ischium,

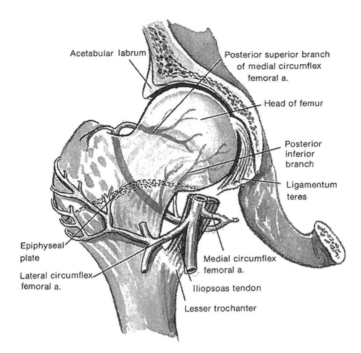

Fig. 5.29 Posterior view of the normal blood supply of the upper end of the femur in an infant. (From Tachdjian MO. Pediatric Orthopedics, 2nd ed, vol 1. Philadelphia: Saunders, 1990. Reprinted with permission)

and pubis. Integrity of this growth plate is essential for acetabular *height* to be normal. The *depth* of the acetabulum is a function of the cartilaginous labrum that circumferentially surrounds the developing acetabulum.

Developmental Dislocation of the Hip

The previous nomenclature "congenital dislocation" was recently changed to "developmental dislocation" in recognition of the fact that some of these hips are located at birth and go on to dislocate in the postnatal period. The incidence of this condition is about 1 per 1,000 live births and is more common in females. Although it is fair to say that the etiology is unknown, it is important to recognize that there are both genetic and environmental factors; hence, it is considered a multifactorial trait. It is also critical to recognize that this is a true dysplasia (i.e., aberrant growth), and NOT simply a femoral head that is not located in the acetabulum (Fig. 5.30). It is important to stress this fact to the parents in an effort to assist them in understanding the pathology.

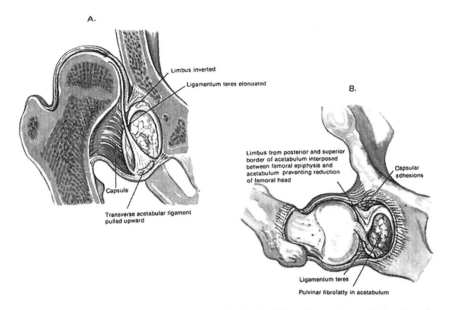

Fig. 5.30 Pathology of the dislocated hip that is irreducible owing to intraarticular obstacles. (**a**) The hip is dislocated. (**b**) It cannot be reduced on flexion, abduction, or lateral rotation. Obstacles to reduction are inverted limbus, ligamentum teres, and fibrofatty pulvinar in the acetabulum. The transverse acetabular ligament is pulled upward with the ligamentum teres. (From Tachdjian MO. Pediatric Orthopedics, 2nd ed, vol 1. Philadelphia: Saunders, 1990. Reprinted with permission)

Early diagnosis is the key to optimal treatment and the best prognosis. First, consider the risk factors:

1. First-born female
2. Breech presentation
3. Positive family history
4. Hip "click"
5. Presence of a muscular torticollis

With these in mind, a careful physical examination of the hips is the logical next step. In the newborn, one should attempt to demonstrate laxity and instability (Fig. 5.31). The Barlow test is performed with the infant supine and the hips flexed. As the hips are brought from the abducted to adducted position, a positive test is noted as the femoral head subluxes posteriorly over the posterior rim of the acetabulum. This would indicate instability. The Barlow is a provocative test: the hip is located and the maneuver dislocates it. Conversely, the Ortolani test is a reduction maneuver; the hip is dislocated and the test reduces it. This is accomplished by

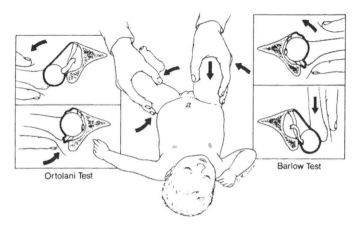

Fig. 5.31 On the *left*, the Ortolani (reduction) test is demonstrated. The Barlow (provocation dislocation) test is shown on the *right*. These tests must be performed on a relaxed infant. (From Sabiston DC Jr. Essentials of Surgery. Philadelphia: Saunders, 1987. Reprinted with permission)

abducting the adducted hip and noting a palpable (but rarely audible) "clunk" as the femoral head reduces over the posterior acetabular rim.

As the child gets older (by 3 months), the dislocated hip tends to become fixed in that position, and the classic signs of instability disappear in favor of those indicating a fixed dislocation deformity. Limited abduction is perhaps the most important finding to note. Examining the child on a firm surface, subtle differences in the degrees of hip abduction may herald a dislocated hip on the restricted side. Similarly,

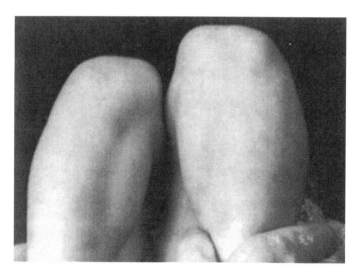

Fig. 5.32 The Galeazzi test is performed by comparison of the relative height of the femoral condyles by holding the hips in flexion. The right femur appears shorter because of a right hip dislocation. This test is usually not helpful in the case of bilateral hip dislocations. (From Sabiston DC Jr. Essentials of Surgery. Philadelphia: Saunders, 1987. Reprinted with permission)

viewing knee height with the child supine and the hips and knees flexed may reveal a positive Allis sign (Fig. 5.32), one knee higher than the other, again indicating a dislocation on the low side.

Imaging studies are important in both diagnosis and treatment. The current popularity of ultrasound is based on the fact that under 3 months of age much of the proximal femur is cartilaginous. Ultrasound has been helpful in the diagnosis of DDH (Fig. 5.33), as well as in defining relatively subtle degrees of acetabular dysplasia. The value of ultrasound after the child is 3 months old decreases, and standard X-rays assume a more central role. Many still feel that a standard

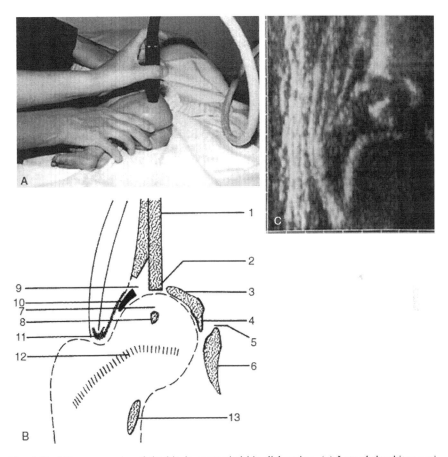

Fig. 5.33 Ultrasonography of the hip in congenital hip dislocation. (**a**) Lateral decubitus position of the infant for ultrasonographic examination of the hip. (**b**) Diagram of structures identified during static non-stress ultrasonography of the hip: (1) iliac bone; (2) the most distal point of the ilium in the roof of the acetabulum; (3) ossified medial wall of the acetabulum; (4) the inferior end of the iliac bone at the triradiate cartilage; (5) triradiate cartilage; (6) ossified ischium; (7) the cartilaginous femoral head; (8) ossific nucleus of the femoral head; (9) cartilaginous roof of the acetabulum; (10) labrum; (11) intertrochanteric fossa; (12) cartilaginous growth plate of the femoral head; (13) ossified metaphysis of the femoral neck. (**c**) Ultrasonogram showing structures. (From Tachdjian MO. Pediatric Orthopedics, 2nd ed, vol 1. Philadelphia: Saunders, 1990. Reprinted with permission)

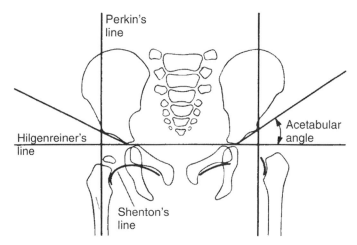

Fig. 5.34 Radiographic features of congenital dislocation of the hip (*left hip dislocated, right hip normal*). There is a delay in ossification of the capital femoral epiphysis. Shenton's line, a smooth continuation of an imaginary line drawn along the femoral neck and superior margin of the obturator foramen, is disrupted. The acetabular angle is increased usually greater than 30°. The proximal medial I margin of the femoral metaphysis is displaced lateral to Perkin's line, a line drawn from the lateral margin of the acetabulum perpendicular to Hilgenreiner's line. (From Sabiston DC Jr. Essentials of Surgery. Philadelphia: Saunders, 1987. Reprinted with permission)

anteroposterior (AP) view of the pelvis with the hips in neutral is the "gold standard" to which all other studies need to be compared (Fig. 5.34). Historically, many classic measurements are made on this X-ray that allow one to determine the location of the femoral head as well as the degree of acetabular dysplasia. In addition, subsequent X-rays are important to monitor the progress of treatment, despite the enthusiasm in some centers to use ultrasound for therapeutic monitoring.

Treatment

Simply stated, the goals are the following:

1. Reduce the femoral head concentrically into the acetabulum.
2. Maintain this reduction.
3. Avoid the complications of doing both.

There is probably no other pediatric orthopedic malady in which there is a greater understatement of treatment. The pitfalls in accomplishing these apparently simple goals qualify more as "land mines." The adage, "The first physician to treat DDH is the last physician with the opportunity to achieve a normal hip," emphasizes the difficulties frequently encountered in the management of this problem. Also implied is the fact that the younger the child is when treatment is initiated, the better the prognosis will be. Indeed, it is generally believed that if treatment is delayed until after the age of walking, it will not be possible to produce a normal hip.

Fig. 3.35 The Pavlik
harness. (From Tachdjian
MO. Pediatric Orthopedics,
2nd ed, vol 1. Philadelphia:
Saunders, 1990. Reprinted
with permission.)

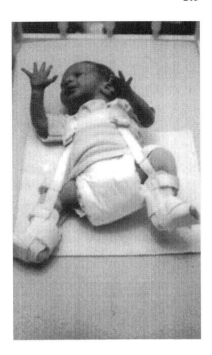

The use of a Pavlik harness (Fig. 5.35) as initial treatment in the infant has become the international standard. For the child under 3 months of age with a frank dislocation or with persistent instability (as documented, for example, by a positive Barlow test in a 3-week-old), appropriate application and use of a Pavlik harness will assure a normal hip in about 80% of cases. The device, however, is not foolproof, with avascular necrosis inferior dislocation and femoral nerve palsy reported as complications, not to mention failure to achieve a reduction. One should be familiar with the appropriate use of this device and NOT randomly apply it as a panacea to all children with hip clicks.

If diagnosis for some reason is delayed and the child presents after 6 months for treatment, more aggressive modalities are generally required to achieve a reduction. Closed reduction under anesthesia, adductor tenotomy, and occasionally prereduction traction are generally employed at this point, with open reduction indicated for those who cannot undergo closed reduction. Immobilization in a spica cast is essential to maintain the reduction.

After 18 months of age, operative approaches are required to reduce the hip and also to reconform the acetabulum. Pelvic osteotomies and proximal femoral osteotomies are utilized in the older age groups. Keep in mind that it is rarely possible to produce a normal hip when treatment is initiated after the age of walking.

The prognosis for DDH is generally very good when the diagnosis is made early and treatment initiated in infancy. With delay in diagnosis and, therefore, in treatment, the prognosis worsens. The complication most dreaded, avascular necrosis, can occur at many points in the treatment algorithm. Despite earlier diagnosis and advances in treatment, many reported series still record about a 10% incidence of avascular necrosis. If it occurs, the prognosis is fair at best.

Perthes' Disease

Idiopathic avascular necrosis of the femoral head in the child was originally described in 1909 by multiple authors: Legg in Boston, Calvé in France, and Perthes in Germany. Unfortunately, all authors interpreted that the observed changes were due to nontuberculous sepsis. Slowly, it was recognized that the cause was, in fact, an avascular event. It has more recently been shown that the changes cannot be produced by a single period of avascularity. Rather, multiple episodes are needed to cause the characteristic pathologic changes. The exact trigger for this vascular disruption has remained elusive.

The affected children are typically males from a lower socioeconomic status, aged 4–9 years, and slightly delayed in skeletal growth. Generally, the child presents with a limp and absence of any systemic symptoms. Clinically, the child will usually have restricted hip motion, especially rotational, and some adductor muscle spasm. Local findings of tenderness and erythema are not seen. Since standard laboratory studies are usually normal, imaging studies are paramount in the diagnosis and treatment of the disease.

Pathologically, the disease progresses through four stages (Fig. 5.36), and these are reflected by the X-rays and magnetic resonance imaging (MRI) scans. Initially, the stage of synovitis, which lasts 2–3 weeks, produces an irritable hip syndrome easily confused with toxic synovitis. The X-rays are negative at this time. Subsequently the stage of avascularity onsets, lasting 2–3 months, during which time the femoral head necrosis occurs. Fragmentation changes of the capital femoral epiphysis herald this stage. Once the avascular event has occurred, the femoral head will revascularize and the process will "heal," resulting in the stage of revascularization. The critical issue is the degree of deformation of the normally spherical femoral head before complete healing occurs. Eccentric mechanical loads applied to the softened, diseased head frequently alter its sphericity. Ultimately, the process burns itself out, leaving the hip in the stage of residua. The healing phase lasts approximately 2 years, at which time only the residual deformity remains as the permanent marker of the disease.

The treatment principles for this disease are really no more advanced than they were 30 years ago. Nevertheless, certain facts seem generally accepted. The prognosis seems to hinge on two basic features. First is the patient's age at onset of the disease. Children under age 5 will do well left untreated, which is the current recommendation. Those over age 8 do poorly, despite treatment. The other factor is the extent of head involvement. Obviously, the head that is completely necrotic is more likely to sustain permanent deformation than a head only partially involved. For children of intermediate age, 5–8 years, the principle of "containment" continues

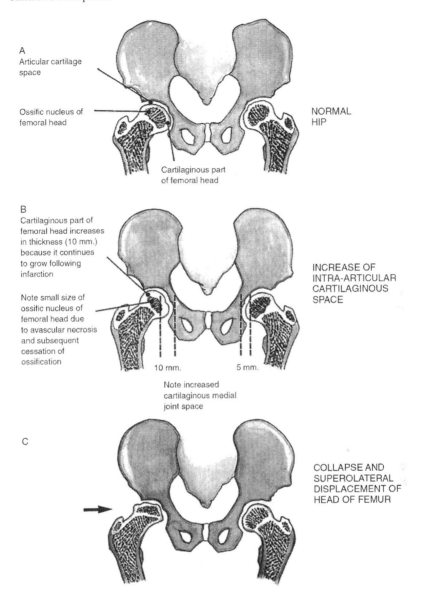

Fig. 5.36 Pathogenesis of deformity of the femoral head in Legg–Calve–Perthes' disease. (**a**) Normal hips. (**b**) Widening of the medial cartilaginous joint space due to hypertrophy of the cartilage covering of the femoral head. Note the smaller ossific nucleus due to cessation of bone growth as a result of avascular necrosis. (**c**) Collapse of the femoral head with superolateral displacement. (**d**) The hip is adducted in weightbearing position. Note in (**e**) the dent in the lateral part of the femoral head blocking concentric reduction of the hip. (**e, f**) Hinged abduction. On abduction of the hip (**f**), the femoral head is displaced further laterally, with increase in the medial joint space. (From Tachdjian MO. Pediatric Orthopedics, 2nd ed, vol 1. Philadelphia: Saunders, 1990. Reprinted with permission)

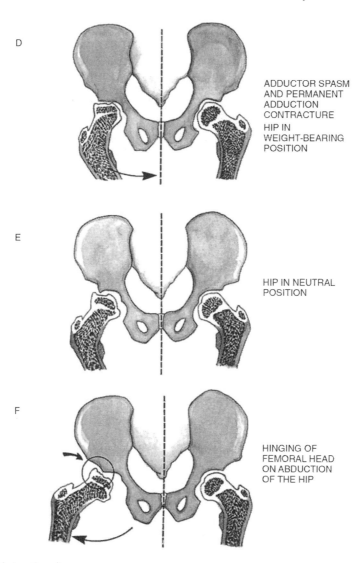

D

ADDUCTOR SPASM
AND PERMANENT
ADDUCTION
CONTRACTURE
HIP IN
WEIGHT-BEARING
POSITION

E

HIP IN NEUTRAL
POSITION

F

HINGING OF
FEMORAL HEAD
ON ABDUCTION
OF THE HIP

Fig. 5.36 (continued)

to be accepted. Conceptually, the thought is to place the softened femoral head concentrically into the acetabulum, which will in turn act as a mold or template as the head revascularizes. This can be accomplished in the smaller child by using an abduction orthosis (Fig. 5.37) and in the larger child by using either a femoral or acetabular osteotomy to improve congruity prior to deformation. The treatment for the older child with an already deformed hip is highly controversial.

In general, the prognosis is good for the younger children, whereas many of those diagnosed after age 9 require total hip replacement in their forties or fifties.

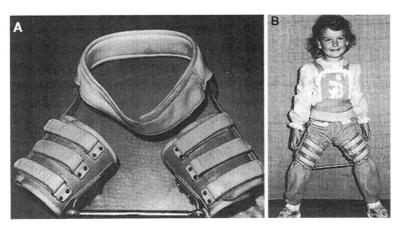

Fig. 5.37 Scottish-Rite hip orthosis. (**a**) Anteroposterior view of the orthosis. (**b**) Anteroposterior view of a patient wearing the orthosis. (From Tachdjian MO. Pediatric Orthopedics, 2nd ed, vol 1. Philadelphia: Saunders, 1990. Reprinted with permission)

Slipped Capital Femoral Epiphysis

Hip pain in the adolescent should always raise suspicion of this entity. In fact, many of these patients present with pain along the medial side of the thigh radiating to the knee. This referred pain in the obturator distribution is quite typical. These children also share a common body habitus: they tend to be quite obese, with delayed secondary sexual characteristics. Many of these children have been limping for several months before they present for evaluation.

Pathologically, the capital femoral epiphysis has "slipped" or translated posteriorly and inferiorly relative to the femoral neck (Fig. 5.38). There are those who prefer to emphasize the fact that the neck is actually moving anteriorly and superiorly relative to the head. This displacement ultimately results in irritated hip which is manifested by a limp, pain, and external rotational deformity of the leg. This deformity is usually readily apparent on physical examination. As the hip is flexed, the leg obligately externally rotates.

There have been multiple suggestions as to the etiology of the slipped capital femoral epiphysis. Many authors feel that these children are hormonally predisposed and with the superimposed stress of obesity, the perichondral ring is no longer able to "girdle" the physis; hence, the slip occurs. Typically, the slip is said to occur through the hypertrophic zone of the plate. Recent studies suggest that the displacement may actually transcend the entire physis. There have been several different attempts to clinically group these patients. Historically, children were said to have chronic slips implying that they had symptoms for over 3 weeks. Acute slipped capital femoral epiphysis was often considered the result of an acute injury and, therefore, frequently considered by some authors to be a fracture through the physis.

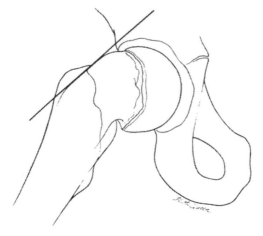

Fig. 5.38 Slipped capital femoral epiphysis is most reliably seen on the lateral radiograph. Posterior migration of the femoral head relative to the neck is seen. A line drawn up the anterior or lateral margin of the femoral neck does not intersect the epiphysis. (From Sabiston DC Jr. Essentials of Surgery. Philadelphia: Saunders, 1987. Reprinted with permission)

When the child had a history of limping and then a superimposed acute injury, the resultant slip was often referred to as an acute on chronic slip.

At the present time, most simply classify slips into stable versus unstable groups. The defining characteristic is the ability of the child to walk. Children with unstable slips are unable to bear weight on the extremity.

Treatment for slipped capital femoral epiphysis (SCFE) is very straightforward: stop the slipping and avoid the complications of doing so. In order to stop the slipping, an "in situ" pinning with a centrally placed compression screw crossing the physis is employed (Fig. 5.39). It is currently important to note that any attempt to reduce the slipped epiphysis is rarely recommended; to do so would subject the head to a high risk of avascular necrosis.

Slips are typically graded based on the degree of displacement and, should severe slipping have occurred, resulting in excessive deformity, most authors would recommend that this deformity be corrected as a second stage once the physis has fused.

The complications of the disease and its treatment can be devastating. Avascular necrosis is primarily a complication of the treatment rather than the disease itself. Aggressive reduction maneuvers and femoral neck osteotomies have both been implicated in the etiology of avascular necrosis. There is literature to suggest, however, that avascular necrosis may be a complication of high-grade slips.

The other concern is chondrolysis. This phenomena, most feel, is a complication of the disease more so than the treatment. It appears to be a particular concern in Afro-Americans, leading some to suggest an immunologic link. Slowly, one observes degradation of the articular cartilage with resultant joint space narrowing and severe hip stiffness.

It should be recognized that this condition primarily affects adolescents. Therefore, when it is diagnosed in a younger child, one should consider specific

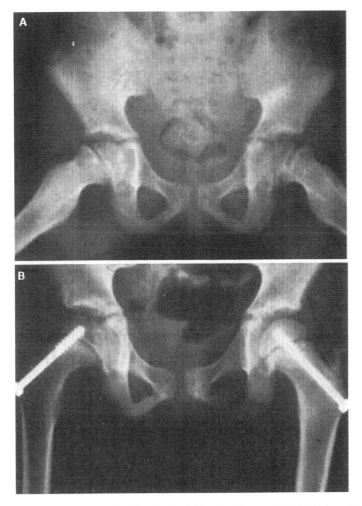

Fig. 5.39 Slipped capital femoral epiphysis of both hips in a 10-year-old girl with hypothyroidism. (**a, b**) Anteroposterior and lateral views of both hips. (From Tachdjian MO. Pediatric Orthopedics, 2nd ed, vol 1. Philadelphia: Saunders, 1990. Reprinted with permission)

endocrine abnormalities or metabolic diseases such as hypothyroidism or chronic renal failure. With early and adequate treatment, specifically pinning "in situ," excellent long-term results can be anticipated.

Transient Synovitis of the Hip

By far and away, the MOST COMMON cause of limp and hip pain in a child is the "irritable hip syndrome," also called "transient" or "toxic synovitis." Frequently, these children will have a history of an upper respiratory infection (URI) or ear infection in the recent past, leading many to believe that this condition is a postinfectious inflammation of the hip.

Clinically, such children are not sick; they remain active, feed well, and are afebrile. Their lab studies, including X-rays, are usually normal. On a typical exam, the hip is irritable, with additional findings of an antalgic limp, decreased range of motion, and pain with log rolling of the leg.

The treatment is supportive and includes nonsteroidal anti-inflammatory drugs (NSAIDs) and activity reduction, the latter being key. Normally, the process is self-limited, with the limp disappearing in 5–7 days. If it persists longer, one should suspect that the child has remained too active.

The Pediatric Knee

Unlike the hip, the affectations that one sees about the knee in a child are, for the most part, all benign and generally respond to simple treatment measures.

Osgood–Schlatter's Disease

Osteochondritis of the tibial tuberosity (Fig. 5.40) is one of the more common causes of knee pain, especially of the preadolescent age group. Although the name implies inflammation, there generally is relatively little present. Essentially, this is a "traction apophysitis," namely, a powerful muscle group pulls on an open growth plate producing an overload strain, resulting irritation of the local tissues.

These children have local swelling and tenderness over the tibial tuberosity without other findings. The key to successful treatment is activity restriction observed acutely at first, followed by activity modification until the plate closes. It is important for the children to accept responsibility for their knee care: decreasing activity, using ice after activity, and occasionally using a lightweight knee sleeve primarily for psychological support. It is equally important to reassure the parents that, no matter how much pain their child has, he or she is not damaging the knee in any permanent way.

Osteochondritis Dissecans

Another osteochondrosis, osteochondritis dissecans, is felt to be an avascular necrosis of a portion of the subchondral bone (Fig. 5.41). Typically, it most commonly affects the medial side of the lateral femoral condyle, adjacent to the intercondylar notch. However, it can occur on any of the condylar surfaces.

Clinically, the child presents with vague knee pain, which is poorly localized. Occasionally, an effusion will be present. The diagnosis is usually made radiographically, especially if an intercondylar notch view is obtained. Generally, short-term

Fig. 5.40 Osgood–Schlatter disease of the left proximal tibia with free ossicle lying anterior to the proximal tibial tubercle. (From Tachdjian MO. Pediatric Orthopedics, 2nd ed, vol 1. Philadelphia: Saunders, 1990. Reprinted with permission)

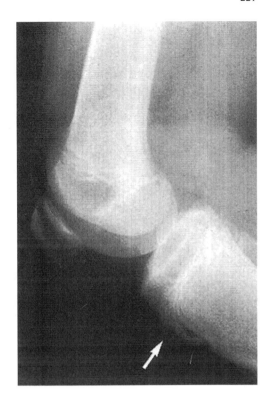

activity restriction, ice, and NSAIDs are adequate to relieve acute symptoms. Many can then be returned to sports. If symptoms continue unabated or recur, arthroscopy should be considered; should a loose fragment be identified, it can be removed or pinned into place.

The Discoid Meniscus

The menisci develop embryologically from a cartilaginous plate referred to as the interzone. The cartilage plates normally thin out to become shaped like the letter "C" on the medial side and the letter "O" on the lateral side of the knee. Should this hollowing out NOT occur on the lateral side, a thick cartilage plate persists as a discoid meniscus (Fig. 5.42). This structure causes the child to have knee pain and occasional effusion beginning about age 3–5 years. Most dramatic is a prominent audible and palpable "clunk" seen when the knee is flexed and extended with some rotation applied. If symptoms warrant, arthroscopic removal of the central portion of the disc is required, contouring it to the normal shape. Complete excision is NOT desirable.

Fig. 5.41 Osteochondritis dissecans of the knee. (From Tachdjian MO. Pediatric Orthopedics, 2nd ed, vol 1. Philadelphia: Saunders, 1990. Reprinted with permission)

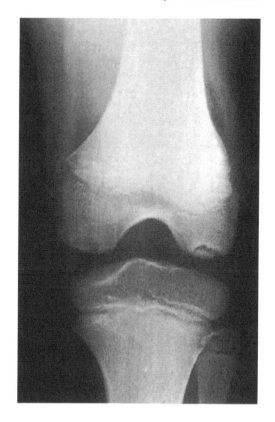

Fig. 5.42 Discoid lateral meniscus. (From Tachdjian MO. Pediatric Orthopedics, 2nd ed, vol 1. Philadelphia: Saunders, 1990. Reprinted with permission)

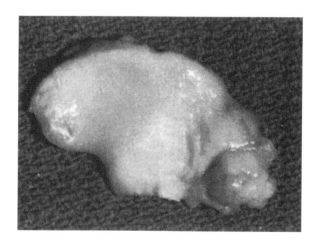

Popliteal Cysts

A localized mass in the popliteal space (Fig. 5.43) occurs more than infrequently in small children. Typically, this is a cyst containing gelatinous fluid. As with any mass, these cysts are a source of great concern to the parents, who can benefit a great deal from reassurance as to the correct diagnosis. These can be seen at a young age, frequently just after the child begins to walk.

Fig. 5.43   Popliteal cyst. Clinical appearance. (From Tachdjian MO. Pediatric Orthopedics, 2nd ed, vol 1. Philadelphia: Saunders, 1990. Reprinted with permission)

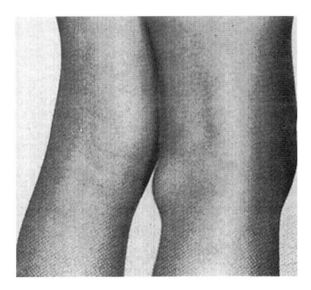

Typically, the cyst presents between the tendon of the semitendinosus and the medial head of the gastrocnemius; thus, it lies medial in the popliteal space. An X-ray should be negative, and an ultrasound will confirm a cystic structure. A more extensive workup should be considered if the mass is atypical – that is, on lateral side, painful, and enlarging.

Because most of these cysts will disappear in time, surgical excision should be reserved for the ones that cause symptoms. It is important to note that in children these are rarely associated with intraarticular pathology, whereas in the adult that association is the norm.

The Pediatric Foot

There are as many developmental variations in foot configuration as there are children who have feet. It seems that no two pairs of feet are exactly alike. The challenge then for the physician is to determine which of these feet are pathologic and which are essentially normal. Although a number of guidelines have been suggested, none is as helpful as the axiom "Feel the foot." The pathologically deformed foot cannot be positioned normally by manual manipulation; hence, it is rigid. Conversely, if the abnormally positioned foot can be reduced to a normal configuration with only modest manual pressure, the foot should be considered flexible and the result of excessive intrauterine molding. It is generally true that most flexible "deformities" are considered "non-disease" and as such require no specific treatment. On the other hand, rigid deformities usually present a definite therapeutic challenge. Foot deformities in children are common and a frequent cause for orthopedic referrals.

The Flatfoot

As the name implies, the longitudinal arch is low to nonexistent. Officially, the foot is pronated, and the heel is typically in valgus or everted. Flatfeet can be flexible or rigid, and the difference is critical. Besides feeling the foot, the other technique that is helpful in differentiating the two is simply to examine the child sitting, standing, and standing on the toes. The rigid flatfoot will remain flat in all three positions, whereas the flexible foot is only flat when standing. When seated (not weightbearing) and when toe-standing, the arch reconstitutes itself and the foot appears to normalize.

Congenital Hypermobile Flatfoot

This is no longer considered an abnormality and is not a cause for exclusion from military service as it once was. Rather, this genetic trait currently is viewed as a normal variant, and the mere finding of it is not an indication for treatment as in years past. Three pain syndromes do occasionally occur which generally respond to simple therapeutic measures:

1. Arch pain: The child with flatfoot will occasionally develop a strain pattern in the arch. This is easily treated with simple, inexpensive, commercially available supports.
2. Calf pain: Typically, this is caused by tight heel cords and can be treated simply with stretching exercises and arch supports.
3. Accessory navicular syndrome: A modest percentage of children will have a separate ossicle in the posterior tibial tendon adjacent to the tarsal navicular. The prominence of this bone may cause symptoms, which generally respond to padding or occasionally excision of the accessory navicular.

The Rigid Flatfoot

The pronated foot that does not correct on toe-standing should be studied for the presence of a tarsal coalition. These bony, cartilaginous, or fibrous bridges are genetically determined and usually can be diagnosed by appropriate X-rays and a computed tomography (CT) scan. Treatment is based on location and severity of symptoms.

Another cause of a rigid flatfoot when seen in a newborn is congenital vertical talus. This germ plasm defect results in abnormal positioning of the talus, with the navicular dorsally dislocated onto the talar neck. As a result, the foot is beyond flat – the arch actually is convex (rather than concave) and frequently referred to as a "rocker bottom deformity." This uncommon pathologic foot requires surgical correction.

Congenital Clubfoot

Similar to DDH, this deformity is multifactorial in origin. Environmental factors applied to a genetically predisposed individual result in this pathologic deformity. As with DDH, it is important to make it clear to the parents that this is NOT a postural deformity. Rather, there is an anatomic abnormality of the talus. Due to the abnormal medial and plantar deviation of the talar neck, there are a number of secondary deformities. The tarsal navicular is dislocated dorsally onto the talar neck; soft tissue contractures develop, and the resultant configuration is characteristic. The forefoot is adducted, the hindfoot is in varus (inverted), and the entire foot is in equinus.

A clubfoot, as is the case with most pathologic feet, is rigid on clinical exam (Fig. 5.44). X-rays can be used to confirm the diagnosis. Since clubfeet are frequently seen in association with other abnormalities, every effort should be made to evaluate the whole child. Syndromes often associated with the presence of clubfeet include myelodysplasia, arthrogryposis, and diastrophic dwarfism. The treatment of these deformed feet in these syndromic children is usually exceedingly difficult. It is probably fair to say that surgery will be required in virtually all cases.

In the case of the "standard" congenital clubfoot, occurring in an otherwise normal child, the recommended initial treatment is stretching and serial casting. The Ponseti method has regained significant popularity. Using this method of manipulation in conjunction with serial casting, many authors are reporting successful correction by closed treatment in 80% of cases. Should closed treatment fail or should recurrent deformity be observed, surgical correction is the usual next step. Most authors recommend surgical correction between 6 and 9 months of age if closed treatment has been unsuccessful. The overall success of various treatment protocols is largely dependent on the initial severity of the deformity. In addition, the need for late procedures to correct residual deformity will similarly be a function of initial severity as well as the success of initial correction techniques. In general, if correction is complete and achieved prior to the age of walking, an excellent prognosis can be anticipated. It is, however, important to point out to the family that congenital clubfoot involves not only the foot, but the soft tissues of the leg itself. Therefore, an overall decrease in the girth of the calf should be expected.

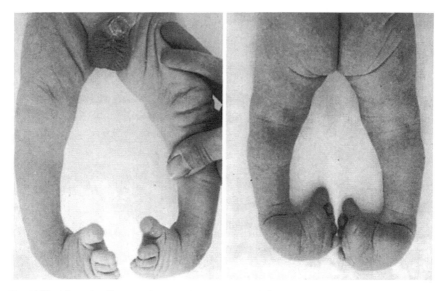

Fig. 5.44 Bilateral talipes equinovarus in a newborn infant. (From Tachdjian MO. Pediatric Orthopedics, 2nd ed, vol 1. Philadelphia: Saunders, 1990. Reprinted with permission)

Metatarsus Adductus

One of the more common problems seen in the child's foot is metatarsus adductus. Many cases are simply the result of excessive uterine cramming and, therefore, are best considered as "non-disease." The supple postural deformities are essentially normal variants and will correct without specific treatment. The clinical problem, however, is that some of these feet are, in fact, pathologic rather than postural and, therefore, do need appropriate care.

Typically, metatarsus adductus presents with forefoot adduction (Fig. 5.45) and supination. When viewed from the plantar surface, the foot with metatarsus adductus has a typical "kidney bean" appearance. Again, on examination it is critical to "feel the foot." By doing so, these feet can be grouped into three clinical types. First, type I (mild): foot is supple and easily corrects with digital stroking of the lateral side of the foot. Type II (moderate): gentle, manual pressure is required on the medial forefoot for correction. Type III (severe): moderate force is required for correction; even so, some cases may not be correctable.

The mild and moderate deformities frequently correct spontaneously and do not require aggressive treatment. Simple shoeing or occasionally serial casts are used in these children to gain initial improvement. A simple way to monitor this improvement is to stand the child on a copying machine at each follow-up visit and reproduce a copy of the plantar surface of the feet. The severe feet and some of the tighter moderate feet clearly deserve serial casting at the very least. Certainly in some cases, when serial casting fails, surgical intervention may be required.

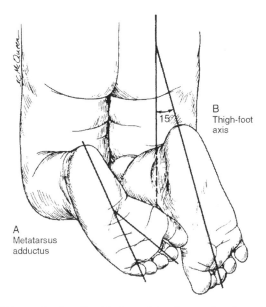

Fig. 5.45 The heel bisector line is utilized in determining the severity of metatarsus (**a**). Deviation of the forefoot causes this line to extend lateral to the second toe. The deviation of the forefoot causes the lateral border of the foot to be convex and the medial border to be concave. The thigh–foot axis (**b**) is used to determine tibial version. The normal thigh–foot axis is external 15°, as demonstrated. (From Sabiston DC Jr. *Essentials of Surgery*. Philadelphia, PA: Saunders; 1987. Reprinted with permission)

Fig. 5.46 Untreated metatarsus deformity in young boy. (From Gartland JJ. Fundamentals of Orthopaedics, 4th ed. Philadelphia: Saunders, 1987. Reprinted with permission)

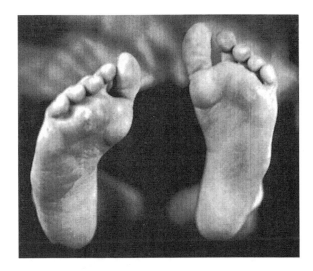

For the vast majority of cases, the prognosis is excellent. Even those children with mild persistent deformity have virtually no functional or cosmetic problems with their feet. Unfortunately, persistent severe metatarsus adductus (Fig. 5.46) can cause problems such as shoe fitting, pain, and cosmetic deformity. Late reconstruction of these feet usually requires osteotomies through the midfoot.

The Pediatric Upper Extremity and Neck

In general, the vast majority of upper extremity problems in children that require orthopedic evaluation are traumatic in origin. Fractures of the elbow and forearm are relatively common and represent some of the most challenging problems in orthopedics. Nontraumatic conditions of the upper extremity are far less common, and those worthy of note are primarily congenital in nature.

Sprengel's Deformity

Congenital elevation of the scapula (Fig. 5.47) is generally due to persistence of a fibrous cartilaginous or bony bar that persists between the spine and the superior medial border of the scapula, that is, an omovertebral bar. This structure prevents the scapula from migrating inferiorly from its embryonic position adjacent to the cervical spine to the normal adult position.

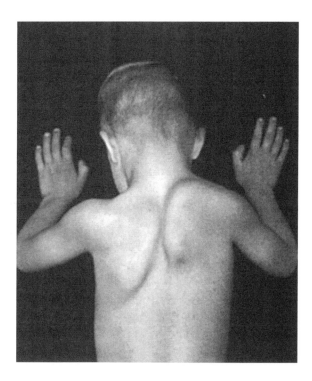

Fig. 5.47 Sprengel's deformity of the right shoulder. The scapula is elevated and hypoplastic, its horizontal diameter being greater than the vertical. (From Tachdjian MO. Pediatric Orthopedics, 2nd ed, vol 1. Philadelphia: Saunders, 1990. Reprinted with permission)

Sprengel's deformity usually presents as asymmetry of the neck or shoulder and physical examination is generally adequate for diagnosis. Since most children have no significant functional deficits, surgical treatment is usually not recommended. Cosmesis is an occasional complaint and can be managed by simple excision of the upper portion of the scapula. If a functional deficit does exist, several operative procedures have been developed to reduce the scapula to its normal position.

Congenital Muscular Torticollis

Although not truly an upper extremity problem, children with this condition present with a wry neck and asymmetry. Physical examination is usually adequate to make the diagnosis and differentiate it from some of the other causes of asymmetry in this region: Klippel–Feil anomaly, congenital scoliosis, and Sprengel's deformity (Fig. 5.48).

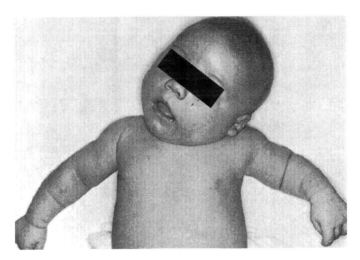

Fig. 5.48 Congenital muscular torticollis on the left. The head is tilted to the left and the chin rotated to the right. (From Tachdjian MO. Pediatric Orthopedics, 2nd ed, vol 1. Philadelphia: Saunders, 1990. Reprinted with permission)

Essentially, the problem is a contracture within the sternocleidomastoid muscle. The exact etiology of this contracture has been the subject of some controversy. Intrauterine hemorrhage within the muscle, local compartment syndrome, and fibrotic bands have all been proposed. Despite the etiology, the net result is a newborn presenting with a torticollis and facial asymmetry. Typically, the head is tilted TO the side of the lesion and the face and chin are turned AWAY from the side of the lesion.

The deformity usually responds to simple physical therapy, stretching by the parents, and positioning the crib to encourage the infant to look TO the side of the lesion, thereby stretching the tight sternocleidomastoid. Occasionally, nonsurgical treatment is not adequate, and operative release is required. This should be done before the child is 18 months to 2 years of age, most importantly, to level the eyes.

Worthy of note is the coincidence of this condition and developmental hip dysplasia. Since 20% of these children have abnormal hips, careful screening in this group is strongly recommended.

Radial Anomalies

The most common long-bone deficiencies in the upper extremity involve the radius (Fig. 5.49). Partial or complete absence of this bone, with or without adjacent hand deficiencies, can be seen as an isolated finding or in association with several syndromes. Franconi's and Vater syndromes should be considered when the radial dysplasia is bilateral. Further workup will usually reveal the renal defect or the thrombocytopenia.

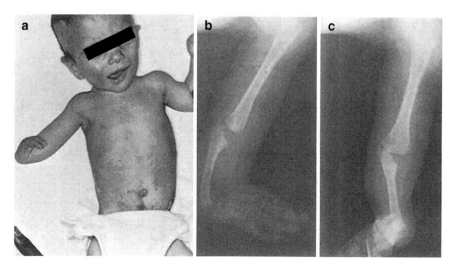

Fig. 5.49 Congenital absence of the radius in an infant. (**a**) Clinical appearance. (**b**) Preoperative radiograms. (From Tachdjian MO. Pediatric Orthopedics, 2nd ed, vol 1. Philadelphia: Saunders, 1990. Reprinted with permission)

The hand tends to deviate to the radial side and is referred to as "radial clubhand." Early treatment is nonoperative and based on stretching and bracing. Later surgical reconstruction of the extremity to improve wrist function is appropriate.

Congenital Trigger Thumb

Perhaps it is best not to use the term "congenital" since the defect is rarely noticed at birth or, for that matter, in the first 6 months. It is usually appreciated when the child begins using the hand for grasping. At this point, the flexed attitude of the interphalangeal joint is noticed by the parents. Initially, stretching will straighten the digit, but as the tendinous nodule of the flexor pollicis longus enlarges, it will no longer slide under the flexor pulley. The thumb is then "stuck" in flexion.

Some will respond to simple stretching, but most require surgical tenolysis after 6–9 months of age. The vast majority of those treated in this way have an excellent result and no recurrence.

Pediatric Trauma

The basic principles of injury to the immature skeleton have been discussed in part elsewhere. The unique features of pediatric fractures are primarily due to the biologic differences between child and adult. Specifically, the presence of an open growth plate, the periosteum, the ability of pediatric bone to plastically deform, and the ability to remodel this deformity are the bases for the fracture patterns typically seen.

The physis is clearly an internal "flaw" in the bone and thus a point of mechanical weakness. Many loading modes are capable of causing failure through the physis. These fractures were classified many years ago by Salter and Harris (Fig. 5.50). Their classification was based on the direction that the fracture line took through the physis and adjacent osseous structures. Purportedly, this classification correlates with prognosis – the higher the number of fracture type, the poorer the prognosis. Although true within certain limits, this is not always the case. For example, a Salter II fracture of the distal radius is a common, benign injury, whereas a Salter II fracture of the distal femur is complicated by a partial physeal arrest in more than 50% of cases. Fractures of the physis heal rapidly in 3–4 weeks, but parents should be warned about potential growth plate arrest. Physeal fractures that cross the plate and/or enter the joint require operative restoration of normal anatomy in an effort to minimize the risk of this complication.

The periosteum (Fig. 5.51), as previously noted, is thicker, more vascular, and more osteogenic than that of an adult. The mechanical benefits provided by the periosteum tend to minimize fracture displacement, act as an aid in reduction, and assist in maintenance of reduction. Biologically, the active osteogenic potential allows fractures to heal in half the time required for a similar bone in the adult.

The biologic plasticity of pediatric bone is responsible for the typical fracture patterns seen in the pediatric diaphysis. The incomplete fractures – greenstick and torus – represent the ability of these bones to bend, but not break all the way through. In general, this phenomena is not seen in the adult bone due to the progressive stiffening of cortical bone that occurs with aging. Occasionally, this feature presents a therapeutic dilemma. In the forearm, a plastically deformed ulna will act as a spring to redeform the already fractured radius. The solution is to complete the fracture of the ulna by osteoclasis. This will allow one to align the forearm acceptably and prevent redeformation.

Finally, the extensive remodeling ability of pediatric bone has corrected many seemingly unacceptable reductions without the need for multiple closed reductions.

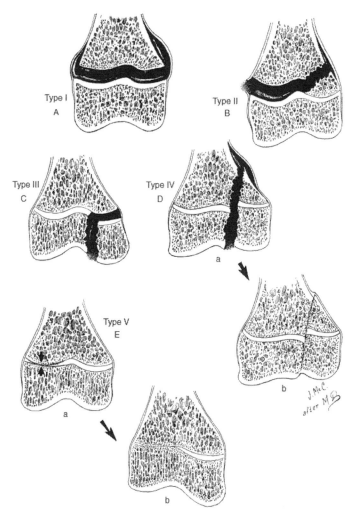

Fig. 5.50 Classification of epiphyseal plate injuries according to Salter and Harris. (Redrawn after Salter RB, Harris WR. Injuries involving the epiphyseal plate. *J Bone Joint Surg.* 1963; 45A:587. In: Tachdjian MO. Pediatric Orthopedics, 2nd ed, vol 1. Philadelphia: Saunders, 1990. Reprinted with permission)

There are limits to the amount of correction that can be anticipated (Fig. 5.52). One should not be overly secure, expecting "Mother Nature" to correct all malposition. In general, angular deformity will remodel to variable degrees. Greater correction can be expected if the deformity is in the plane of motion of the joint. Similarly, the closer the fracture to the joint, the more complete will be the correction. Translational deformity (i.e., displacement) at all levels tends to completely remodel. Rotational malalignment does NOT remodel; therefore, it is important to

Fig. 5.51 The basis of remodeling. (From Rang M. In: Rang M ed. *Children's Fractures*, 2nd ed. Philadelphia, PA: Lippincott; 1983. Reprinted with permission)

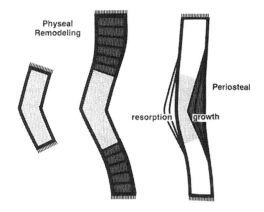

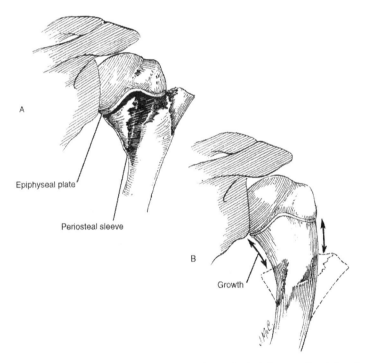

Fig. 5.52 Diagram showing remodeling process of a malunited fracture involving the proximal humeral physis. (From Tachdjian MO. Pediatric Orthopedics, 2nd ed, vol 1. Philadelphia: Saunders, 1990. Reprinted with permission)

correct all rotatory deformity. Complications of pediatric fractures are uncommon with adequate treatment; however, when they do occur, management is frequently problematic. The reason for this is the growth remaining in the skeleton. Any injury compromising the growth mechanics of a long bone will only compound itself over time as the deformity appears to worsen. Periarticular fractures and physeal fractures tend to present more problems in this regard than do those in the diaphysis.

The treatment principles, then, are directed toward fracture reduction and maintenance while avoiding complications – goals similar to those in the adult. Operative treatment of certain physeal injuries is common, and there is now current interest in operative treatment of more diaphyseal fractures, especially of the femur, in an effort to decrease length of hospital stay. Regardless of the reduction approach, the need for immobilization is undisputed. Children by definition are noncompliant; premature removal of immobilizing devices usually has disastrous results. One need *not* be concerned about joint stiffness or a cast-induced atrophy in children. It is far more important to continue the immobilization until the fracture is healed. Physical therapy following cast removal is rarely needed since the activity level of a normal child, unhampered by a cast, is more than adequate to mobilize the extremity. It is especially important NOT to subject the child with an elbow injury to a well-meaning, but overaggressive physical therapist. This will only aggravate the joint stiffness and retard resolution.

In summary, children's fractures mandate management goals similar to the adult: reduction, maintenance, and avoidance of complications. However, due to generally permissive biologic mechanisms, the tolerances in treatment are much greater. Successful results require adequate recognition of the unique qualities of the pediatric skeleton and the special problems that may follow trauma to it.

Battered Child Syndrome

No discussion of pediatric skeletal trauma would be complete without mention of this syndrome. The sociologic implications are extensive for the patient, the family, and the physician. Child abuse rarely occurs as an isolated event, and the result of returning the child to the home may be disastrous. It then becomes important to recognize the signs and symptoms of "nonaccidental" trauma. Failure to recognize or suspect this syndrome has often resulted in continued abuse.

As the name implies, this is a "syndrome," meaning the diagnosis is usually based on finding a constellation of manifestations. The diagnosis rarely can be made on the basis of an isolated fracture; rather, several fractures in multiple stages of healing will more reliably indicate abuse over time. The syndrome typically presents with findings in multiple areas, including the following:

1. *General neglect.* Beware the child who fails to make eye contact with parents or physician. The child who is dirty and uncared for and who exhibits evidence of psychological and nutritional neglect should raise one's suspicions.
2. *Skin and soft tissue injury.* "Imprinting" of the skin due to blows with specific objects, such as belt buckles, coat hangers, and ropes, should be searched out. Evidence of cigarette and radiator burns can commonly be found. Eye-ground hemorrhages and forehead hematomas indicate "shaken baby syndrome."

3. *Craniocerebral injury*. Subdural or epidural hematomas with or without nonparietal skull fractures are highly suggestive of abuse.
4. *Skeletal injury* (Fig. 5.53)

   a. Rib fractures. Multiple fractures especially in a line typically indicate a kicking injury.
   b. Metaphyseal-epiphyseal fractures. "Bucket-handle" and "teardrop" fractures of the metaphyseal region generally suggest shaking the child while holding the limb.
   c. Diaphyseal fractures. Spiral fractures of the distal humerus and fractures of the femoral shaft in a nonambulatory child are the most typical of abuse. Other long-bone injuries occurring as an isolated finding should not generate a referral to child protective services.

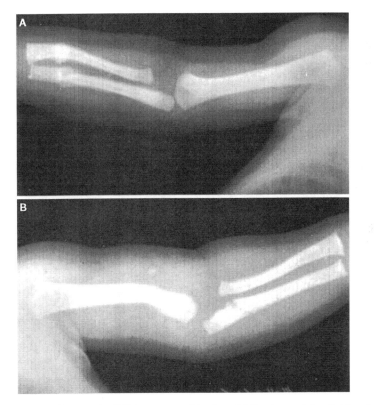

Fig. 5.53 Multiple fractures in different stages of healing. (**a**) Fractures of the distal end of the right radius and ulna with callus at the fracture site and smooth periosteal new bone formation along the shaft. (**b**) Fracture of the left humerus and proximal end of the ulna with minimal reaction. There is also a metaphyseal avulsion of the distal end of the radius. (From Akbarnia BA, Adbarnia NO. The role of (the) orthopedist in child abuse and neglect. *Orthop Clin North Am*. 1976;7(3):739. Reprinted with permission)

This tragic problem is becoming more commonly diagnosed in recent years, primarily due to heightened societal awareness of the problem. Physicians need to be vigilant and knowledgeable of the hallmarks of the syndrome; only then can they meet their legal reporting requirements, thereby saving a child from return to an abusive environment.

Evaluation of a Limp

The limping child is a relatively common problem, and yet one that is difficult to evaluate. Multiple etiologies, the child's difficulty in localizing pain, and a vague history make it essential that the physician has a systematic approach to this problem. Rather than order multiple unpleasant and expensive diagnostic studies, it is usually more valuable to carefully observe and examine the child, especially in a sequential fashion.

Generically, a limp is any uneven or laborious gait or, for that matter, any alteration in normal gait sequence. Normal gait classically occurs in two phases for each extremity: stance and swing. The stance phase is initiated at heel strike for a given limb and terminated with toe-off of that extremity. Stance accounts for 60% normally, leaving 40% of the cycle for swing when the foot is off the ground. Three classic aberrations of the gait cycle have been described in children:

1. Antalgic limp: Pain is the etiology of this gait aberration. Due to pain in the limb with ground contact, the stance phase is shortened and the patient unloads the extremity more quickly. Many etiologies will cause an antalgic limp, such as a fracture in the foot or toxic synovitis of the hip.
2. Trendelenburg limp (gluteus medius lurch): Frequently referred to as an abductor lurch, this pattern is due to the incompetence of the abductor lever arm to stabilize the pelvis (Fig. 5.54). If one remembers that a moment is created by a force acting over a distance, it can be appreciated that altering either factor will cause a Trendelenburg limp:
   a. Force alteration: Muscle weakness, as seen in polio
   b. Distance alteration: Shortened lever arm, as seen in DDH or malunited femoral neck fracture
3. Short leg limp: Leg-length discrepancy of significance will be manifested as an apparent limp with the pelvis dropping on the short side (Fig. 5.55).

A careful history should investigate a past traumatic event, systemic symptoms, and the effect on activity. Physical findings such as fever, focal findings of swelling, limitation of motion, and muscle spasm should be sought. Age itself may be a clue to the etiology since each group seems particularly prone to certain ailments.

Fig. 5.54 Gluteus medius
lurch. (From Tachdjian MO.
Pediatric Orthopedics, 2nd
ed, vol 1. Philadelphia:
Saunders, 1990. Reprinted
with permission)

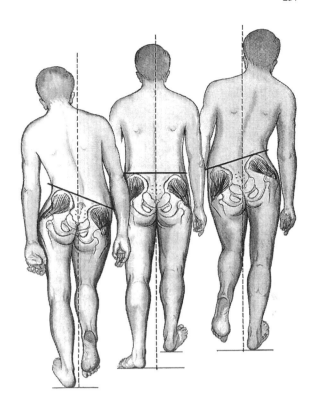

1- to 3-year-old: trauma, infection, DDH, new shoes
5- to 9-year-old: transient synovitis, Perthes' disease, JRA, Lyme disease
Over 12 years: SCFE

Extending the diagnostic workup, one should first consider standard X-rays,
especially of the hips. Routine hemogram is frequently beneficial. A three-phase
bone scan is a reasonable second-line study, especially if localization is necessary.
Unfortunately, it is not possible to specifically outline the studies to be routinely
obtained. Reaching the correct diagnosis is all too often the result of coinciding
historical data, physical findings, laboratory data, and a "gut" sense. Several diagnostic algorithms have been proposed that emphasize the basic factors in evaluating
pediatric limp:

Is there a history of trauma?
Are there systemic symptoms?
Are there focal findings?

By answering there questions, a workup can be fashioned that should ultimately
reveal the etiology.

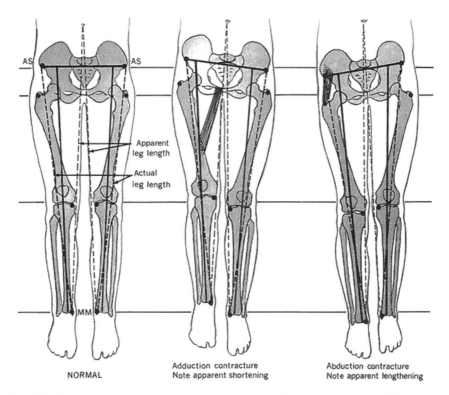

Fig. 5.55 Measurement of actual and apparent leg lengths. AS, anterior iliac spine; MM, medial malleolus. (From Tachdjian MO. Pediatric Orthopedics, 2nd ed, vol 1. Philadelphia: Saunders, 1990. Reprinted with permission)

Conclusions

Children are different. They are not small adults. Biologically and mechanically their musculoskeletal systems predispose them to patterns of injury and disease unique to their age group. By understanding these differences, one can antici-pate some of the patterns, thereby permitting appropriate treatment and minimizing complications.

The seven categories of disease – vascular, infections, tumor, arthritis, metabolic, injury, and neurodevelopmental – all produce changes in the skeleton that reflect the unique feature of childhood: *growth*. Simple insults can be made worse over time due to aberrational growth and conversely potentially disas-trous insults can be palliated by the innate remodeling potential of the pediatric skeleton.

Pediatric Spine: William C. Lauerman

Scoliosis

Scoliosis refers to abnormal curvature of the spine when viewed in the coronal plane. The human spine is normally straight when viewed from behind, but, because of the potential implications of unnecessarily labeling a child as "having" scoliosis, minor deviations from normal (less than 10°) may be considered within normal limits. Scoliosis has been discussed in the medical and orthopedic literature since antiquity and is widely believed by the lay population and medical professionals to be a debilitating or disabling condition, resistant to treatment, and with a grave prognosis. Advances in both operative and nonoperative treatment in the last 40 years, as well as a better understanding of the natural history of scoliosis, have removed much of the stigma from this condition.

A variety of conditions may cause or be associated with scoliosis (Table 5.2). The most common type of scoliosis is referred to as idiopathic, meaning that the cause of the disorder is unknown. Hereditary factors have been implicated, and research is ongoing as to other possible causes of idiopathic scoliosis. While it is likely that the development of idiopathic scoliosis is multifactorial, genetic, hormonal, biochemical, biomechanical, and neuromuscular abnormalities continue to be investigated. Idiopathic scoliosis can be broken down by age at diagnosis: curvature of the spine diagnosed up to age 3 years is defined as infantile idiopathic

Table 5.2 Etiology of scoliosis

Idiopathic
Congenital
Neuromuscular
    Polio
    Cerebral palsy
    Posttraumatic (spinal cord injury)
    Spinal muscular dystrophy
    Muscular dystrophy
    Friedrich's ataxia
    Charcot–Marie–Tooth disease
    Syringomyelia
    Myelomeningocele
    Arthrogryposis
Neurofibromatosis
Marfan's syndrome
Ehlers–Danlos syndrome
Juvenile rheumatoid arthritis
Spine or spinal cord tumor
Postlaminectomy
Thoracic cage defect/deficiency
Osteochondrodystrophy (dwarfism)
Osteogenesis imperfecta

scoliosis, a diagnosis between the ages of 4 and 10 is juvenile idiopathic scoliosis, and curves diagnosed after the age of 10, or the onset of adolescence, is referred to as adolescent idiopathic scoliosis. Most cases of idiopathic scoliosis are identified during the adolescent growth spurt and are therefore considered adolescent curves.

Numerous other conditions either cause or are associated with scoliosis and must be considered when evaluating an individual for scoliosis. Congenital abnormalities of the vertebrae, resulting in congenital scoliosis or congenital kyphosis, represent some of the more common etiologies of spinal deformity. Neuromuscular disorders such as polio, cerebral palsy, muscular dystrophy, spinal muscular atrophy, or myelomeningocele are frequently associated with spinal deformity. Other conditions, such as neurofibromatosis or Marfan's syndrome, may result in spinal deformity and scoliosis is also seen secondary to intraspinal anomalies such as syringomyelia (cystic degeneration of the central aspect of the spinal canal) or a tethered spinal cord. There is also a known association between scoliosis and certain congenital conditions, such as congenital heart disease.

Estimates of the prevalence of scoliosis depend on the threshold for definition. While 1.5–3% of the population are believed to have curves over 10°, only 0.2–0.3% of the normal population have curves over 30°, a magnitude where treatment is typically instituted. The natural history of idiopathic scoliosis has been well established. Most curves are identified in early adolescence. Progression is variable and is more likely in younger patients, in skeletally immature patients (in particular, premenarchal girls), and in larger curves. Finally, while mild curves are as common in boys as in girls, progressive curves and curves requiring treatment are far more common in girls.

The implication of scoliosis in adulthood entails consideration of curve progression, pain, disability, and mortality. It has been established that an idiopathic curve of greater than 50°, in particular a right thoracic curve (which is the most common type of idiopathic curve), is at significant risk for progression even in adulthood. While curve progression is a possibility, the presence of scoliosis does not necessarily place the patient at risk for back pain. Some patients with scoliosis appear to have pain related to the curve, but it has been demonstrated that patients with idiopathic scoliosis are not at any increased risk, when compared to the general population, for the development of disabling low back symptoms. Similarly, pulmonary dysfunction and significant functional disability are relatively rare occurrences.

The mortality rate of individuals with idiopathic scoliosis does not differ significantly, with the possible exception of severe (greater than 100°) curves present since childhood, from that of the general population. Finally, scoliosis does not have an adverse impact on a woman's ability to bear children, nor is the curve more likely to progress during pregnancy than at other times.

Management

The management of a child with documented or suspected scoliosis begins with a thorough evaluation. Most cases are picked up during school screening or by the patient's primary care physician. The Adam's forward bend test is the key to checking a child for possible scoliosis. Asymmetry of the spine and trunk is identified by asking the child to bend forward at the waist with the knees straight and the hands hanging toward the floor (Fig. 5.56). The observer is seated behind the patient. Asymmetry of the ribs from right to left is considered a positive test and merits further evaluation by an orthopedist. Other possible signs of scoliosis include pelvic or shoulder asymmetry or asymmetry of the waist creases. Evaluation for scoliosis, including the Adam's forward bend test, should be a routine part of a pediatrician's well-child physical examination and is very sensitive for picking up most cases of scoliosis.

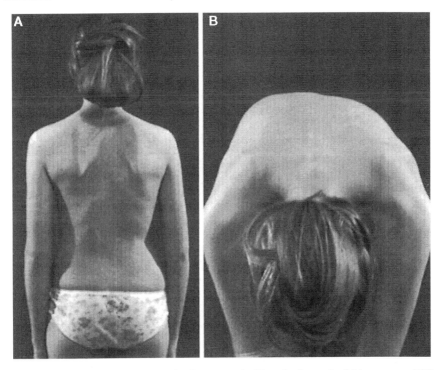

Fig. 5.56 Careful examination by a school nurse resulted in early diagnosis of this curvature (10°). Note the spine asymmetry in the flexed position (**b**)

In evaluating the patient with possible scoliosis, important historical points include a family history of spinal deformity, any abnormality or delay in reaching developmental milestones, and associated neurologic symptoms involving the lower extremities or urogenital system, including gait abnormalities, paresthesias, and recent onset of enuresis. Physical examination includes the above evaluation as well as a thorough inspection of the skin, looking for café au lait spots, palpation of the spine, looking for an occult spina bifida, and examination of the lower extremities, looking for calf or foot atrophy or asymmetry. Neurologic examination should also be carried out, including assessment of deep tendon reflexes, superficial skin reflexes, and testing for Babinski's sign. Any sign or symptom suggestive of central nervous system abnormality merits a more detailed workup, possibly including imaging of the brain stem, spinal cord, or cauda equina.

Radiographic evaluation is carried out on any patient suspected of having significant scoliosis. A standing posteroanterior view (PA) of the full spine, including the pelvis, will demonstrate the presence or absence of significant deformity. The pelvis is inspected for evidence of skeletal maturity, manifested by closure of the iliac apophysis. In some cases, obtaining a wrist film for bone age may be helpful. Because there is a known association between scoliosis and spondylolisthesis (see below), a lateral X-ray of the spine should be obtained, including visualization down to the sacrum.

Treatment options available for the growing child with scoliosis include observation, bracing, and surgery. Previous attempts at curve control utilizing physical therapy, chiropractic, exercises, or electrical stimulation have proven ineffectual and are not to be recommended. Observation, with repeat radiographs every 4–6 months, is appropriate in the child with scoliosis less than 25–30°. Curves that have been documented to progress beyond 25° or curves measuring beyond 30° at first presentation, in a child with significant growth remaining, are commonly treated with a brace.

For many years the standard orthosis for the treatment of scoliosis was the Milwaukee brace, which had documented effectiveness in controlling curves measuring between 25 and 40°. Patient resistance to the use of the Milwaukee brace, including the neck and chin ring, has resulted in the now widespread use of underarm orthoses such as the Boston or Wilmington brace. These braces have proven equally effective at controlling most thoracic and thoracolumbar idiopathic curves, avoiding the need for surgery in approximately 80% of cases, and have become the current standard for the management of curves of moderate magnitude in skeletally immature patients. Unfortunately, successful bracing means preventing any further progression of the scoliosis but does not usually result in permanent improvement in the curve. Further, there is good evidence that bracing is not effective in boys, for reasons that are not entirely clear, and is now usually reserved for girls with appropriate curves.

When a curve exceeds 40 or 45° it becomes increasingly difficult to control with an external orthosis. Because of this, as well as the increasing risk of progression into adulthood with curves greater than 50°, surgery is generally recommended for curves that progress into the range of 40–50°. The commonly accepted indications for surgical treatment of scoliosis include adolescents with curves documented to have progressed beyond 40–45°, adolescents with curves at presentation exceeding 45–50°, and on occasion, adults with either documented curve progression, disabling pain, or both. The goals of the surgical treatment of scoliosis include the arrest of progression, achievement of a solidly fused, balanced spine, and improvement in the curve with associated improvement in cosmetic appearance. While upward of 50% curve correction can routinely be obtained in the adolescent, the more important goals of surgery are achieving a solid fusion, well balanced over the sacrum, and extending from the top to the bottom of the curve.

The surgical treatment of scoliosis constitutes, first and foremost, a spinal fusion. The most common approach to this fusion is posterior, although certain curves are amenable to anterior fusion. Since the introduction of the Harrington rod in the

1950s, instrumentation of the spine at the time of fusion has become well accepted. Improved rates of correction and fusion, as well as a diminished need for postoperative immobilization, have more than offset the risks incurred. Spinal instrumentation has evolved over the last quarter of a century and newer implants, utilizing multiple points of fixation along the spine, are more easily contoured to help the surgeon restore physiologic alignment in three planes. Postoperative immobilization is rarely needed when these newer implants are utilized (Fig. 5.57).

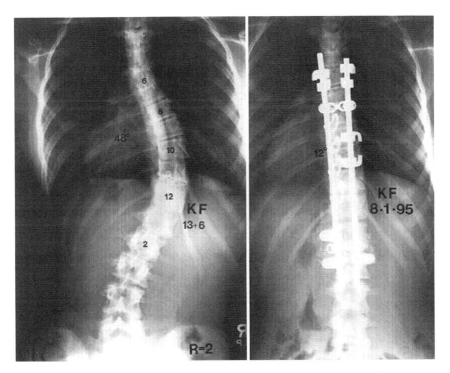

Fig. 5.57 A 13-year-old girl with progressive idiopathic scoliosis measuring 48°. Following surgery, a posterior spinal fusion with segmental instrumentation and iliac crest bone graft, her curve corrected to 12°. She went on to a solid fusion with no loss of correction

In the adolescent with idiopathic scoliosis, curve correction using modern techniques averages 50–70%. About 95–98% of patients go on to solid fusion with less than 10% loss of correction. Infection and thromboembolic disease are occasional complications of spinal instrumentation and fusion, although they are seen more commonly in adults than in adolescents. The most feared complication of surgery for scoliosis, paraplegia, is rare in the absence of a known risk factor such as kyphosis, congenital scoliosis, or a preoperative neurologic deficit, but it is a recognized occurrence. Neurophysiologic monitoring of intra-operative spinal cord function is now commonplace and appears to decrease the risk of irreversible neurologic catastrophe.

Congenital Scoliosis

Individuals with congenital abnormality of the spine represent an unusual, but well-defined subset of patients with spinal deformity. Failure of formation (hemivertebrae), failure of segmentation (bars), and mixed deformities are seen. The prognosis varies depending upon the type of anomaly present, but the patient with congenital scoliosis, in particular with a failure of segmentation, is certainly at higher risk for progression than the patient with an idiopathic curve. There is a known association between congenital spine deformity and congenital anomalies of the urogenital system and all patients with congenital scoliosis or kyphosis should be referred for imaging of the genitourinary (GU) system. Congenital heart disease is also more common in this population, although a normal history and physical examination of the heart is considered sufficient to rule out a significant cardiac abnormality.

In addition to the increased risk of progression, which approaches 100% in curves involving a unilateral unsegmented bar, congenital curves have proven to be resistant to bracing. While progressive congenital scoliosis in a growing child is still routinely treated with an orthosis, the orthopedic surgeon, the pediatrician, and the patient and family need to be aware that there is a high risk for further progression necessitating surgical intervention. Congenital deformities can, on occasion, result in quite severe curves in very young children, but postponing surgery in this setting only results in a more difficult reconstructive problem at a later date.

Neuromuscular Deformity

Neuromuscular or paralytic causes of scoliosis include polio, cerebral palsy, muscular dystrophy, posttraumatic paraplegia, and myelomeningocele. At one time polio was the most common cause of scoliosis in this country, and it continues to be so in much of the Third World. Neuromuscular curves have a characteristic long, C-shaped appearance. Extension of the curve into the pelvis, with pelvic obliquity on sitting or standing, is common and complicates both surgical and nonsurgical treatment. The risk of scoliosis varies among these conditions, but may be as high as 60–70%. All neuromuscular curves have a propensity, once progression ensues, for rapid collapse of the spine into a severe curve. Because of the respiratory difficulty associated with many of these conditions, it is imperative to screen patients carefully for scoliosis, to monitor them closely for progression, and to institute early and aggressive treatment when indicated.

Brace treatment with a well-molded, total contact thoracolumbosacral orthosis (TLSO) is instituted for curves measuring beyond 30° in the growing patient. Progression despite adequate bracing, resulting in progressive loss of function, is believed in most cases to be an indication for surgery in this patient population. In these patients, surgical treatment is fraught with a high rate of complications, including instrumentation failure secondary to osteoporosis, increased rates of infection, and postoperative respiratory failure.

Kyphosis

Kyphosis refers to forward curvature, or rounding, of the spine when viewed from the side. Kyphosis is normal in the mid and upper thoracic spine, with a normal range of thoracic kyphosis from 20 to 45° in children and adolescents. Excessive kyphosis, as measured on a standard lateral radiograph exceeding 45–50°, has several possible etiologies.

The child or adolescent presenting with hyperkyphosis of the thoracic spine is frequently accompanied by a parent giving a long history of "poor posture." While postural kyphosis is not uncommon, other causes of the deformity should be considered. The most prominent among these is juvenile kyphosis, known as "Scheuermann's disease." Although the etiology of Scheuermann's disease remains unknown, several theories have been proposed, including avascular necrosis of the cartilaginous ring apophysis of the vertebral body, the presence of Schmorl's node (herniation of intravertebral disc material through the endplate), endocrine or nutritional abnormalities, and metabolic bone disease. Congenital kyphosis is a rare condition that must be ruled out, due to the possibility of severe progression and subsequent neurologic abnormality. As in congenital scoliosis, congenital kyphosis can result from failure of formation or failure of segmentation. In contrast to congenital scoliosis, however, congenital kyphosis secondary to failure of formation (congenital hemivertebrae) is the more malignant type, with an exceedingly high rate of progression. Congenital kyphosis in association with a hemivertebrae has the highest rate of neurologic impairment of any of the spinal deformities. Tuberculosis should also be considered in the child or adolescent with excessive kyphosis, particularly if there is a history of travel outside the United States or a positive family history.

Scheuermann's kyphosis is the most common form of nonpostural kyphosis. The criteria for diagnosis in the thoracic spine include excessive thoracic kyphosis with associated radiographic abnormalities including vertebral wedging of greater than 5° at three consecutive vertebrae, endplate irregularity, and the presence of Schmorl's nodes (Fig. 5.58). The reported prevalence of this disorder varies among authors, but is approximately 1%. The female to male ratio varies from 1.4:1 to 2:1. Although the postural abnormality may be identified earlier, radiographic changes are usually not seen until 11–12 years of age.

Most cases of thoracic hyperkyphosis represent primarily cosmetic abnormalities. Mild postural kyphosis will frequently resolve spontaneously, or following a thoracic extension exercise program. The natural history of Scheuermann's disease

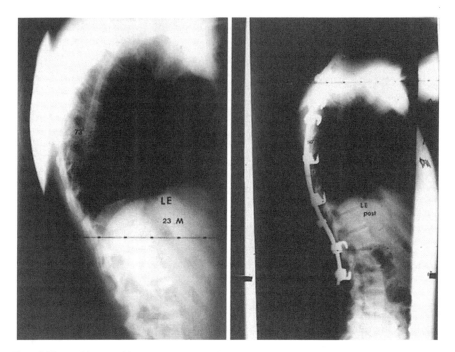

Fig. 5.58 A 23-year-old young man with persistent thoracic back pain secondary to Scheuermann's kyphosis. Because of failure to improve after a 1-year course of exercises and NSAIDs, he underwent a posterior fusion with segmental instrumentation and bone grafting, which resulted in excellent pain relief

has only recently been elucidated. Most patients with Scheuermann's kyphosis lead normal lives, with no functional limitations and an incidence of disabling back pain that is not increased over the normal population. There is some evidence, however, that adults with kyphosis in excess of 65–70° may have an increased incidence of thoracic back pain and mild to moderate functional limitations. Neurologic complications secondary to Scheuermann's disease are rare, but have been reported. There is no evidence that cardiopulmonary dysfunction is a complication of this condition.

Management of the patient with hyperkyphosis begins with a thorough physical examination. The increase in normal thoracic kyphosis is best appreciated when viewed from the side and frequently coexists with increased lumbar lordosis. Differentiation between Scheuermann's disease and postural kyphosis is facilitated by viewing the patient, in the forward flexed position, from the side. Patients with postural kyphosis have a smooth, round curve which reverses on voluntary extension. The typical deformity in Scheuermann's kyphosis involves a sharp, angular gibbus that does not correct on extension of the spine. A minimal scoliosis of the spine may also be noticed on forward bending and is a common finding in patients with juvenile kyphosis. A thorough neurologic examination is mandatory to rule out spastic paraparesis, which would suggest other possible diagnoses including congenital kyphosis, intraspinal anomaly, or thoracic disc herniation. Standing PA and lateral radiographs of the entire spine are obtained. Kyphosis is measured using the Cobb technique and the lateral X-ray is scrutinized for findings of Scheuermann's disease, as described above. A mild scoliosis is frequently seen radiographically. In addition, it is important to check for the presence of lumbosacral spondylolisthesis, which has been reported to be increased in prevalence in patients with Scheuermann's disease.

Patients with hyperkyphosis can be treated with observation, bracing, or surgery. Observation, frequently accompanied by a program of thoracic extension exercises, is utilized in patients with postural kyphosis or without evidence of clear-cut progression in cases of Scheuermann's disease. Bracing is indicated for patients with structural kyphosis who have clear-cut evidence of progression of the curve and have at least 18 months of growth remaining. Because underarm orthoses are ineffective in this condition, Milwaukee brace treatment, or an orthosis applying pads at the clavicles, is required in most cases. Unlike scoliosis, Scheuermann's kyphosis responds in many cases with long-lasting curve improvement, typically about 10°, following successful brace treatment. It should be noted, however, that patients with larger curves, in excess of 70–75°, frequently lose correction following cessation of bracing.

Because of the usually benign natural history of Scheuermann's kyphosis, surgery is rarely indicated. Bracing should be attempted in most patients with adequate growth remaining, since long-lasting curve improvement may result. Surgery is usually reserved for individuals who do not respond to brace treatment, who have curve progression in the brace, or who have severe curves, usually in excess of 80–90°, which are not likely to respond to bracing and represent a potentially significant functional and cosmetic deformity. Surgery is also undertaken, on occasion, in adults with intractable thoracic back pain that does not respond to a nonoperative program of exercise and nonsteroidal anti-inflammatory medication. These individuals usually have curves in excess of 65–70°.

Surgery for the patient with Scheuermann's kyphosis consists of a spinal fusion with instrumentation. The fusion extends from just above to just below the area of kyphosis, typically over 10–12 levels. Flexible curves, which can be reversed to 55° or less on hyperextension, may be treated with a posterior spinal fusion with compression instrumentation. More severe or more rigid curves are treated with anterior discectomies and release of the hypertrophied anterior longitudinal ligament, followed by posterior fusion with instrumentation. Surgery typically results in excellent curve correction ranging from 30 to 50% in most series of combined anterior and posterior surgery, which usually reduces the kyphosis into the normal range. Cosmetic improvement is significant, but when the surgery is undertaken for pain relief the results are uncertain. Complications of surgery include infection, implant failure, and neurologic injury. Junctional kyphosis, the development of kyphosis above or below the end of the fusion, may be seen as well. It should be stressed that the surgical treatment of Scheuermann's kyphosis is rarely employed and the surgeon, the patient, and the patient's parents need to view the natural history of this disorder in the context of the magnitude of the surgery required, and the risks entailed.

Spondylolisthesis

"Spondylolisthesis" refers to the forward slippage of one vertebrae on that below it. First described by Herbiniaux, a Belgian obstetrician, this condition has been extensively studied and reported. Spondylolisthesis is most common in the lower lumbar spine, particularly at L5–S1, and is a common cause of back pain in children and adolescents (Fig. 5.59).

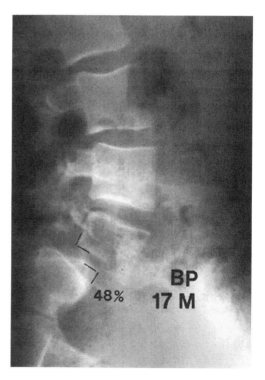

Fig. 5.59 A 17-year-old boy with a 48% (grade II) isthmic L5–S1 spondylolisthesis

Spondylolisthesis has been classified by Newman (Table 5.3). The most common types are Type II, isthmic, and Type III, degenerative. Degenerative spondylolisthesis occurs in middle-age and older adults as a result of degenerative changes in the discs and facet joints allowing subluxation. It most commonly occurs at L4–L5 and is often associated with spinal stenosis. The most common type of spondylolisthesis is Type II or isthmic spondylolisthesis. This is caused by a defect in the pars interarticularis at L5, resulting in slippage at L5–S1. The pars defect, referred to as spondylolysis, is believed to be a stress or fatigue fracture and occurs in most

Table 5.3 Classification of spondylolisthesis

Type I	Dysplastic – congenital dysplasia of the S1 superior articular facet, or L5 inferior facet
Type II	Isthmic – a defect in the pars interarticularis a. Stressor fatigue fracture b. Elongated but intact pars c. Acute traumatic pars fracture
Type III	Degenerative – degenerative changes in the disc and facet joints allowing subluxation
Type IV	Traumatic – acute fracture, other than in the pars (e.g., facet, pedicle), allowing anterolisthesis
Type V	Pathologic – attenuation of the posterior elements, with subluxation, secondary to abnormal bone quality (e.g., osteogenesis imperfecta, neurofibromatosis)
Type VI	Postsurgical – anterolisthesis that occurs or worsens following compressive laminectomy

affected individuals when they are between the ages of 4 and 7. Spondylolysis is present in 5–6% of the normal adult population; 75–80% of these individuals also demonstrate spondylolisthesis. Spondylolisthesis is twice as common in males as in female and is more common in whites than in blacks. It is also seen more commonly in athletes who participate in sports demanding frequent hyperextension, such as gymnasts or football lineman.

In children and adolescents, spondylolysis or spondylolisthesis may present as back pain, frequently associated with hamstring spasm. Other less common causes of back pain in the pediatric population include disc space infection, benign tumors such as osteoid osteoma, or lumbar disc herniation. Isthmic spondylolisthesis can also be, and more commonly is, a cause of back pain in the adult. Patients with isthmic spondylolisthesis are reported to have an increased prevalence of disc degeneration, back pain, and sciatica, with the onset of symptoms occurring anywhere during adulthood. Because back pain is such a ubiquitous complaint, the relationship between a patient's complaint of back or leg pain and the presence of spondylolisthesis is often difficult to determine.

Evaluation of the patient with spondylolisthesis begins with a thorough history and physical. In the adult, a history of back pain during adolescence may be helpful. While acute pars fractures are occasionally seen, there is usually no distinct history of trauma given. The patient typically presents with low back pain, which radiates into the buttock and, on occasion, down the leg in a dermatomal distribution. Physical examination may demonstrate tenderness in the area of the L5–S1 facet joint. Often a characteristic, painful "catch" in extension is elicited. The most telltale sign in the adolescent is hamstring spasm, which can be quite severe. In patients with a high-grade slip, flattening of the buttocks and a transverse abdominal crease may be seen. Neurologic findings are rare, although in more advanced cases L5 findings may be seen.

Plain radiographs should be obtained in the standing position. Most pars defects are visible on the lateral radiograph. If the diagnosis is uncertain, oblique views

Fig. 5.60 A pars defect (spondylolysis) at L4, seen on this oblique radiograph as a "collar" on the neck of the "Scotty dog"

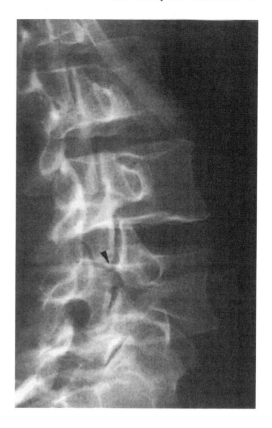

increase the sensitivity of plain radiography. The posterior arch has been described as a "Scotty dog" on the oblique view, and a pars defect appears as a "collar" on the neck of the Scotty dog (Fig. 5.60). Radionuclide bone scanning [single photon emission computed tomography (SPECT) scan] or fine-cut CT scanning may be used to diagnose occult defects in the pars interarticularis and MRI imaging is useful to identify nerve root compression in the L5–S1 foramen in patients with significant leg pain.

The treatment of patients with spondylolysis or spondylolisthesis depends on the degree of slippage as well as the patient's symptoms. The percent slip ranges from 0 to 100% and has been broken down as grades I (0–25%), II (25–50%), III (50–75%), and IV (75–100%). It is not uncommon for pediatric patients to be diagnosed with spondylolisthesis following an episode of minor trauma and then to become asymptomatic. In the skeletally immature patient who is asymptomatic, activity guidelines are based on the degree of slippage. In patients with a grade I slip, full activity is allowed with annual radiographic follow-up. Skeletally immature individuals with grade II spondylolisthesis are advised to avoid contact sports or repetitive hyperextension activities such as are seen in gymnastics. Operative treatment is usually recommended for skeletally immature patients with progressive slippage or with grades III or IV spondylolisthesis.

Symptomatic patients are initially treated with activity modification and nonsteroidal anti-inflammatory medication. Since many of these patients are athletes, temporarily holding them out of their sport will frequently result in improvement in symptoms. The patient is then begun on a program of Williams' flexion exercises and gradually increased activity. Persistent symptoms sometimes respond to bracing, and treatment with a brace or cast is advocated by some when an acute pars fracture is suspected. The majority of patients, both pediatric and adult, respond quite well to nonoperative treatment, although a return to high-level competitive sports is sometimes impossible.

Operative treatment is recommended for patients with progressive spondylolisthesis, for skeletally immature patients with spondylolisthesis exceeding 50%, and for patients with persistent, incapacitating pain. The overwhelming majority of surgical patients fall into the latter category. The hallmark of the surgical treatment of spondylolisthesis is spinal fusion. Inter-transverse fusion between the transverse processes of L5 in the sacral alae, utilizing iliac crest bone graft, has a high rate of success with a low complication rate. In adult patients with significant buttock and leg pain, or in individuals with neurologic deficits secondary to root compression, removal of the loose posterior arch of L5 and decompression of the exiting L5 nerve root are recommended. Fusion is routinely performed in addition to decompression in these cases. Many authors recommend pedicle screw instrumentation as an adjunct to spinal fusion; instrumentation is routine in adults, in patients with spondylolisthesis greater than 25%, and in individuals with documented instability. Finally, operative reduction of the spondylolisthesis is advocated by some in cases of severe spondylolisthesis, usually exceeding 60–70% slippage, with a concomitant cosmetic deformity. The results of surgery are usually quite rewarding, particularly in the pediatric population. Complications of surgery include failure of fusion, progressive slippage, persistent or recurrent pain, and neurologic injury. Complication rates are higher in adults, in higher grades of spondylolisthesis, and when reduction is attempted.

Suggested Reading

1. MacEwen GD. *Pediatric Fractures.* Malvern, PA: Williams & Wilkins; 1993.
2. Staheli L. *Fundamentals of Pediatric Orthopaedics.* New York, NY: Raven; 1992.
3. Wenger D, Rang M. *Art and Practice of Children's Orthopaedics.* New York, NY: Raven; 1993.

Chapter 6
Sports Medicine

John J. Klimkiewicz

Introduction

The emphasis presently placed on physical fitness in society in terms of overall health is at an all-time high. Participation in both organized as well as recreational sports has escalated over the past several decades as a result. This increase in participation has led to an emphasis on treating injuries associated with sporting activities. The advances within medicine regarding the diagnosis of these injuries, such as magnetic resonance imaging (MRI), as well as arthroscopy for their treatment, have improved results only to focus more attention within this field. A number of skilled physicians and other health professionals have developed interests regarding the specific care of athletes. The goal of sports medicine as a subspecialty is the prevention of injury, diagnosis and treatment of athletic injury, and returning athletes to pre-injury activity with no acute or long-term sequelae. The purpose of this chapter will be to focus on the biologic tissues involved in sporting injuries, highlighting the patterns in which they are injured. An overview will then follow regarding the evaluation and treatment principles as they relate to the management of athletes and sport-specific injuries.

Patterns of Injuries

Injuries within the field of sports medicine can be generally classified into one of two categories: *microtrauma* and *macrotrauma*. Microtraumatic injuries are those that typically are associated with overuse injury by the athlete such as many of the tendinopathies or stress fractures that are common in long-distance runners. Microtraumatic injuries are the result of repetitive stresses leading to structural

J.J. Klimkiewicz (✉)
Division of Sports Medicine, Department of Orthopedic Surgery, Georgetown University Medical Center, 3800 Reservoir Road NW, Pasquerilla Healthcare Center (PHC), Ground Floor, Washington, DC 20007, USA
e-mail: jjk4@gunet.georgetown.edu; kajklim@mac.com

S.W. Wiesel, J.N. Delahay (eds.), *Essentials of Orthopedic Surgery*,
DOI 10.1007/978-1-4419-1389-0_6, © Springer Science+Business Media, LLC 2010

breakdown of the tissue in question. Macrotrauma, on the other hand, involves a single traumatic episode resulting in injury to a specific region. A downhill skier fracturing the tibia and a soccer player cutting and injuring the anterior cruciate ligament are two examples of macrotraumatic injury. In these instances, the force imparted to a specific tissue is greater than that the tissue is able to withstand, resulting in catastrophic mechanical failure of the tissue in question.

Musculoskeletal Tissues

Tendons

Tendons are strong, inextensible tissue that attaches muscle to the bone. They are composed of closely packed, well-aligned collagen bundles within a matrix of pro-teoglycan. Fibroblasts are the predominant cell type and are arranged in parallel orientation between the bundles of collagen fibers. The tendon fibroblasts act to produce both collagen and proteoglycan within the tendon unit. Collagen is a major constituent of tendon. Type I collagen comprises 86% of a healthy tendon's dry weight, while type III is found in lesser amounts. It is the high concentration of collagen in combination with its parallel orientation that gives tendons their high tensile strength. Collagen chains are linked together to form fibrils that, in turn, are bound together by a proteoglycan matrix to form a fascicle, the primary unit in tendon structure. Fascicles, in turn, are bound by the endotenon, a layer of elastin-containing loose connective tissue that supports the blood, lymphatic, and neural supply to the tendon unit. It is the endotenon that is contiguous with both the muscle fibers and periosteum at the musculotendinous and tendo-osseous junctions, respectively.

Acute tendon injuries may be direct, occurring as a result of laceration or contusion, or indirect, occurring secondary to tensile overload. Both are examples of macrotrauma. Tensile overload is a common injury within the field of sports medicine (i.e., patellar tendon, achilles tendon ruptures). In majority of these cases, because most tendons can withstand tensile forces greater than can be exerted by their muscular or bony attachments, avulsion fractures and muscle–tendon junction ruptures are far more common than midsubstance ruptures of tendon.

Chronic tendon overload represents the classic microtraumatic injury in sports medicine. These injuries occur at the sites of high exposure to repetitive tensile overload. Examples are given in Table 6.1. Whether or not inflammation has a role in the early stages of these overuse injuries is unclear. However, in cases that are not responsive to short periods of rest with persistence of symptoms, similar findings can be seen histologically, reflecting a more degenerative process. Disruption of collagen fibrils, hyaline degeneration, proliferation of vasculature are classic in these entities and termed angioplastic fibroplasia, and result in tendonosis or breakdown of the corresponding tendinous unit. At this stage it is clear that this is not an inflammatory process, as no acute or chronic inflammatory infiltrates are demonstrable on

Table 6.1 Common sites of sports-related tendon overload

Site of injury	Sport
Achilles tendon	Running
Iliotibial band	
Flexor hallicus longus tendon	Dancing
Patellar tendon	Basketball, volleyball
Quadriceps tendon	
Supraspinatus tendon	Swimming, softball, baseball
Extensor carpi radialis brevis tendon	Golf, racquet sports
Flexor pronator origin	
Abductor pollicus longus tendon	Rowing
Extensor pollicus brevis tendon	

these histologic specimens. Tendonosis is also observed in cases of spontaneous rupture and may be clinically silent until rupture occurs. An example is an achilles tendon rupture seen in middle-aged athletes participating in strenuous sports.

Ligaments

Ligaments are short bands of connective tissue that serve to connect two osseous structures. Like tendons, these are very organized hierarchical structures with high tensile strengths. Ligaments are likewise composed of bundles of type I collagen fibers, which make up approximately 70% of its dry weight. Small amounts of elastin are combined with fibroblasts in a complex extracellular matrix. This collagen matrix comprises a series of fibers forming a subfascicular unit. Multiple subfascicular units are then bound together to form a fasciculus. These fasciculi can in turn be oriented in a simple longitudinal fashion such as the medial collateral ligament of the knee or can spiral to form a more helical structure such as the anterior and posterior cruciate ligaments of the knee.

At their attachments to bone, the transition from ligament to bone occurs gradually in a series of distinct phases. These phases range from ligament to fibrocartilage, from fibrocartilage to mineralized fibrocartilage, and from mineralized fibrocartilage to bone. The size of each zone varies from ligament to ligament and is related to its structural properties. Collagen fibers, known as Sharpey's fibers, run in continuity throughout this zone of transition and have an important role in securing the ligament to bone. While somewhat similar to tendons in their microscopic organization and composition, ligaments and tendons are structurally and biochemically different. Ligaments contain a lower percentage of collagen and a higher percentage of extracellular matrix. There is also a more random alignment of collagen fibers than their tendinous counterparts.

Unlike injuries to tendons that can be both acute and chronic processes, ligamentous injuries occur as a result of acute trauma and represent a macrotraumatic process. When a stress is applied to a ligament, a sprain occurs, whose severity

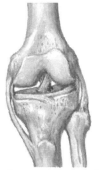 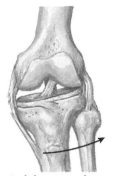 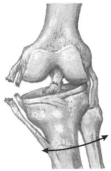

1st-degree sprain. Localized joint pain and tenderness but no joint laxity

2nd-degree sprain. Detectable joint laxity plus localized pain and tenderness

3rd-degree sprain. Complete disruption of ligaments and gross joint instability

Fig. 6.1 Classification of ligamentous injuries (sprains). (Netter images reprinted with permission from Elsevier. All rights reserved)

(grades I–III) depends on the amount of stress applied (Fig. 6.1). A grade I sprain represents the least traumatic episode when some ligamentous fibers are torn on a microscopic level. Structural integrity of the ligament, however, is maintained. An example of this is a common ankle sprain where traditionally the anterior talofibular ligament is injured. In a grade II sprain, some fibers are macroscopically torn in combination with microscopic damage resulting in a stretching of the ligament. While the biomechanical properties of the ligament are compromised in this scenario, some structural integrity of the ligament remains. An example of this injury is an injury to the medial collateral ligament to the knee. On application of a valgus force, the knee demonstrates increased laxity as compared to the other side, but an endpoint is present at the ligament, signifying some integrity to this structure remains. In a grade III sprain, the ligament structure fails, with no structural integrity of the ligament remaining. After rupture of the anterior cruciate ligament, there is both an increase in anterior translation when an anterior force is applied to the tibia and a non-existent endpoint. This represents a complete failure.

Intra- and extra-articular ligaments differ in their response to acute trauma. This is influenced by a difference in the local vascular supply of these entities, as well as the degree of the injury, and whether or not a significant gap forms between the two ends of ligamentous rupture. Typically extra-articular ligaments have a high potential for healing and gradually heal with predominantly type I collagen within a 6- to 12-week time frame. Maturation of this ligament scar can take up to 1 year in cases, despite histologic evidence of healing as early as 6 weeks. Contrastingly, intra-articular ligaments such as the anterior cruciate ligament have a poor healing potential. In cases of complete disruption of this structure, dissociation of the midsubstance "mop ends" results in significant gap formation with the inhibition of the healing process. These differences result in different treatment approaches to these injuries as extra-articular ligamentous injuries are frequently treated conservatively, while intra-articular injuries are typically treated surgically secondary to a poor healing response.

Muscle

Injuries of skeletal muscle and the musculotendinous junction commonly lead to prolonged clinical disability. Muscle strains alone account for up to 50% of injuries in particular sports.

Active force generation within the muscle depends on its contractile apparatus. The contractile apparatus is composed of actin and myosin myofilaments that are arranged into functional units called sarcomeres. Muscle contraction consists of an energy-dependent process of cross-bridge unlinking and advancement of the myofilaments within the sarcomere. Either aerobic or anaerobic processes provide cellular energy for this process. Muscle fibers may be characterized by their capacity for aerobic respiration. Oxidative (red) fibers are characterized by sustained slow contractions, while glycolytic (white) fibers contract rapidly under anaerobic conditions. Fiber-type composition varies significantly between muscular groups and among different individuals. The force of muscle contraction is directly related to its cross-sectional area, which is reflective of its number of parallel contractile elements.

Muscular injury can result from direct mechanical deformations that occur in muscular strains, contusions, and lacerations or from indirect mechanisms such as vasculature or neurologic injury as seen in cases of acute and chronic (exercise-induced) compartment syndromes.

Muscular strains involve either partial or complete disruption of the muscle–tendon unit. This represents a macrotraumatic process. Clinical and experimental observations suggest that most muscular strain injuries involve the muscle–tendon junction. Common examples involve hamstring and adductor strains surrounding the hip. This usually occurs with passive stretch or with lengthening during muscular contraction (eccentric contraction). Complete injuries are often associated with muscle retraction, hematoma formation, and local inflammation, while lesser degree strains involve more microscopic failure. Functional recovery is dependent on the coordinated specific repair of the contractile elements with their surrounding connective tissues and neurovascular structures. This process can take up to 6 months in some cases. While after injury individual muscular fibers may contract normally after repair and regeneration, whole muscle contractile function rarely is normal after gross skeletal muscular injury.

Less common are muscular contusions that are a result of direct trauma. In these cases such as quadriceps contusion, skeletal muscle damage results from non-penetrating, sudden, high-energy force directed to the muscular group in question. These forces can result in the temporary or permanent loss of vascular and neurologic function secondary to direct trauma imparted to the musculature. These injuries are often characterized by a large associated hematoma. Ultimate recovery is often related to the magnitude of original injury. A relatively infrequent complication of this is myositis ossificans. In this case, normal mesenchymal cells involved in the healing process differentiate into osteoblasts, resulting in the formation of bone. This abnormal bone often results in a prominence in the injured area with subsequent symptoms.

Articular Cartilage

Often associated with trauma surrounding a particular joint are injuries and more long-term degeneration of the articular cartilage. When diffuse and occurring over a period time, this process can result in osteoarthritis (microtrauma); however, there is an additional subset of these injuries that are more focal and result from a direct injury, often referred to as osteochondral injuries (macrotrauma). Although highly desirable, functional restoration of injury to articular cartilage remains one of the most challenging of orthopedic problems within the sports medicine field.

Articular cartilage composition and thickness varies from joint to joint and is directly age dependent. The tissue typically is composed of 75–80% water and dense extracellular matrix consisting of 50–75% of type II collagen and 15–30% of proteoglycan macromolecules. Water and proteoglycans make up its extracellular matrix. A remarkable characteristic of articular cartilage is its acellularity as chondrocytes occupy less than 10% of this tissue. These cells maintain the extracellular matrix and aid in cellular homeostasis. The collagen provides tensile strength to articular cartilage while the proteoglycans and extracellular matrix provide its more important compressive role.

Structurally, articular cartilage is highly organized into four zones of depth from the articular surface to the underlying subchondral bone (Fig. 6.2). Zone 1, also called the *superficial layer*, makes up approximately 10% of cartilage, determines its load-bearing ability, and serves as a gliding surface. Within this layer chondrocytes arranged with collagen fibers are parallel to the joint surface to provide high tensile strength and stiffness. Zone 2 is a *transitional layer* and is composed of chondrocytes and randomly oriented collagen fibers. It has a higher concentration of proteoglycan and lower concentration of collagen as compared to zone 1. Zone 3, or *deep layer*, is composed of collagen fibers and clusters of chondrocytes oriented perpendicular to the underlying subchondral plate, providing compressive strength. Zone 4, the *calcified layer*, acts to join the deep zone of uncalcified cartilage to the subchondral bone. There are few cells within this layer. It contains the tidemark adjacent to the subchondral bone.

| Zones | Collagen Orientation | Chondrocyte Appearance |

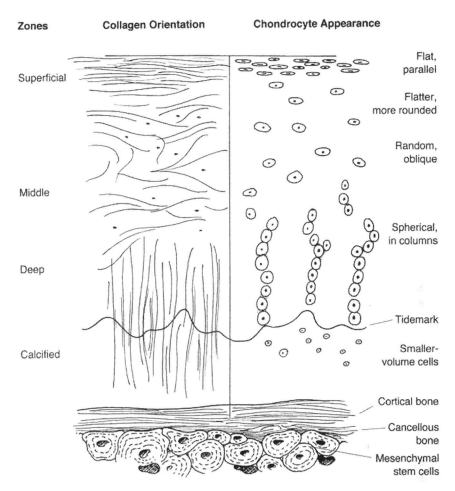

Fig. 6.2 Morphology of articular cartilage. (From Browne JE, Branch TP. Surgical alternatives for treatment of articular cartilage lesions. *J Am Acad Orthopaed Surg*, 2000;8(3):180–189. Copyright 2000 American Academy of Orthopaedic Surgeons. Reprinted with permission)

Articular cartilage is an avascular as well as aneural tissue. As an avascular tissue, it exchanges gases, nutrients, and waste products through a process of diffusion through tissue fluid or synovium. This poor blood supply results in poor reparative capability in the event of acute injury or chronic wear.

Injuries to articular cartilage are best described by the Outerbridge classification system (Fig. 6.3). This system characterizes the injury to articular cartilage based on its qualitative appearance at the time of surgery: grade I, softening with swelling; grade II, fragmentation and fissuring; grade III, fragmentation and fissuring down to subchondral bone; grade IV, exposed subchondral bone. Grade I/II lesions are thought to involve superficial injury and are best left untreated while grade

Fig. 6.3 Outerbridge
classification. (From Browne
JE, Branch TP. Surgical
alternatives for treatment of
articular cartilage lesions.
J Am Acad Orthopaed Surg.
2000;8:180–189. Reprinted
with permission)

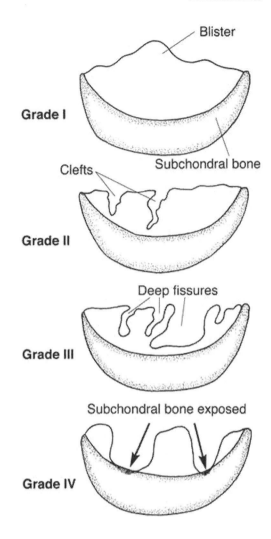

III/IV lesions represent full thickness cartilaginous injuries and are best treated surgically.

Meniscus

The meniscus of the knee is formed of a combination of fibrocartilage with some proteoglycan present. The collagen fibers are type I and are arranged in a predominantly circumferential orientation. It is this orientation that gives this tissue its unique loading characteristics and function within the knee. This highly structured network provides the ability of the meniscus to allow the compressive forces of joint loading to be dissipated circumferentially along these parallel collagen fibers, termed "hoop stresses." The meniscus biomechanically transmits a compressive force to one that is tensile in nature and absorbed within the meniscus. Injury to the meniscus results in a decreased ability to perform its function, resulting in higher compressive forces being transmitted across the knee joint.

Like articular cartilage, the vascularity of the meniscus is poor. Only the peripheral one-third of the meniscus receives a blood supply and therefore the potential for healing after injury is limited. Location and type of meniscal tearing in a symptomatic knee determine one's ability for potential healing. Meniscal injuries are best categorized by the location of the tear as well as the morphology of the tear. The location can be best described in reference to the blood supply of the meniscus. *Red–red* tears involve the peripheral one-third of the meniscus and have excellent healing potential. *Red–white* tears involve a zone of the meniscus with good blood supply on the peripheral aspect of the tear and poor blood supply on the more central portion and have intermediate healing potential. *White–white* tears involve those tears completely in the avascular zone with poor healing potential. Morphologic classification of meniscal tears is demonstrated in Fig. 6.4.

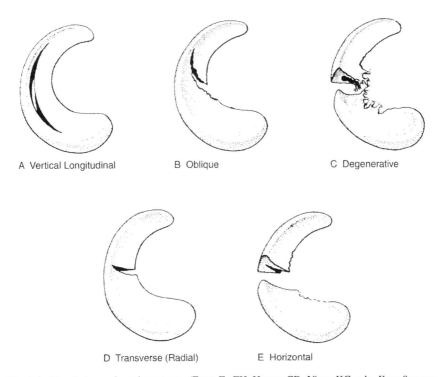

A Vertical Longitudinal   B Oblique   C Degenerative

D Transverse (Radial)   E Horizontal

Fig. 6.4 Morphology of meniscus tears. (From Fu FH, Harner CD, Vince KG, eds. *Knee Surgery*, vol. 1. Philadelphia, PA: Williams & Wilkins; 1994. Reprinted with permission)

Evaluation of Common Sports Medicine Injuries

The principles involved in the initial evaluation of the injured athlete focus on history and physical examination in combination with auxiliary tests and are similar in comparison to other orthopedic injuries. This subspecialty differs from that of a general orthopedic setting in two distinct manners. One large difference in the management of the athlete is the ability to provide prompt, "on-the-field" attention as a result of game time coverage by the sports medicine physician. This allows one to often visualize the injury directly and distinguish as to whether the mechanism was a direct result of blunt trauma as compared to a more indirect mechanism (i.e., cutting injury). Additionally, it provides one with a golden window of time to evaluate the injury before the effects of swelling and subsequent pain and spasm complicate the physical exam. It often allows the opportunity to make the diagnosis without the need for auxiliary tests that are often required when evaluating these injuries on a more subacute basis. Furthermore, the sports medicine physician is often asked about the safety of returning to play in light of a specific injury. Knowledge of the common injuries, as well as the sporting activities themselves, is important in making these decisions. The following sections will focus on the history as well as physical exam in the sports medicine setting. Specifics regarding the injuries are elaborated on in their respective chapters.

History

The history in many sporting injuries is straightforward and related to acute trauma. Examples include twisting the ankle when coming down for a rebound, feeling the shoulder "pop out" when being tackled, or hearing a "pop" within one's knee on cutting cross-field. Important in this history is the mechanism of injury, as this often relates very closely with the structure injured. When this is more ambiguous upon questioning the athlete, input from other players, trainers, and coaches, as well as game time film can be invaluable in determining the mechanism of injury. Other injuries within this field are a result of microtrauma, or overuse, and have no specific mechanism of injury. Examples can include plantar fasciitis of the foot or shin splints. For these insidious conditions, it is important to obtain the specifics of recent activity, including changes in recent activity (number of miles run per week), shoe wear or other equipment, or the surface involved (track to road, flat surface to hills, etc.). Other pertinent details include whether or not this problem has occurred before, and if so, how it happened, what type of treatment was rendered, and what was the outcome. Previous problems may alert the clinician to a different treatment problem to prevent recurrence of the injury. Examples include the management of "first time" as opposed to recurrent shoulder dislocations.

Symptoms that occur with activity and improve with rest are typical of overuse injuries. Nocturnal awakening usually indicates more serious injury or an underlying systemic disorder. Such a distinction is important in distinguishing shin splints from a stress fracture in a long-distance runner. Are there any specific activities that might cause symptoms? In the athlete with intermittent knee symptoms, pain in the anterior aspect of the knee that is worse with stair climbing or with prolonged sitting suggests problems related to the patellofemoral joint. Symptoms that occur predictably with cutting and pivoting activities, accompanied by swelling and instability, suggest an internal derangement of the knee such as a meniscus injury or tear of the anterior cruciate ligament.

Physical Examination

The specific examination depends on the nature of the symptoms and the region affected. Each anatomic region and orthopedic condition has pertinent special tests. All physical examinations, however, should begin with inspection and observation of the extremity. After acute injury, one should compare the injured joint in question to its opposite side. Inspection for skin changes such as ecchymoses, abrasions, and associated swelling can be important clues in distinguishing macrotrauma from a microtraumatic event. Determining range of motion of the joint in question, both actively and passively, is imperative. First, have the athlete move the joint in question and observe for associated pain or asymmetry as compared to the opposite side. Examples include a patient who presents with shoulder pain of insidious onset whose active and passive range of motion is asymmetric and limited on the affected side, suggesting an adhesive capsulitis as a diagnosis. This is compared to a rotator cuff injury where passive range of motion would be full despite a limited active range of motion secondary to pain. Other examples would be the active inability to extend one's knee after an acute injury, despite nearly full passive range of motion. This suggests an injury (rupture) of the extensor mechanism that can be seen in patellar tendon or quadriceps tendon ruptures.

Strength assessment is an important component to the exam of any joint-related injury. During strength assessment, weakness may be due to direct injury to a musculotendinous unit responsible for joint function. However, pain, guarding, or reflex inhibition of muscular contraction can also be responsible for perceived weakness on examination. The ability of the sports medicine professional to examine the athlete in the acute setting shortly after the injury (before pain and swelling set in) is especially helpful in obtaining an accurate assessment of strength. Although relatively uncommon, injuries to nerve and vasculature structures can and do occur and should be ruled out as a precipitating cause of injury especially in the acute setting. Their examination is an essential component of a complete physical exam.

On initial examination, one should always keep an open mind for referred symptoms. In addition to examining the joint in question, one should also focus particularly on the adjacent joints, as well as the spine, for a contributing role in the symptoms. Examples include a slipped capital femoral epiphysis (SCFE) of the hip in an adolescent with knee pain or a cervical disc herniation as a cause for shoulder discomfort.

Applying special examination techniques specific to the area in question and suspected diagnosis completes the physical examination. These techniques can be found in their respective chapters according to the area in question. Examples of special tests include impingement signs in case of shoulder pain or apprehension in the case of shoulder instability as the arm is placed in a position of abduction and external rotation (Fig. 6.5).

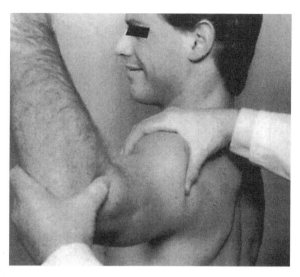

Fig. 6.5 Examining for anterior instability, the apprehension test is performed by placing the shoulder in a provocative position of abduction and external rotation. Gentle anterior pressure is placed on the humeral head in this position, seeking to elicit patient apprehension as an indication of shoulder instability. (From Hawkins RJ, Bokor DJ. Clinical evaluation of shoulder problems. In: Rockwood CA, Matsen FA eds. *The Shoulder*, vol. 1. Philadelphia, PA: Saunders; 1990:149–177. Reprinted with permission)

Special Tests

X-Rays

Radiographs are mandatory in any athlete with a history of trauma where macrotraumatic injury is in question. As a rule, microtraumatic injuries do not usually demonstrate radiographic findings when a soft tissue component is suspected as a cause for pain. One exception, however, is when an osseous component is thought to be a cause for pain in the absence of trauma (i.e., stress fracture). In this setting X-rays are helpful as an initial screening tool. When negative, other special tests such as MRI or bone scintigraphy can be especially helpful.

Specifically obtained stress views can be useful in assessing joint integrity. Common examples include stress views taken for grade III sprains of the acromioclavicular joint (Fig. 6.6).

Fig. 6.6 (**a**) Technique of stress radiography in accentuating the deformity in acromioclavicular (AC) joint injuries. (**b**) Using 10–15 lb weights, the distance between the superior aspect of the coracoid and the undersurface of the clavicle is measured and compared to the opposite side to determine the competency of the coracoclavicular ligaments. (From Rockwood CA, Green DP, eds. *Fractures*, 2nd ed, vol. 3. Philadelphia, PA: Lippincott; 1984. Reprinted with permission)

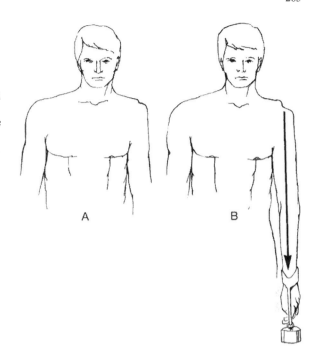

A   B

Magnetic Resonance Imaging

Revolutionizing the ability to visualize soft tissues and establish diagnoses noninvasively, MRI is an exceptional diagnostic tool. In addition to demonstrating precise anatomic detail, MRI provides a precise physiologic window with which to see various inflammatory, metabolic, and traumatic conditions. It is helpful in diagnosing both microtraumatic and macrotraumatic injuries. Variation in software techniques allows precise imaging of osseous structures, tendons, ligaments, menisci, and articular cartilage. The addition of intra-articular contrast has been especially helpful in the shoulder and hip in the diagnosis of injuries to the labral structures. MRI has emerged as the most common imaging modality within the field of sports medicine. Its use, however, should be utilized judiciously secondary to cost as well as age-related changes found in asymptomatic individuals. Its use also should not overshadow a thorough history and physical exam.

Bone Scintigraphy

Bone scans generate images based on dynamic physiology rather than static structure. Increased tracer uptake can occur due to a number of conditions and is pathognomonic for any one particular injury. Interpretation should be carried out in the context of history, physical examination, and routine X-rays. For example, in

Fig. 6.7 Bone scan of the
tibia in a runner with leg pain
reveals focal uptake at the
junction of the mid- and distal
third tibia, consistent with a
stress fracture. (From DeLee
JC, Drez Jr D, eds.
*Orthopaedic Sports
Medicine: Principles and
Practice*, vol. 2. Philadelphia,
PA: Saunders; 1994.
Reprinted with permission)

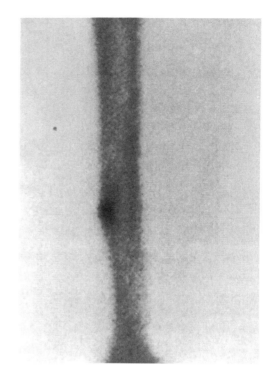

a runner with progressively increasing leg pain in which a bone scan displays focal
uptake in the mid-tibia, a stress fracture is likely (Fig. 6.7).

Arthroscopy

Most commonly applied to the knee, shoulder, ankle, elbow, and hip, arthroscopy is
the gold-standard tool for definitive diagnosis and treatment of joint-related injuries.
Its utility in diagnosis is especially helpful in situations where all other diagnostic
testing has not been successful in establishing a diagnosis. Its overwhelming use in
the field of sports medicine, however, is predicated on the treatment of joint injuries
once a diagnosis is reached. For more complex problems, arthroscopy often serves
as an invaluable diagnostic tool.

Treatment of Sports Injuries

Treatment of macrotraumatic and microtraumatic injuries follows an algorithmic
approach. The goals of treatment are to reduce pain, inflammation, swelling, and

stiffness initially, followed by an increase in strength and function to allow expeditious return to normal function and athletic activity. Treatment can be divided into three distinct but overlapping phases: immediate, early, and definitive.

Macrotraumatic Injuries

Immediate

Immediate treatment begins at the time of injury and involves the pneumonic "RICE" (rest, ice, compression, and elevation). Immobilization of the joint in the early stages after an injury, in combination with RICE, acts to limit the initial swelling. By accomplishing this purpose, local soft tissue edema and pain are minimized. This often allows the treating physician an accurate physical exam, leading to a good working diagnosis and the need for definitive tests can also be determined.

Early

Early treatment involves establishing a definitive diagnosis and minimizing the sequelae of trauma, including joint stiffness and muscle atrophy. Often additional testing is required at this stage to help formulate both the diagnosis and the definitive treatment plan.

Late

Most macrotraumatic sports injuries are successfully treated non-operatively, with physical rehabilitation necessary to provide normal strength and motion. Specific indications for operative management vary with the injury in question, its outcomes with different treatment options, as well as the athlete's goals and expectations both on and off the athletic field. Surgical intervention may involve traditional open techniques or, more commonly, an arthroscopic approach in order to limit the morbidity imposed by a surgical approach.

Microtraumic Injuries

Immediate

Rest, in the treatment of overuse injury, does not necessarily require crutches, cast, or sling, but it does mean activity modification. Any activity that causes the athlete's symptoms should be avoided. The tissues involved must be allowed to rest in order to heal and resolve the inflammatory process causing the symptoms. Often for the athlete, this involves restriction from his/her sport.

Early

During the period of activity modification, a number of techniques can be helpful to further relieve pain and inflammation in order to restore normal function. This can begin with the use of non-steroidal anti-inflammatory drugs (NSAIDs). Various modalities such as ice, heat, electrical stimulation, ultrasound, and massage can all be of some help in decreasing pain and associated swelling.

Late

Although activity modification is the mainstay of treatment, a prolonged period of inactivity can result in muscular atrophy as well as overall de-conditioning. Definitive treatment for these injuries often involves a dedicated physical therapy program aimed at restoring the athlete's strength and endurance required for a return to sport. Focus on the athlete's biomechanics is also an essential component in treating overuse injuries to prevent their recurrence. Attention to the specifics of the supporting structures is often helpful in this regard. Alignment problems are often identified in this phase of treatment for lower extremity injuries. Fabrication of a shoe lift orthotic for a previously unrecognized leg length discrepancy or a medial longitudinal arch support for over-pronation can lead to a more successful return to activity. Sometimes videotape analysis of the activity or technique is helpful to identify, correct, and prevent poor biomechanics.

Occasionally, overuse injuries do not respond to non-operative measures and surgical correction is required. Conditions that are occasionally associated with failure of conservative treatment include lateral epicondylitis, shoulder impingement, and patellar/achilles tendonitis. Failure of conservative treatment in these cases involves long courses (often 6 months to 1 year) of conservative management. Rarely, stress fractures are in high-risk areas (i.e., hip) or fail to respond to adequate immobilization and require surgical intervention.

Summary and Conclusion

As the numbers of active individuals continue to grow, so does the field of sports medicine. Emphasis at present within this field focuses on the prevention of injuries as well as minimizing the effects of surgery through less invasive approaches such as arthroscopy. As knowledge within this field continues to grow, accomplishing the goal of a successful return to sport both safely and expeditiously becomes a feasible reality. Appreciation of the basic science as it relates to these injuries and the means in which they are treated is essential in bridging the gap between the practice of clinical medicine and the successful return to the athletic field.

Suggested Reading

1. DeLee JC, Drez D Jr, Miller MD, eds. *Orthopaedic Sports Medicine: Principles and Practice.* 2nd ed. Philadelphia, PA: WB Saunders Company; 2001.
2. Garrick JG, Webb DR. *Sports Injuries: Diagnosis and Management.* Philadelphia, PA: WB Saunders Company; 1990.
3. Griffin LY, ed. *Orthopaedic Knowledge Update: Sports Medicine.* Rosemont, IL: American Academy Orthopaedic Surgeons; 1994.
4. McGinty JB, ed. *Operative Arthroscopy.* 2nd ed. Philadelphia, PA: Lippincott-Raven; 1996.

Chapter 7
The Spine

William C. Lauerman, Steven C. Scherping, Jr., and Sam W. Wiesel

The majority of adults, at some point in their lives, are affected by disorders of the spine. Every physician should have a basic knowledge of the potential pathology and be able to distinguish a serious problem from a minor condition. Disastrous sequelae such as paralysis can occur if this differentiation is not appreciated. This chapter will first address the cervical spine and then present the lumbar spine. In each area, the history, physical, and appropriate diagnostic studies will be reviewed. Next, a standardized protocol or algorithm for the diagnosis and management of these patients will be described. Finally, several of the most common conservative treatment modalities will be presented with special attention given to their efficacy.

Cervical Spine

Disorders of the neck are ubiquitous. Significant problems can arise from various types of arthritis as well as trauma. In each instance, recovery or improvement is the usual outcome, but poor results can occur with paraplegia and/or death as the most disastrous. Every physician should be familiar with the signs and symptoms of the various diagnostic entities that occur in the cervical spine and be able to identify the serious problems that require immediate attention.

History

The location of the pain is the major point to obtain from a patient's history. The majority of patients complain of localized symptoms in the neck, with and without referral of pain between the scapulae or shoulders. The pain is described as vague, diffuse, axial, nondermatomal, and poorly localized. The pathogenesis of this type

W.C. Lauerman (✉)
Division of Spine Surgery, Department of Orthopedic Surgery, Georgetown University Medical Center, Washington, DC 20007, USA
e-mail: lauermaw@gunet.georgetown.edu

S.W. Wiesel, J.N. Delahay (eds.), *Essentials of Orthopedic Surgery*,
DOI 10.1007/978-1-4419-1389-0_7, © Springer Science+Business Media, LLC 2010

of complaint is attributed to structures innervated by the sinuvertebral nerve or the nerves innervating the paravertebral soft tissues and is generally a localized injury.

Another group of patients will complain of neck pain with the addition of arm involvement. This arm pain is secondary to nerve root irritation and is termed radicular pain. The degree of nerve root involvement can vary from a monoradiculopathy to multiple levels of involvement. It is described as a deep aching, burning, or shooting arm pain, often with associated paresthesias. The pathogenesis of radicular pain can derive from soft tissue (herniated disc), bone (spondylosis), or a combination of the two.

Finally, a third group of patients will complain of symptoms secondary to cervical myelopathy, which is compression of the spinal cord and usually secondary to degenerative changes. The clinical complaints vary considerably. The onset of symptoms usually begins after 50 years of age, and males are more often affected. Onset is usually insidious, although there is occasionally a history of trauma. The natural history is that of initial neurologic deterioration followed by a plateau period lasting several months. The resulting clinical picture is often one of an incomplete spinal lesion with a patchy distribution of deficits. Disability varies with the number of vertebrae involved and with the degree of changes at each level.

Common presenting symptoms of cervical myelopathy include numbness and paresthesias in the hands, clumsiness of the fingers, weakness (greatest in the lower extremities), and gait disturbances. Abnormalities of micturition are seen in about one-third of cases and indicate more severe cord involvement. Symptoms of radiculopathy can coexist with myelopathy and confuse the clinical picture. Sensory disturbances may show a patchy distribution. Spinothalamic tract (pain and temperature) deficits may be seen in the upper extremities, the thorax, or the lumbar region and may be in a stocking or glove distribution. Posterior column deficits (vibration and proprioception) are more commonly seen in the feet than in the hands. Usually there is no gross sensory impairment, but a diminished sense of appreciation of light touch and pinprick. A characteristic broad-based, shuffling gait may be seen, signaling the onset of functionally significant deterioration.

Physical Examination

The physical examination should begin with observation of the cervical spine and upper torso unencumbered by clothing. The physical findings are of two different types. One set can be categorized as nonspecific and found in most patients with neck pain, but will not help to localize the type or level of the pathological process. A decreased range of motion is the most frequent nonspecific finding. It can be secondary to pain or, structurally, to distorted bony or soft tissue elements in the cervical spine. Hyperextension and excessive lateral rotation, however, will usually cause pain—even in a normal individual.

Tenderness is another nonspecific finding that can be quite helpful. There are two types of tenderness that must be considered. One is diffuse, elicited by compression of the paravertebral muscles, and is found over a wide area of the posterolateral muscle masses. The second type of tenderness is more specific and may help localize the level of the pathology. It can be localized by palpation over each intervertebral foramen and spinous process.

The next goal of the physical exam is to isolate the level or levels in the cervical spine responsible for the symptomatology. The exam is also important to rule out other sources of pain, which include compression neuropathies, thoracic outlet syndrome, and chest or shoulder pathology.

The major focus of the exam is directed at finding a neurologic deficit (Table 7.1). A motor deficit (most commonly weak triceps, biceps, or deltoid)

Table 7.1 Cervical radiculopathy symptoms and findings

Disk level	Nerve root	Symptoms and findings
C2–C3	C3	*Pain*: Back of neck, mastoid process, pinna of ear *Sensory change*: Back of neck, mastoid process, pinna of ear *Motor deficit*: None readily detectable except by EMG *Reflex change*: None
C3–C4	C4	*Pain*: Back of neck, levator scapula, anterior chest *Sensory change*: Back of neck, levator scapula, anterior chest *Motor deficit*: None readily detectable except by EMG *Reflex change*: None
C4–C5	C5	*Pain*: Neck, tip of shoulder, anterior arm *Sensory change*: Deltoid area *Motor deficit*: Deltoid, biceps *Reflex change*: Biceps
C5–C6	C6	*Pain*: Neck, shoulder, medial border of scapula, lateral arm, dorsal forearm *Sensory change*: Thumb and index finger *Motor deficit*: Biceps *Reflex change*: Biceps
C6–C7	C7	*Pain*: Neck, shoulder, medial border of scapula, lateral arm, dorsal forearm *Sensory change*: Index and middle fingers *Motor deficit*: Triceps *Reflex change*: Triceps
C7–T1	C8	*Pain*: Neck, medial border of scapula, medial aspect of arm and forearm *Sensory change*: Ring and little fingers *Motor deficit*: Intrinsic muscles of hand *Reflex change*: None

Source: From Boden S, Wiesel SW, Laws E, et al. *The Aging Spine*. Philadelphia, PA: Saunders; 1991:46. Reprinted with permission

or diminished deep tendon reflex is most likely an objective finding in a patient with a radiculopathy. Although less reproducible, manual tests and maneuvers that increase or decrease radicular symptoms may be helpful. In the neck compression test, the patient's head is flexed laterally, slightly rotated toward the symptomatic side, and then compressed to elicit reproduction or aggravation of the radicular symptoms. The axial manual traction test is performed in the presence of radicular symptoms in the supine position. With 20–25 lbs of axial traction, a positive test is the decrease or disappearance of radicular symptoms. All of these tests are highly specific (low false-positive rate) for the diagnosis of root compression, but the sensitivity (false-negative rate) is less than 50%.

Myelopathic physical findings should also be specifically checked. These patients can have a gait disturbance, so they should be observed walking. The extent of motor disability can vary from mild to severe. Pyramidal tract weakness and atrophy are more commonly seen in the lower extremities and are the most common abnormal signs. The usual clinical findings in the lower extremities are spasticity and weakness.

Weakness and wasting of the upper extremities and hands may also be due to combined spondylotic myelopathy and radiculopathy. In this situation, the patient usually complains of hand clumsiness. A diminished or absent upper-extremity deep tendon reflex can indicate compressive radiculopathy superimposed on spondylotic myelopathy.

Sensory deficits in spinothalamic (pain and temperature) and posterior column (vibration and proprioception) function should be documented. Usually there is no gross impairment of sensation; rather, a patchy decrease in light touch and pin-prick is seen. Hyperreflexia, clonus, and positive Babinski's signs are seen in the lower extremities. Hoffman's sign and hyperreflexia may be observed in the upper extremities.

Diagnostic Studies

In evaluating any pathologic process, one will usually have a choice of several diagnostic tests. The cervical spine is no exception. This section will deal with the most common ones that are routinely used. In general, all of these tests play a confirmatory role. In other words, the core of the information derived from a thorough history and physical examination should be the basis for a diagnosis; the additional tests are obtained to confirm this clinical impression. Trouble develops when these tests are used for screening purposes since most of them are overly sensitive and relatively nonselective. Thus, the studies discussed should never be interpreted in isolation from the overall clinical picture.

Plain Radiographs

Radiographic evaluation of the cervical spine is helpful in assessing patients with neck pain and the routine study should include anteroposterior, lateral, oblique and odontoid views. Flexion-extension X-rays are necessary in defining stability. The generally accepted radiographic signs of cervical disc disease are loss of height of the intervertebral disc space, osteophyte formation, secondary encroachment of the intervertebral foramina, and osteoarthritic changes in the apophyseal joints.

It should be stressed that the identification of some pathology on plain cervical X-rays does not, per se, indicate the cause of the patient's symptoms. In several series, large numbers of asymptomatic patients have shown radiographic evidence of advanced degenerative disc disease. At approximately age 40, some degeneration (narrowing) can be expected, particularly at the C5–C6 and C6–C7 levels. This is considered to represent a normal aging process. The difficult problem with regard to radiographic interpretation is not in the identification of these changes, but rather in determining how much significance should be attributed to them.

Radiographic abnormalities of alignment in the cervical spine may also be of clinical significance, but they need to be correlated with the whole clinical picture; listhesis or slipping forward or backward (retrolisthesis) of one vertebra upon the vertebra below it is such a finding.

If instability is suspected, functional X-rays may be taken. These view the spine from the side, with the head flexed (bent forward) or extended (arched back); the spine normally flexes equally at each spinal level. If one vertebral level is unstable, that particular vertebra moves more or less and disrupts the symmetry of motion. Again, this finding must be correlated with the whole clinical picture as its mere presence may be asymptomatic.

Magnetic Resonance Imaging

Magnetic resonance imaging (MRI) provides an image on film that is obtained by measuring the differences in proton density between the various tissues evaluated. With the use of the computer, multiplanar images are obtainable. It is a safe test since it uses neither ionizing radiation nor invasive contrast agents.

The technical advances for MRI have rapidly changed. The distinction between soft tissues and bone and the relationship of both to the neural foramen are excellent (Fig. 7.1). MRI can also accurately detect rare conditions such as infection, tumor, or intrinsic abnormalities of the spinal cord. An excellent test, MRI can be combined with plain films to permit an accurate noninvasive evaluation of a cervical radiculopathy or myelopathy. It is currently the diagnostic study of choice in the cervical spine.

The MRI should be used as a confirmatory test to substantiate a clinical impression. It should not be used as a screening test since there are many false-positive as well as false-negative results. Thus, some normal people will have abnormal MRI findings, whereas some abnormal people will be found to have normal MRIs.

Myelography

A myelogram is performed by injecting a water-soluble dye into the spinal sac so that the outline of the sac itself, as well as each nerve root sleeve, can be evaluated.

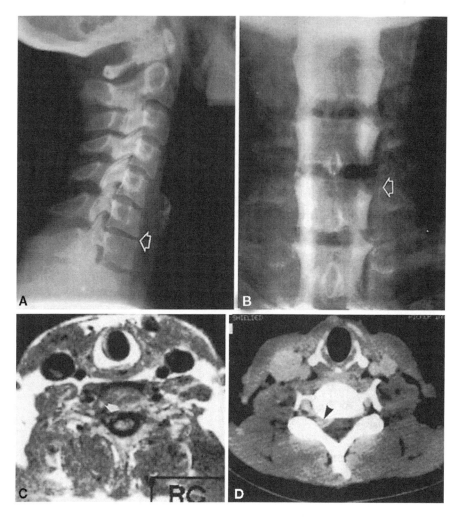

Fig. 7.1 This 33-year-old male presented with right triceps weakness, C7 radicular pain, and absent triceps reflex. (**a**) Lateral radiograph of C6–C7 shows loss of disc height (*arrow*). (**b**) Anteroposterior myelogram confirms right C7 root sleeve cutoff. (**c**) Axial magnetic resonance imaging (*left*) and computerized tomography (*right*) show occlusion of the right C6–C7 foramen (*arrows*). (From Boden S, Wiesel SW, Laws E, et al. *The Aging Spine.* Philadelphia, PA: Saunders; 1991. Reprinted with permission)

If there is pressure upon the nerve root or dural sac from either a bony spur or a disc herniation, it will be seen as a constriction on the X-ray picture. Complications from myelography are rare and it can be performed on an outpatient basis. The major disadvantages are its invasive nature, radiation exposure, and the lack of diagnostic specificity. Water-soluble myelography does provide excellent contrast for subsequent examination by computerized tomography (Fig. 7.1).

Computerized Tomography

Computerized tomography (CT) permits one to create cross-sectional imaging of the cervical spine at any desired level. It is currently used after the instillation of water-soluble dye, which is termed a CT-myelogram. The advantages of CT-myelography include excellent differentiation of bone and soft tissue (disc or ligament) lesions, direct demonstration of spinal cord and spinal cord dimensions, assessment of foraminal encroachment, and visualization of regions distal to a myelographic blockade.

Unfortunately, when combined with myelography, CT becomes an invasive procedure and involves radiation exposure. It does, however, provide very good information and is especially useful for patients who, for a variety of reasons, cannot undergo MRI investigation.

Electromyography

Electromyography (EMG) is an electric test that confirms the interaction of nerve to muscle. The test is performed by placing needles into muscles to determine if there is an intact nerve supply to that muscle. The EMG is particularly useful in localizing a specific abnormal nerve root. It should be appreciated that it takes at least 21 days for an EMG to show up as abnormal. After 21 days of pressure on a nerve root, signs of denervation with fibrillation can be observed. Before 21 days, the EMG will be negative in spite of nerve root damage. It should be noted that there is no quantitative interpretation of this test. Thus, it cannot be said that the EMG is 25 or 75% normal.

The EMG is an electronic extension of the physical examination. Although it is 80–90% accurate in establishing cervical radiculopathy as the cause of pain, false-negative results do occur. If cervical radiculopathy affects only the sensory root, the EMG will be unable to demonstrate an abnormality. A false-negative examination can occur if the patient with acute symptoms is examined early (4–28 days from onset of symptoms). A negative study should be repeated in 2–3 weeks if symptoms persist. The accuracy of the EMG increases if both the paraspinal and extremity muscles innervated by the suspected root demonstrate abnormalities.

The EMG is not part of the routine evaluation of the cervical spine. It is indicated to confirm a clinical impression or to rule out other sources of pathology, such as peripheral neuropathies or compressive neuropathies in the upper extremities.

Clinical Conditions

There are many conditions that may present as neck pain, with or without arm pain, in any particular individual. However, there are several that are quite common and will be presented in detail.

Neck Sprain-Neckache

Neck sprain, while a misnomer, describes a clinical condition involving a nonradiating discomfort or pain about the neck area associated with a concomitant loss
of neck motion (stiffness). While the clinical syndrome may present as a headache,
most often the pain is located in the middle to lower part of the back of the neck.
A history of injury is rarely obtained, but the pain may start after a night's rest or
on simply turning the head. The source of the pain is most commonly believed to
be the ligaments about the cervical spine and/or the surrounding muscles. The axial
pain may also be produced by small annular tears without disc herniation or from
the facet joints.

The pain associated with a neck sprain is most often a dull aching pain, which
is exacerbated by neck motion. The pain is usually abated by rest or immobilization. The pain may be referred to other mesenchymal structures derived from a
similar sclerotome during embryogenesis. Common referred pain patterns include
the scapular area, the posterior shoulder, the occipital area, or the anterior chest
wall (cervical angina pectoris). Those referred pain patterns do not connote a true
radicular pain pattern and are not usually mechanical in origin.

Physical examination of patients with neckache usually reveals nothing more
than a locally tender area or areas, usually just lateral to the spine. The intensity of
the pain is variable and the loss of cervical motion correlates directly with the pain
intensity. The presence of true spasm, defined as a continuous muscle contraction,
is rare except in severe cases where the head may be tilted to one side (torticollis).

Since the radiograph in cervical sprain is usually normal, a plain X-ray is usually not warranted on the first visit. If the pain continues for more than 2 weeks
or the patient develops other physical findings, then an X-ray should be taken to
rule out other more serious causes of the neck pain such as neoplasia or instability.
The prognosis for these individuals is excellent since the natural history is one of
complete resolution of the symptoms over several weeks. The mainstay of therapy
includes rest and immobilization, usually in a soft cervical orthosis. Although medications such as antiinflammatory agents or muscle relaxants may aid in the acute
management of pain, they do not seem to alter the natural history of the disorder.

Acute Herniated Disc

A herniated disc is defined as the protrusion of the nucleus pulposus through the
fibers of the annulus fibrosus (Fig. 7.2). Most acute disc herniations occur posterolaterally and in patients around the fourth decade of life when the nucleus is
still gelatinous. The most common areas of disc herniation are C5–C6 and C6–C7,
whereas C7–T1 and C3–C4 are infrequent. Disc herniation of C2–C3 is very,
very rare. Unlike the lumbar herniated disc, the cervical herniated disc may cause
myelopathy in addition to radicular pain due to the presence of the spinal cord in
the cervical region.

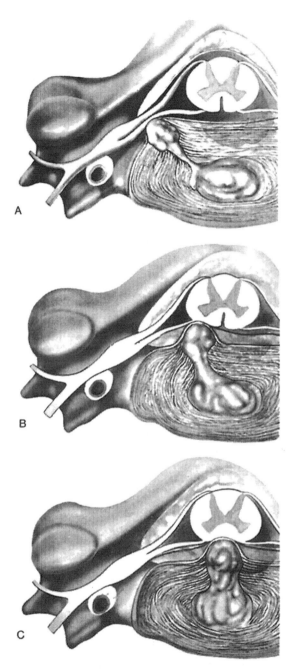

Fig. 7.2 Types of soft disk protrusion. (**a**) Intraforaminal, most common. (**b**) Posterolateral, produces mostly motor signs. (**c**) Midline, may manifest as myelopathy. (Modified from DePalma AF, Rothman RH. *The Intervertebral Disc*. Philadelphia, PA: Saunders; 1970. From Wiesel S, Delahay J eds. *Essentials of Orthopaedic Surgery*. 2nd ed. Philadelphia, PA: Saunders; 1997. Reprinted with permission)

The disc herniation usually affects the root numbered lowest for the given disc level; for example, a C3–C4 disc affects the C4 root, C4–C5 the fifth cervical root, C5–C6 the sixth cervical root, C6–C7 the seventh nerve root, and C7–T1 the eighth cervical root. Unlike the lumbar region, the disc herniation does not involve other roots, but more commonly presents some evidence of upper motor neuron findings secondary to spinal cord local pressure.

Not every herniated disc is symptomatic. The presence of symptoms depends on the spinal reserve capacity, the presence of inflammation, the size of the herniation, as well as the presence of concomitant disease such as osteophyte formation.

Clinically, the patient's major complaint is arm pain, not neck pain. The pain is often perceived as starting in the neck area, but then radiates from this point down the shoulder, arm, forearm and usually into the hand, commonly in a dermatomal distribution. The onset of the radicular pain is often gradual, although there can be a sudden onset associated with a tearing or snapping sensation. As time passes, the magnitude of the arm pain will clearly exceed that of the neck or shoulder pain. The arm pain may vary in intensity from severe enough to preclude any use of the arm without severe pain to a dull cramping ache in the arm muscles with use of the arm. The pain is usually severe enough to awaken the patient at night.

Physical examination of the neck usually shows some limitation of motion and on occasion the patient may tilt the head in a "cocked robin" position (torticollis) toward the side of the herniated cervical disc. Extension of the spine will often exacerbate the pain since it further narrows the intervertebral foramina. Axial compression, Valsalva maneuver, and coughing may also exacerbate or re-create the pain pattern.

The presence of a positive neurologic finding is the most helpful aspect of the diagnostic workup, although the neurologic exam may remain normal despite a chronic radicular pattern. Even when a deficit exists, it may not be temporally related to the present symptoms, but to a prior attack at a different level. To be significant, the neurologic exam must show objective signs of reflex diminution, motor weakness, or atrophy. The presence of subjective sensory changes is often difficult to interpret and require a coherent and cooperative patient to be of clinical value. The presence of sensory changes alone is usually not enough to make a diagnosis firm.

Nerve root sensitivity can be elicited by any method which increases the tension of the nerve root. Radicular arm pain is often increased by the Valsalva maneuver or by directly compressing the head. While these signs are helpful when present, their absence alone does not rule out radicular pain.

The provisional diagnosis of a herniated disc is made by the history and physical examination. The plain X-ray is usually nondiagnostic, although occasionally disc space narrowing at the suspected interspace or foraminal narrowing on the oblique films will be seen. The value of the films is largely to exclude other causes of neck and arm pain. The MRI is a confirmatory examination and should not be used as a screening test since misinformation may ensue.

The treatment for most patients with a herniated disc is nonoperative since the majority of patients respond to conservative treatment over a period of months. The efficacy of the nonoperative approach depends heavily on the doctor–patient relationship. If a patient is well informed, insightful, and willing to follow instructions, the chances for successful nonoperative outcome are greatly improved.

The cornerstone to the management of a cervical herniated disc is rest and immobilization. The use of a soft cervical orthosis greatly increases the likelihood that the patient will rest. Patients should markedly decrease their physical activity for at least 2 weeks and wear the cervical orthosis at all times (especially at night). After the acute pain begins to abate, patients should gradually wean off the orthosis. Most persons will be able to return to work, or at least light duty, in a month.

Drug therapy is an important adjunct to rest and immobilization. Antiinflammatory medications, analgesics, and muscle relaxants have historically been used in the acute management of these patients. Since it is commonly believed that the radicular pain is in part inflammatory, the use of aspirin or other nonsteroidal antiinflammatory medications seems to be appropriate. All these medications have gastrointestinal side effects, but are generally well tolerated for brief periods.

Analgesic medication is only rarely needed if the patient is compliant. However, if the pain is severe enough, a brief course of oral codeine may be prescribed. Muscle relaxants and the benzodiazepines are truly tranquilizers and central nervous system depressants. As such, they have at best a limited role in the management of the acute herniated disc patient. While it is true that these medications help patients relax and get their needed rest, the potential for an addictive effect adding to any psychosocial problems patients may have is not, in the majority of patients, worth the long-term risk for the short-term gain.

Cervical Spondylosis

What was once commonly referred to as cervical degenerative disc disease more recently has been called cervical spondylosis. Cervical spondylosis is a chronic process defined as the development of osteophytes and other stigmata of degenerative arthritis as a consequence of age-related disc disease. This process may produce a wide range of symptoms. However, it should be stressed that an individual may have significant spondylosis and be asymptomatic.

Cervical spondylosis is believed to be the direct result of age-related changes in the intervertebral disc. These changes include desiccation of the nucleus pulposus, loss of annular elasticity, and narrowing of the disc space with or without disc protrusion or rupture. In turn, secondary changes include overriding of facets, increased motion of the spinal segments, osteophyte formation, inflammation of synovial joints, and even microfractures. These macro- and microscopic changes can result in various clinical syndromes (spondylosis, ankylosis, central or foraminal spinal stenosis, radiculopathy, myelopathy, or spinal segmental instability).

The typical patient with symptomatic cervical spondylosis is over the age of 40 and complaining of neckache. Not infrequently, however, these patients will have very few neck pain symptoms and will present with referred pain patterns: occipital headaches; pain in the shoulder, suboccipital and intrascapular areas and the anterior chest wall; or other vague symptoms suggestive of anatomic disturbances (e.g., blurring of vision, tinnitus). In patients with predominantly referred pain, a past history for neck pain is usually obtained.

Physical examination of the patient with cervical spondylosis is often associated with a dearth of objective findings. The patient will usually have some limitation of neck motion associated with midline tenderness. Not infrequently, palpation of the referred pain areas will also produce local tenderness and should not be confused with local disease. The neurologic examination is normal.

Anteroposterior (AP), lateral, and oblique radiographs of the cervical spine in cervical spondylosis show varying degrees of changes. These include disc space narrowing, osteophytosis, foraminal narrowing, degenerative changes of the facets, and instability. As previously discussed, these findings do not necessarily correlate with symptoms. In large part, the radiograph serves to rule out other more serious causes of neck and referred pain such as tumors. Further diagnostic testing is usually not warranted.

Cervical spondylosis alone is treated by nonoperative measures. The mainstay of treatment for the acute pain superimposed on the chronic problem is rest and immobilization. In addition, oral antiinflammatory medications such as aspirin are beneficial. Often these medications will need to be administered on a chronic basis or at least intermittently. Trigger-point injections with local anesthetics (lidocaine) and corticosteroids (triamcinolone) may be therapeutic as well as diagnostic. Once the pain abates, the immobilization (usually a soft cervical collar) should be discontinued and the patient maintained on a series of cervical isometric exercises. Further counseling with regard to sleeping position, automobile driving, and work is in order. Manipulation and traction are rarely needed and may, in fact, be deleterious to the patient.

Cervical Spondylosis with Myelopathy

When the secondary bony changes of cervical spondylosis encroach on the spinal cord, a pathologic process called myelopathy develops. If this involves both the spinal cord and nerve roots, it is called myeloradiculopathy. Radiculopathy, regardless of its etiology, causes shoulder or arm pain.

Myelopathy is the most serious sequelae of cervical spondylosis and the most difficult to treat effectively. Less than 5% of patients with cervical spondylosis develop myelopathy and they are usually between 40 and 60 years of age. The changes of myelopathy are most often gradual and associated with posterior osteophyte formation (called spondylitic bone or hard disc) and spinal canal narrowing (spinal stenosis). Acute myelopathy is most often the result of a central soft disc herniation.

The characteristic stooped, wide-based, and somewhat jerky gait of the aged summarizes the chronic effects of cervical spondylosis with myelopathy. The spinal cord changes may develop from single- or multiple-level disease and as such may not present in a singular or standard manner. A typical clinical presentation of chronic myelopathy begins with the gradual notice of a peculiar sensation in the hands, associated with clumsiness and weakness. The patient will also note lower extremity symptoms that may antedate the upper extremity findings, including difficulty walking, peculiar sensations, leg weakness, hyperreflexia, spasticity, and clonus. The upper extremity findings may start out unilaterally and include hyperreflexia, brisk Hoffman's sign, and muscle atrophy (especially of the hand muscles). Neck pain, per se, is not a prominent feature of myelopathy. Sensory changes can evolve at these levels and are often a less reliable index of spinal cord disease. The protean nature of the signs and symptoms of cervical myelopathy, along with its potential for severe functional impairment, merits a high index of suspicion in patient evaluation.

Radiographs of the cervical spine in these patients will often reveal advanced degenerative disease, including spinal canal narrowing by prominent posterior osteophytosis, variable foraminal narrowing, disc space narrowing, facet joint arthrosis, and instability. Congenital stenosis of the cervical canal is frequently seen, predisposing the patient to the development of myelopathy. The myelogram is diagnostic, exhibiting a washboard appearance to the dye column with multiple anterior and posterior defects. The posterior defects are secondary to facet arthrosis and buckling of the ligamentum flavum. The MRI is also quite striking and diagnostic.

In general, myelopathy is a surgical disease, but it is not an absolute indication for surgical decompression. Conservative therapy consisting of immobilization and rest with a soft cervical orthosis offers a viable option to the myelopathic patient who is not a good operative risk. The goals of surgery in the myelopathic patient are to decompress the spinal canal to prevent further spinal cord compression and vascular compromise. If the myelopathy is progressive despite a trial of conservative treatment, surgery is clearly indicated. These indications may vary slightly from surgeon to surgeon because of the lack of absolute or definitive clinical data.

Rheumatoid Arthritis

Rheumatoid arthritis affects 2–3% of the population. About 60% of patients with rheumatoid arthritis will exhibit signs and symptoms of cervical spine involvement, whereas up to 86% will have radiographic evidence of cervical disease. Cervical spine involvement, secondary to the erosive, inflammatory changes of rheumatoid arthritis (synovitis), is divided into three categories: (1) atlantoaxial instability, (2) basilar invagination, and (3) subaxial instability. Atlantoaxial instability is the most common and most serious of the instability patterns affecting 20–34% of hospitalized patients. The evaluation of a patient with rheumatoid arthritis is difficult due to the multiple system involvement. The physical examination should start with a careful neurologic evaluation to rule out upper motor neuron disease before moving to neck range of motion or other vigorous maneuvers that may harm the patient.

The patient with cervical spine involvement from rheumatoid arthritis most often has neck pain located in the middle posterior neck and occipital area. The range of motion is decreased and crepitance or a feeling of instability may be noted. The neurologic changes can be variable and difficult to elicit in the context of diffuse rheumatoid changes. The evaluation of the patient with cervical rheumatoid arthritis begins with plain radiographs of the neck, which may reveal osteopenia, facet erosion, disc space narrowing, and subluxation of the lower cervical spine (stepladder appearance). To determine that atlantoaxial disease is present, dynamic flexion-extension views of the lateral upper cervical spine are required.

Basilar invagination is defined as upper migration of the odontoid projecting into the foramen magnum. The addition of a CT scan with and without contrast material in the upper cervical spine can provide valuable information as to the relationship of the bony elements to the spinal cord. Subaxial subluxations are identified by dynamic flexion-extension films.

The majority of these patients, despite rather dramatic disease patterns, can be successfully managed nonoperatively. While the natural history of rheumatoid arthritis predicts a high incidence of involvement of the cervical spine, it is estimated that only a few patients die from medullary compression associated with significant atlantoaxial disease. Although atlantoaxial disease worsens with time, only 2–14% of patients exhibit neurologic progression.

The mainstay in nonoperative therapy is the cervical orthosis. Although this does not fully immobilize the atlantoaxial interval, it does produce symptomatic relief. Some authors have advocated intermittent home traction, but this must be used only with great caution under a physician's direction. Medications have a definite role in the nonoperative management of rheumatoid disease. Initial management includes aspirin in high dosages monitored by serum drug levels. Secondary agents such as methotrexate, chloroquine, or oral steroids are best administered under the direction of a rheumatologist.

Cervical Hyperextension Injuries

Hyperextension injuries of the neck occur most often when the driver of a stationary car is struck from behind by another vehicle. The driver is usually relaxed and unaware of the impending collision. The sudden acceleration of the struck vehicle pushes the back of the car seat against the driver's torso. This pushes the driver's torso forward and his or her head is thrown backward, causing hyperextension of the neck. This occurs very quickly after impact. If no head rest is present, the driver's head is hyperextended past the normal limit of stretch of the soft tissues of the neck. This injury has been descriptively termed whiplash because of the hyperextension of the head.

The sternocleidomastoid muscle, the scalenes, and the longus colli muscles may be mildly or severely stretched or, at worst, torn. Muscle tears of the longus colli muscles might involve injury to the symptomatic trunk unilaterally or bilaterally, resulting in Horner's syndrome, nausea, or dizziness. Further hyperextension may injure the esophagus, resulting in temporary dysphagia and injury to the larynx, causing hoarseness. Tears in the anterior longitudinal ligament may cause hematoma

formation with resultant cervical radiculitis (arm pain) and injury to the intervertebral disc. In the recoil-forward flexion that occurs when the car stops accelerating,
the head is thrown forward. This forward flexion of the head is usually limited by
the chin striking the chest and does not usually cause significant injury. However, if
the head is thrown forward and strikes the steering wheel or the windshield, a head
injury can occur.

The driver is often unaware that he or she has been injured. The driver suffers
little discomfort at the scene of the accident and often does not even wish to go
to the hospital. Later that evening or the next day, 12–14 h after the accident, the
patient begins to feel stiffness in the neck. Pain at the base of the neck increases
and is made worse by head and neck movements. Soon any movement of the head
or neck causes excruciating pain. The anterior cervical muscles are often tender to
the touch. The patient may have pain on mouth opening or chewing, hoarseness or
difficulty swallowing, and will seek medical care.

The physical examination must be detailed and complete. Abrasions on the forehead would suggest that forward flexion led to the head striking the steering wheel
or windshield. A dilated pupil might suggest a case of Horner's syndrome secondary
to the injury of the sympathetic chain or it might be a sign of significant intracranial
injury if the patient's level of consciousness is altered. Point tenderness in front of
the ear would suggest injury to the temporomandibular joint and tenderness to touch
in the suboccipital area would suggest the head struck the back of the seat.

A complete neurological examination is crucial. Any evidence of objective neurological deficit merits immediate diagnostic tests to determine the cause. Although
by definition hyperextension cervical injury causes damage only to the soft tissue
structures of the neck, plain radiographs of the cervical spine should be obtained in
all cases. Unsuspected fracture—dislocations of the cervical spine, facet fractures,
odontoid fractures, or spinous process fractures—might be otherwise missed in the
neurologically intact patient. Cervical spondylosis will be demonstrated on plain
radiographs as well. Of course, if objective neurologic deficits are present, then
further diagnostic aids are necessary, (e.g., head CT, spine CT, myelogram, MRI).

Since the majority of patients have no neurologic deficits, a reasonable medical
routine is based on the premise of resting the involved injured soft tissues. A soft
cervical collar helps significantly in relieving muscle spasm and preventing quick
head turns. The collar should not be worn for more than 2–4 weeks, lest the recovering muscles start weakening from nonuse. Heat is helpful and should be applied
by a heating pad, hot showers, or hot tub soaks. If neck pain is severe, a short period
of bed rest may be necessary. Mild analgesics, nonsteroidal antiinflammatory drugs
(NSAIDs), and muscle relaxants are all helpful and are generally indicated. Narcotic
analgesics should be avoided if at all possible. Activity should be restricted as determined by the severity of the symptoms. Generally, driving should be avoided for the
acute symptomatic period. After approximately 2 weeks of this regimen, significant
improvement should be noted. If not, two more weeks of continued conservative
care with the addition of some light home-cervical traction should be employed. If
symptoms persist at 4 weeks post-injury, some further testing is necessary before
emotional overlay is considered the cause. If headaches persist, a cranial MRI scan
should be done. If normal at 4 weeks, the patient can be assured that no intracranial

abnormality is present. If arm or shoulder pain persists, an MRI should be considered. If these tests are normal, the patient can be assured that no compression of neural structures is present.

Cervical Spine Algorithm

The task of the physician, when confronted with the cervical spine patient, is to integrate his or her complaints into an accurate diagnosis and to prescribe appropriate therapy. Achieving this goal depends on the accuracy of the physician's decision-making ability. Although specific information is not available for every aspect of neck pain, there is a large body of data to guide us in handling these patients. Using this knowledge, which has already been presented, an algorithm for neck pain has been designated.

Webster defines an algorithm as "a set of rules for solving a particular problem in a finite number of steps." It is, in effect, an organized pattern of decision making and thought processes which can be found useful, in this instance, in approaching the universe of cervical spine patients. The algorithm can be followed in sequence (Fig. 7.3) and is also presented in table form (Table 7.2).

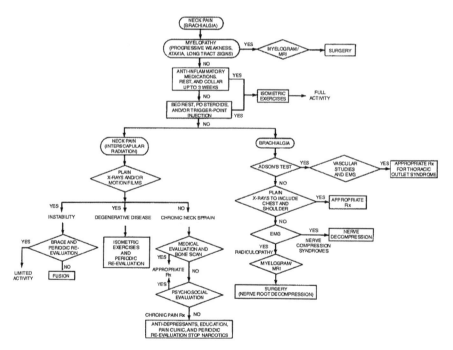

Fig. 7.3 Cervical spine algorithm (From Wiesel SE, Feffer HI, Rothman RH. *Neck Pain*. Charlottesville, VA: Michie; 1988, permission granted by LexisNexis Matthew Bender)

Table 7.2 Differential diagnosis of neck pain

Evaluation	Neck strain	Herniated nucleus pulposus	Instability	Degenerative disc disease	Myelopathy	Tumor	Spondylo-arthropathy	Metabolic	Infection
Predominant pain (arm vs. neck)	Neck	Arm	Neck	Neck	Neck	Neck	Neck	Neck	Neck
Constitutional symptoms						+	+	±	+
Compression test		+							
Neurologic exam		+			+				
Plain radiographs			±	+	±	±	+	+	±
Lateral motion radiographs			+	+	+				
CAT scan		+			±	+			+
Myelogram		+			+				
Bone scan						+	+	±	+
ESR							+		+
Ca/P/alk phos						+		+	

Ca/P/alk phos calcium, phosphate, and alkaline phosphatase, *CAT* computerized axial tomography, *ESR* erythrocyte sedimentation rate

The primary objective for the physician is to return patients to their normal function as quickly as possible. In the course of achieving this goal, the physician must be concerned with other circumstances, which include making efficient and precise use of diagnostic studies, minimizing the use of ineffectual surgery, and making therapy available at a reasonable cost to society. The algorithm follows well-delineated rules, established from the consensus of a broad segment of qualified spine surgeons. It allows the patient to receive the most helpful diagnostic and therapeutic measures at optimal times.

The algorithm begins with the universe of patients who are initially evaluated for neck pain, with or without arm pain. Patients with major trauma, including fractures, are not included. After an initial medical history and physical examination—and assuming that the patient's symptoms are originating from the cervical spine—the first major decision is to rule in or out the presence of a cervical myelopathy.

The character and severity of the myelopathy depend on the size, location, and duration of the lesion. Ventrolateral lesions encroach on the nerve roots and lateral aspects of the spinal cord, producing all the manifestations accompanying nerve root compression. The chief radicular signs are weakness, loss of tone, and volume of the muscles of the upper extremity, while the pressure on the spinal cord may produce pyramidal tract signs and spasticity in the lower extremities.

Midline lesions intrude on the central aspect of the anterior portion of the spinal cord. They produce no signs of nerve root compression. Both lower extremities are primarily involved and the most common problem relates initially to gait disturbance. As the disease progresses, bowel and bladder control may be affected.

Once a diagnosis of cervical myelopathy is made, surgical intervention should be considered without delay. The best results are attained in patients with one or two motor units involved and with myelopathy of a relatively short duration. The longer pressure is applied to the neural elements, the poorer the results. A cervical MRI or CT-myelogram should be obtained in these patients to precisely define the neural compression and an adequate surgical decompression should be performed as soon as possible to achieve the best results.

After cervical myelopathy has been ruled out, the remaining patients, who constitute an overwhelming majority, should be started on a course of conservative management. At this stage of the patient's course, a specific diagnosis, whether it be a herniated disc or neck strain, is not important because the entire group is treated in the same fashion.

Conservative Treatment

The primary mode of therapy in both acute and chronic cervical spine disease is immobilization. In the acute neck injuries, immobilization allows for healing of torn and attenuated soft tissues, whereas in chronic conditions immobilization is aimed at reduction of inflammation in the supporting soft tissues and around the nerve roots of the cervical spine.

Immobilization is best achieved by the use of a soft felt collar. It needs to be properly fitted and comfortable for the patient. Initially, the collar is worn 24 h a day. The patient must understand that during sleep the neck is totally unprotected from awkward positions and movement and that, therefore, the collar is most important.

The other mainstay of the initial treatment is drug therapy. It is directed at reducing inflammation, especially in the soft tissues. There are a variety of anti-inflammatory medications available; however, there is no one drug that has proven to be significantly better than all the others. The dosage must be adequate to achieve a therapeutic blood level. The efficacy of this treatment regimen is predicated on the patient's ability to understand the disease process and the role of each therapeutic modality. The vast majority of patients will respond to this approach in the first 10 days, but a certain percentage will not heal rapidly.

At this juncture, a local injection into the area of maximal tenderness should be considered. Localized tender areas in the paravertebral musculature and trapezii will be found in many individuals and are referred to as trigger points. Marked relief of symptoms is often achieved dramatically by infiltration of these trigger points with a combination of lidocaine (Xylocaine) and 1 mL of a steroid preparation. The object of the injection is to decrease the inflammation in a specific anatomic area. The more localized the trigger point, the more effective this form of therapy.

The patient should be treated conservatively for up to 6 weeks. The majority of cervical spine patients will get better and should be encouraged to gradually increase their activities. The goal is a return to their normal lifestyles. An exercise program should be directed at strengthening the paravertebral musculature, not at increasing the range of motion.

The pathway along this top portion of the algorithm is reversible. Should regression occur, with exacerbation of symptoms, the physician can resort to more stringent conservative measures. The majority of patients with neck pain will respond to therapy and return to a normal life pattern within 2 months of the beginning of their problem. If the initial conservative treatment regimen fails, symptomatic patients are divided into two groups. The first is comprised of people who have neck pain as a predominant complaint, with or without interscapular radiation. The second group is made up of those who complain primarily of arm pain (brachialgia).

Neck Pain Predominant

After 6 weeks of conservative therapy with no symptomatic relief, plain roentgenograms with lateral flexion-extension films are carefully examined for abnormalities. One group of patients will have objective evidence of instability. In the lower cervical spine (C-3 through C-7), instability is identified by horizontal translation of one vertebra on another of more than 3.5 mm or of an angulatory difference of adjacent vertebrae of more than 11°. The majority of patients with instability will respond well to further nonoperative measures, including a thorough explanation of the problem and some type of bracing. In some cases, these measures will fail and a surgical fusion of the involved spinal segments will be necessary.

Another group of patients complaining mainly of neck pain will be found to have degenerative disease on their plain X-ray films. The roentgenographic signs include loss of height of the intervertebral disc space, osteophyte formation, secondary encroachment of the intervertebral foraminae, and osteoarthritic changes in the apophyseal joint. The difficulty is not in identifying these abnormalities on the roentgenogram, but in determining their significance.

Degeneration in the cervical spine can be a normal part of the aging process. In a study of matched pairs of asymptomatic and symptomatic patients, it was concluded that large numbers of asymptomatic patients show roentgenographic evidence of advanced degenerative disease. The most significant roentgenographic finding relevant to symptomatology was found to be narrowing of the intervertebral disc space, particularly between C5–C6 and C6–C7. There was no difference between the two groups as far as changes at the apophyseal joints, intervertebral foraminae, or posterior articular process.

These patients should be treated symptomatically with antiinflammatory medication, support, and trigger-point injections as required. In the quiescent stages, they should be placed on isometric exercises. Finally, they should be reexamined periodically because some will develop significant pressure on the neurologic elements (myelopathy).

The majority of patients with neck pain will have normal roentgenograms. The diagnosis for this group is neck strain. At this point, with no objective findings, other pathology must be considered. These patients should undergo a bone scan and medical evaluation. The bone scan is an excellent tool, often identifying early spinal tumors or infections not seen on routine roentgenographic examinations. A thorough medical search may also reveal problems missed in the early stages of neck pain evaluation. If these diagnostic studies are positive, the patient is treated appropriately. If the above workup is negative, the patient should have a thorough psychosocial evaluation. This is predicated on the belief that a patient's disability is related not only to his or her pathologic anatomy, but also to the perception of pain and the stability in relationship to his or her sociologic environment. Drug habituation, alcoholism, depression, and other psychiatric problems are frequently seen in association with neck pain. If the evaluation reveals this type of pathology, proper measures should be instituted to overcome the disability.

Should the outcome of the psychosocial evaluation prove to be normal, the patient can be considered to have chronic neck pain. One must be aware that other outside factors such as compensation and/or litigation can influence a patient's perception of his or her subjective pain. Patients with chronic neck pain need encouragement, patience, and education from their physicians. They need to be detoxified from narcotic drugs and placed on an exercise regimen. Many will respond to antidepressant drugs such as amitriptyline (Elavil). All of these patients need periodic reevaluation to avoid missing any new or underlying pathology.

Arm Pain Predominant (Brachialgia)

Patients who have pain radiating into their arm may be experiencing their symptoms secondary to mechanical pressure and inflammation of the involved nerve roots. This mechanical pressure may arise from a ruptured disc or from bone secondary to degenerative changes. Other pathologic causes of arm pain should be carefully considered. Extrinsic pressure on the vascular structures or on the peripheral nerves is most likely imitators of brachialgia. Pathology in the chest and shoulder should also be ruled out.

A careful physical examination should be conducted. If there is any question about these findings, appropriate roentgenograms and an EMG should be obtained. If any of these are positive for peripheral pressure on the nerves or other pathology, the appropriate therapy should be administered.

Should all of these studies prove negative and the EMG is consistent, the patient is considered to have brachialgia. One must carefully reevaluate the patient who has a neurologic deficit and/or a positive EMG; those who have either should undergo an MRI. If the MRI is positive and is consistent with the physical findings, surgical decompression should be considered at this juncture.

It has been repeatedly documented that unequivocal evidence of nerve root compression must be found at surgery for it to be effective. One must have a strong confirmation of mechanical root compression from the neurologic exam and a confirming study before proceeding with any surgery. The indications for surgery are the subjective complaint of arm pain and a neurologic deficit or positive EMG. An MRI must confirm the pathology. If the patient does not have these, there is inadequate clinical evidence to proceed with surgery. For patients who have met these criteria for cervical decompression, the results will usually be satisfactory: 95% can expect good or excellent outcomes.

Conservative Treatment Modalities

Most patients with neck pain will achieve relief from a conscientious program of conservative care. As the algorithm indicates, all patients with either chronic or acute neck pain (except those with severe myelopathy) deserve an initial period of conservative therapy. There are a multitude of treatment modalities available, but many of them are based on empiricism and tradition. The purpose of this section is to discuss the rationale behind the use of some of the more common nonoperative therapeutic measures.

Immobilization

The cornerstone of conservative therapy is immobilization of the cervical spine. The goal of immobilization is to rest the neck so that healing of torn and/or attenuated soft tissues in acute cervical injuries can take place. In the chronic situation, the purpose of immobilization is to reduce any inflammation.

Immobilization can best be achieved by the use of a soft cervical collar that holds the head in a neutral or slightly flexed position. It is very important that the collar is fitted properly. If the neck is held in hyperextension, the patient is usually quite uncomfortable and does not derive any benefit from its use. In acute neck injuries, the collar should be worn on a full-time basis, night and day, until the acute pain subsides. This may sometimes take as long as 4–6 weeks, and the patient should be aware of this time course from the outset of treatment so that the physician will not feel pressured to discontinue immobilization before the proper time.

Drug Therapy

There are different groups of medications that have proved helpful in the treatment of neck pain: antiinflammatory drugs, analgesics, and muscle relaxants. They are used as an important adjunct to adequate immobilization.

Antiinflammatory drugs are used because it is felt that inflammation in the soft tissues is a major contributor to pain production in the cervical spine. This is especially true for those patients with symptoms secondary to a herniated disc. The arm pain that these people experience is due not only to the mechanical pressure from the ruptured disc, but also to the inflammation in and around the involved nerve roots. Usually, if one can get rid of the inflammation, the patient's pain will markedly decrease.

There is a spectrum of antiinflammatory agents available, but none has been proven superior. The authors' usual treatment plan is to begin the patient on adequate doses and if the response is not satisfactory after 2 weeks, switch to another. Most patients will get significant relief from one of the agents presently available. It should be stressed that antiinflammatory medications are utilized in conjunction with immobilization; they do not replace adequate rest.

Analgesic medication is also very important during the acute phase of neck pain. The goal is to keep the patient comfortable. Most patients will respond to the equivalent of 30–60 mg of codeine every 4–6 h. If stronger medication is required, the patient should be monitored very closely. In some cases, narcotics will be abused by the patient and addiction will become a problem to some degree. The treating physician must maintain control of the patient's drug use at all times.

Injuries to the cervical spine frequently result in painful muscle spasm. A vicious cycle is established, whereby pain leads to muscle spasm, which leads to ischemia and a further increase in pain. Once the cycle is established, it tends to be self-perpetuating. An effective muscle relaxant frequently breaks this painful cycle and allows more comfort and an increased range of motion in the cervical spine. Methocarbamol or carisoprodol in adequate doses is the drug recommended as they are safe and quite effective.

Traction

Cervical traction has been used for many years. Today, opinions regarding its effectiveness range from that of it being a valuable clinical therapy to the conclusion that it is ineffective and/or potentially harmful.

There is no uniform idea as to how traction actually works and there are a number of methods of actually applying the traction. The three major ways of administering traction are mechanical, manual, and home traction. Many feel that manual traction is preferred due to the interaction between the therapist and patient and the potential specificity of individually varying the traction.

In certain situations, cervical traction is contraindicated. Malignancy, cord compression, infectious disease, osteoporosis, and rheumatoid arthritis are the major disorders for which cervical traction should *not* be employed. It is also felt that when there is a herniated disc present, either in the midline or laterally, traction should not be considered.

The authors feel that cervical traction is useful when a collar has proved ineffective in those patients with a cervical strain or a hyperextension injury. The major benefit is felt to be continued rest and a home traction device is preferred. When used in this situation, only minimal amounts of weight (4–6 lbs) should be utilized and the direction of pull should be in slight flexion. As already mentioned, there are other ways of applying traction, but to date there is no valid scientific evidence available that traction in and of itself is effective.

Trigger-Point Injection

Many patients will complain of a very localized tender spot in the paravertebral area. In some of these cases, relief of the discomfort can be achieved with the infiltration of the trigger point with a combination of Xylocaine and a steroid preparation or Xylocaine by itself. There have been no true randomized clinical trials to study the efficacy or trigger-point injections, but from empirical evidence, they seem to work on some patients. It is interesting to note that although the pharmacologic effects of these drugs may wear off in 2–3 h, the relief may last indefinitely.

Before actually injecting a patient, a history of allergy to the drugs to be used should be obtained. The more localized the trigger point, the more effective the injection tends to be. An area of diffuse tenderness does not respond very well to this approach.

Manipulation

Manipulation of the cervical spine should be approached very carefully. In the United States, this is mainly performed by chiropractors, although other health care professionals are involved. The goal of manipulation is to correct any malalignment of the spinal structures, which is assumed to be the etiology of the patient's pain. There is no real scientific evidence that manipulation of the cervical spine is effective in the treatment of acute or chronic neck problems.

Exercises

After a patient's acute symptoms have cleared and there is no significant pain or spasm, an exercise regimen is reasonable. The exercises should be directed at strengthening the paravertebral musculature and not at increasing the range of motion. Motion will return with the disappearance of pain. The exercises are isometric in nature. They are performed once a day with increasing repetitions. It should be appreciated that at present there are no scientific studies demonstrating that isometric exercises or any other type of cervical exercises will reduce the frequency of recurrent neck pain episodes. Empirically, they do appear to have a positive psychologic effect and give the patient an active part in his treatment program.

Lumbar Spine

Low back pain occurs much more commonly than neck pain. The lifetime incidence of low back pain is estimated to be 65%. Every physician will be either personally affected (family/friends) or professionally challenged by this problem.

History

A general medical review, especially in the older patient, is imperative. Metabolic, infectious, and malignant disorders may initially present to the physician as low back pain.

The location of the pain is one of the most important historical points. The majority of patients just have back pain with or without referral into the buttocks or posterior thigh. Referred pain is defined as pain in structures which have the same mesodermal origin. These patients have a localized injury and the referral of pain into the buttocks or thigh does not signify any compression on the neural elements. This type of pain is described as dull, deep, and/or boring.

Another group of patients complains of pain that originates in their back, but travels below the knee into the foot. It is described as sharp and lancinating. It may be accompanied by numbness and tingling. This pain is termed radicular pain or a radiculopathy. A radiculopathy is defined as a mechanical compression of an inflamed nerve root where the pain travels along the anatomic course of the nerve. The compression can be secondary to either soft tissue (disc) or bone. The most common nerve roots affected are L-5 and S-1—levels that account for pain traveling below the knee. Finally, one should inquire about changes in bowel or bladder habits. Occasionally, a large midline disc herniation may compress several roots of the cauda quina (Fig. 7.4). This is termed cauda equina compression. (CEC) syndrome. Urinary retention and incontinence of bowel or bladder are, along with severe pain, the major symptoms.

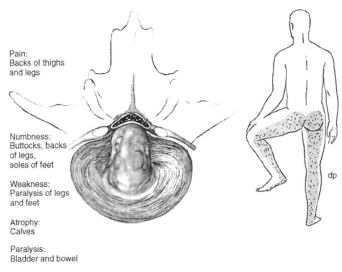

Pain:
Backs of thighs
and legs

Numbness:
Buttocks, backs
of legs,
soles of feet

Weakness:
Paralysis of legs
and feet

Atrophy:
Calves

Paralysis:
Bladder and bowel

dp

Fig. 7.4 Massive herniation at the level of the third, fourth, or fifth disc may cause severe compression of the cauda equina. Pain is confined chiefly to the buttocks and the back of the thighs and legs. Numbness is widespread from the buttocks to the soles of the feet. Motor weakness or loss is present in the legs and feet with loss of muscle mass in the calves. The bladder and bowels are paralyzed. DP, distribution of pain and paresthesia. (From DePalma AF, Rothman RH. *The Intervertebral Disc.* Philadelphia, PA: Saunders; 1970. Reprinted with permission)

Physical Examination

The physical examination is directed at finding the location of the pain. All patients with low back pain can have some nonspecific findings which vary in degree depending on the severity of the condition. These include a list to one side, tenderness to palpation and percussion and a decreased range of motion of the lumbar spine. The above findings can be present in both radiculopathy and referred pain patients. Their presence denotes that there is a problem, but does not identify the etiology or level of the problem. The neurologic examination may yield objective evidence of nerve root compression if present (Table 7.3). A thorough neurologic evaluation of the lower extremities should be conducted on each patient, particularly to check the reflexes and motor findings. Sensory changes may or may not be

Table 7.3 Clinical features of herniated lumbar discs

L3–L4 disc	L4 nerve root
Pain	Lower back, hip, posterolateral thigh, across patella, anteromedial aspect of leg
Numbness	Anteromedial thigh and knee
Weakness	Knee extension
Atrophy	Quadriceps
Reflexes	Knee jerk diminshed
L4–L5 disc	L5 nerve root
Pain	Sacroiliac region, hip, posterolateral thigh, anterolateral leg
Numbness	Lateral leg, first webspace
Weakness	Dorsiflexion of great toe and foot
Atrophy	Minimal anterior calf
Reflexes	None, or absent in posterior tibial tendon reflex
L5–S1 disc	S1 nerve root
Pain	Sacroiliac region, hip, posterolateral thigh/leg
Numbness	Back of calf; lateral heel, foot, and toe
Weakness	Plantar flexion of foot and great toe
Atrophy	Gastrocnemius and soleus
Reflexes	Ankle jerk diminished or absent

Source: From Boden S, Wiesel SW, Laws E, et al. *The Aging Spine*. Philadelphia, PA: Saunders; 1991:177. Reprinted with permission

present, but because of overlap in the dermatomes of spinal nerves, it is difficult to identify specific root involvement.

In patients with radiculopathies, there are several maneuvers that tighten the sciatic nerve and, in so doing, further compress an inflamed lumbar root against a herniated disc or bony spur. These maneuvers are generally termed tension signs or a straight leg-raising test (SLRT). The conventional SLRT is performed with the patient supine. The examiner slowly elevates the leg by the heel with the knee kept straight (Fig. 7.5). This test is positive when the leg pain below the knee is reproduced or intensified; the production of back and/or buttock pain does not constitute a positive finding. The reliability of the SLRT is age-dependent. In a young patient, a negative test most probably excludes the possibility of a herniated disc. After the age of 30, however, a negative SLRT no longer reliably excludes the diagnosis.

Finally, the physical examination should evaluate some specific problems that can present as low back pain. This includes a peripheral vascular examination, hip joint evaluation, and abdominal examination.

Diagnostic Studies

As in the cervical spine, diagnostic tests should be used to confirm the core of information gathered from a thorough history and physical examination. Several lumbosacral imaging modalities are currently available including plain films, myelography, CT, and MRI.

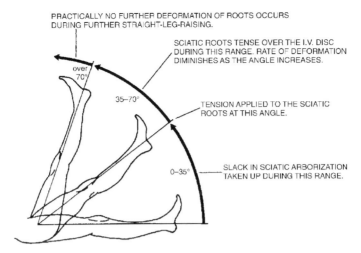

PRACTICALLY NO FURTHER DEFORMATION OF ROOTS OCCURS
DURING FURTHER STRAIGHT-LEG-RAISING.

SCIATIC ROOTS TENSE OVER THE I.V. DISC
DURING THIS RANGE. RATE OF DEFORMATION
DIMINISHES AS THE ANGLE INCREASES.

over 70°

35–70°

TENSION APPLIED TO THE SCIATIC
ROOTS AT THIS ANGLE.

0–35°

SLACK IN SCIATIC ARBORIZATION
TAKEN UP DURING THIS RANGE.

Fig. 7.5 The dynamics of the straight leg-raising test. (Modified from Fahrni WH. Observations on straight leg-raising, with special reference to nerve root adhesions. *Can J Surg.* 1966;9. Reprinted by permission)

To evaluate the true clinical value of any diagnostic study, one must know its sensitivity (false-negatives) and specificity (false-positives). The specificity, or false-positive rate, is usually measured in a population of symptomatic patients who have undergone surgery; however, often there is a much higher rate of false-positives when an asymptomatic group is studied. The accuracy of any single test increases when it is combined with a second or third diagnostic study. The physician's challenge is to select diagnostic tests on the basis of their performance characteristics so that the correct diagnosis is obtained with the least cost and morbidity. The studies most frequently utilized in the diagnostic assessment of low back pain will be described and critically analyzed with this in mind.

Plain Radiographs

The diagnosis of disc herniation can usually be made on the basis of a history and physical examination. Plain radiographs of the lumbosacral spine must be obtained in the appropriate setting to rule out other pathologic conditions such as infection or tumor. Plain radiographs are valuable for seeking the diagnosis of spinal stenosis, spondylolisthesis, gross segmental instability, or fracture.

The radiograph must be of excellent quality and taken with attention to detail. In general, three views are all that are required to assess the lumbosacral spine: an AP view, a lateral view, and a coned-down lateral view of the lower two interspaces. On occasion, two oblique views are also taken to identify subtle spondylolysis or pars interarticularis defects. However, oblique views provide limited information and should not be routinely included.

Although plain films are useful for surveying the bony elements of the spine and paraspinal soft tissues, the contents of the spinal canal, including cord, dura, ligaments, and encroaching disc, are not visualized. In addition, bony lesions may not be apparent until 50% of the cancellous bone has been destroyed.

Finally, degenerative changes such as disc space narrowing, traction osteophytes, vacuum-disc phenomenon, and end-plate sclerosis are quite prevalent in older individuals. Unfortunately, these radiographic findings have been shown to correlate poorly with clinical symptoms.

Magnetic Resonance Imaging

Magnetic resonance imaging is the diagnostic modality of choice when trying to evaluate the different tissues in the spine (Fig. 7.6). It is especially good for observing disc pathology. MRI with gadolinium-diethylenetriaminopentaacetic acid (DTPA) contrast enhancement is superb for demonstrating intraspinal tumors and for distinguishing recurrent disc herniation from scar tissue. As discussed with other diagnostic imaging modalities, MRI also has been shown to have a significant clinical false-positive rate in asymptomatic individuals. In one prospective and blinded study, 22% of the asymptomatic subjects under age 60 and 57% of those over age 60 had significantly abnormal scans. In addition, the prevalence of disc degeneration on the T2-weighted MRI scans was found to approach 98% in subjects over the age of 60.

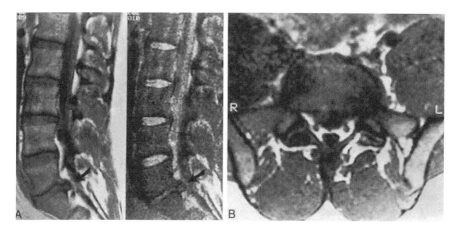

Fig. 7.6 (a) Magnetic resonance imaging (MRI) scan of a herniated disc, sagittal view. T1-weighted image (*left*) demonstrates a herniated disc (*arrow*) at the L5–S1 level. The T2-weighted image (*right*) shows loss of the normal white signal within the nucleus pulposus (*arrow*), a sign of degenerative disc disease. (From Boden SD, Davis DO, Dina TS, et al. Abnormal lumbar spine MRI scans in asymptomatic subjects: A prospective investigation. J Bone Joint Surg. 1990;72A:403–408. Reprinted with permission.) (b) MRI scan of a herniated disc, axial view. T1-weighted image at the L5–S1 disc space demonstrates a large, central herniated disc with lateral displacement of both S1 nerve roots and posterior displacement of the cauda equine. (From Boden S, Wiesel SW, Laws E, et al. *The Aging Spine*. Philadelphia, PA: Saunders; 1991. Reprinted with permission)

Myelography

Myelography is employed for evaluating neural compression when an MRI cannot be used. Dye is injected into the dural sac and mixes with the spinal fluid. The outline of the contents of the spinal canal can be visualized on X-ray; any extradural mass, such as a herniated disc, will show up as a filling defect in the dye column (Fig. 7.7), while an intrathecal mass will appear as an outward protrusion.

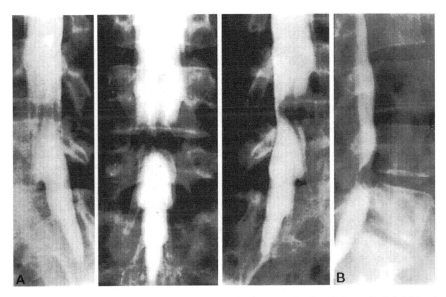

Fig. 7.7 This metrizamide myelogram illustrates a large central disc herniation at the L4–L5 level. (**a**) Anterior–posterior and oblique views reveal this prominent defect more marked on the *right*. (**b**) This lateral view illustrates a "double-density" prominent ventral indentation of the dye column. (From Rothman RH, Simeone FA. *The Spine*, 2nd ed. Philadelphia, PA: Saunders; 1982. Reprinted with permission)

The myelogram is an invasive procedure and should not be taken lightly. Complications include severe headache, nausea, vomiting and, although rare, even seizures. Prior to the utilization of the water-soluble dye metrizamide, the oil-based agent Pantopaque had a much higher incidence of complications and was known to cause a crippling arachnoiditis. Newer contrast agents are now available that are reported to have fewer side effects.

Computed Tomography

Computed tomography is a very versatile and widely available noninvasive modality for evaluating abnormalities of the lumbosacral spine. Multiple cross-sectional (axial) images of the spine are made at various levels and, with reformatting, coronal, sagittal, and three-dimensional images may be created. The CT scan demonstrates not only the bony spinal configuration, but also the soft tissue in graded shading, so that ligaments, nerve roots, free fat, and intervertebral disc protrusions can be evaluated as they relate to their bony environment (Figs. 7.8 and 7.9).

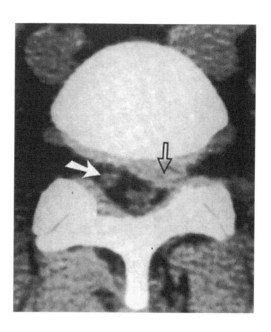

Fig. 7.8 Posterolateral disc herniation. A posterolateral disc herniation at L5–S1 on the left (*open arrow*) is encroaching on epidural fat and compressing the S1 nerve root. Notice the uninvolved S1 nerve root on the right (*white arrow*), which is surrounded by epidural fat. (From Kricun ME. *Imaging Modalities in Spinal Disorders*. Philadelphia, PA: Saunders, 1988. Reprinted with permission)

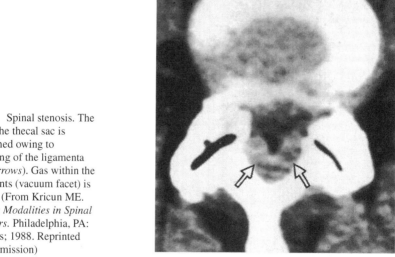

Fig. 7.9 Spinal stenosis. The size of the thecal sac is diminished owing to thickening of the ligamenta flava (*arrows*). Gas within the facet joints (vacuum facet) is evident. (From Kricun ME. *Imaging Modalities in Spinal Disorders*. Philadelphia, PA: Saunders; 1988. Reprinted with permission)

The CT scan is an extremely valuable diagnostic tool when it is used appropriately to confirm the patient's clinical findings. However, recent studies reveal the pitfalls of making clinical decisions on the basis of isolated CT scan findings. Despite many reports in the literature indicating that CT scanning has a mean accuracy of 90% in symptomatic patients, 34% of asymptomatic patients had abnormal CT scans when reviewed by three independent expert interpreters. The implication is that a patient with a negative history and physical examination for a spinal lesion has a one in three chance of having an abnormal CT scan. If the decision for surgery is based only on scan results, there is a 30% chance that the patient will undergo an unnecessary and unsuccessful operation. However, if the patient's clinical picture correlates with the CT scan abnormalities, CT can be a useful confirmatory diagnostic tool.

Electrodiagnostic Testing

The EMG is performed by placing needles into muscles to determine if there is an intact nerve supply to that muscle. An abnormal EMG can demonstrate impaired nerve transmission to a specific muscle and isolate the nerve root involved. Initially, the EMG will be negative in spite of nerve entrapment and will only show muscle irritability. After 3 weeks of significant pressure on a nerve root, signs of denervation with fibrillation can be observed.

The EMG, like all of the other confirmatory tests already discussed, is not a screening tool. In fact, when dealing with the average low back problem, the EMG rarely provides any information that cannot be derived from a careful physical examination. It may even confuse the picture, since an EMG may be abnormal from diabetic neuropathy, previous peripheral nerve entrapment, or trauma. In cases in which the correlation of clinical signs and imaging is equivocal, especially with chronic unexpected sciatica, nerve conduction studies and EMG may be helpful. Electromyography can also detect the involvement of a secondary nerve root in cases of complex back injury preoperatively, sometimes prompting a more extensive operation.

Clinical Conditions

There are a number of conditions that can present as low back pain in any particular individual. However, the following four are the most common of those typically evaluated by orthopedic surgeons and will be discussed in detail: back strain, herniated disc, spinal stenosis, and spondylolisthesis.

Back Strain-Lumbago

The vast majority of people who have low back discomfort suffer from a nonradiating type of low back pain called back sprain or lumbago. The etiology is not always clear, but is probably a ligamentous or muscular strain secondary to either a specific traumatic episode or the continuous mechanical stress of a postural inad-equacy. These may also include patients with a small tear in the annulus fibrosus, which would account for the frequent prior history of low back pain in patients with a ruptured disc.

These patients' main complaint is back pain and it can be limited to one spot or cover a diffuse area of the lumbosacral spine. At times, there may be a refer-ral of pain to the buttocks or posterior thigh since the lower back, buttocks, and posterior thigh all originate from the same embryonic tissue, or mesoderm. Such referral of pain does not necessarily connote any mechanical compression of the neural elements and should not be called sciatica.

The usual findings are limited to local tenderness over the involved area and muscle spasm; however, the attacks will vary in intensity and can conveniently be divided into three categories: mild, moderate, and severe. Those placed in the mild group have subjective pain without objective findings and should be able to return to customary activity in less than a week. The moderate group is characterized by a limited range of spinal motion and paravertebral muscle spasm as well as pain and these patients should be able to resume full activity in less than 2 weeks. The severe group includes those patients who are tilted forward or to the side. They have trouble ambulating and can take up to 3 weeks to become functional again.

Since a normal X-ray is a standard occurrence with a patient complaining of back strain, a radiographic study is usually not necessary on the first visit if the physician feels comfortable with the diagnosis; however, if the response to treatment does not proceed as expected, films should be taken to rule out other more serious problems such as spondylolisthesis or tumor. The authors' usual recommendation is that if a patient fails to respond to conservative treatment for an acute attack of low back pain after a period of 2 weeks, then a routine lumbosacral spine X-ray series is clinically indicated.

The authors' preferred treatment for low back strain is the functional restoration approach. The mainstay of treatment is controlled physical activity, with the judi-cious use of trunk flexibility and strengthening exercises as the acute phase subsides. Often, particularly in the obese patient with weak abdominal muscles, a lightweight lumbosacral corset is useful in helping to mobilize those encumbered by low back strain.

Herniated Disc

A herniated disc can be defined as the herniation of the nucleus pulposus through the torn fibers of the annulus fibrosus. Most disc ruptures occur during the third and fourth decades of life while the nucleus pulposus is still gelatinous. The per-forations usually arise through a defect just lateral to the posterior midline where the posterior longitudinal ligament is weakest. The two most common levels for disc herniation are L4–L5 and L5–S1. These two discs account for 95% of all lum-bar disc herniations; pathology at the L2–L3 and L3–L4 levels can occur, but is relatively uncommon.

Disc herniations at L5–S1 will usually compromise the first sacral nerve root. A lesion at the L4–L5 level will most often compress the fifth lumbar root, while a herniation at the L3–L4 more commonly involves the fourth lumbar root. It should be pointed out, however, that variations in root configuration as well as in the position of the herniation itself can modify these relationships. An L4–L5 disc rupture can at times affect the first sacral as well as the fifth lumbar root and, in extreme lateral herniations, the nerve ending exiting at the same level as the disc will be involved.

Not everyone with a disc herniation has significant discomfort. A large herniation in a capacious canal may not be clinically significant since there is no compression of the neural elements, while a minor protrusion in a small canal may be crippling since there is not enough room to accommodate both the disc and the nerve root.

Clinically, the patient's major complaint is pain. Although there may be a prior history of intermittent episodes of localized low back pain, this is not always the case. The pain not only is present in the back, but also radiates down the leg in the distribution of the affected nerve root. It will usually be described as sharp or lancinating, progressing from the top downward in the involved leg. Its onset may be insidious or sudden and associated with a tearing or snapping sensation in the spine. Occasionally, when the sciatica develops, the back pain may resolve since once the annulus has ruptured, it may no longer be under tension. Finally, the sciatica may vary in intensity; it may be so severe that patients will be unable to ambulate and will feel that their back is "locked." Conversely, the pain may be limited to a dull ache that increases in intensity with ambulation.

On physical examination, there is usually a decreased range of motion in flexion, and patients will tend to drift away from the involved side as they bend. On ambulation, the patient walks with an antalgic gait, holding the involved leg flexed so as to put as little weight as possible on the extremity.

Although neurologic examination may yield objective evidence of nerve root compression, these findings are often undependable since the involved nerve is often still functional. In addition, such deficit may have little temporal relevance since it may relate to a prior attack at a different level. To be significant, reflex changes, weakness, atrophy, or sensory loss must conform to the rest of the clinical picture.

When the first sacral root is compressed, the patient may have gastrocnemius-soleus weakness and be unable to repeatedly rise up on the toes of that foot. Atrophy of the calf may be apparent and the ankle (Achilles) reflex is often diminished or absent. Sensory loss, if any, is usually confined to the posterior aspect of the calf and lateral side of the foot.

Involvement of the fifth lumbar nerve root can lead to weakness in extension of the great toe and, less often, to weakness of the evertors and dorsiflexors of the foot. An associated sensory deficit can appear over the anterior leg and the dorsomedial aspect of the foot down to the great toe. There are usually no primary reflex changes, but, on occasion, a diminution in the posterior tibial reflex can be elicited. The absence of this reflex, however, must be asymmetrical for it to have any clinical significance.

With compression of the fourth lumbar nerve root, the quadriceps muscle is affected. The patient may note weakness in knee extension, and it is often associated with instability. Atrophy of the thigh musculature can be marked. A sensory loss may be apparent over the anteromedial aspect of the thigh and the patellar tendon reflex is usually diminished.

Nerve root sensitivity can be elicited by any method that creates tension; however, the SLRT is the one most commonly employed. As discussed before, a positive test reproduces the patient's pain down the leg. The reproduction of back pain is not considered positive.

The initial diagnosis of a herniated disc is ordinarily made on the basis of the history and physical examination. Plain X-rays of the lumbosacral spine will rarely add to the diagnosis, but should be obtained to help rule out other causes of pain, such as infection or tumor. Other tests such as the EMG, the computerized axial tomography (CAT) scan, and MRI are confirmatory by nature and can be misinformative when they are used as screening devices.

The treatment for most patients with a herniated disc is nonoperative since 80% of them will respond to conservative therapy when followed over a period of 5 years. The efficacy of nonoperative treatment, however, depends upon a healthy relationship between a capable physician and a well-informed patient. If a patient has insight into the rationale for the prescribed treatment and follows instructions, the chances of success are greatly increased.

One of the most important elements in the nonoperative treatment is controlled physical activity. Patients should markedly decrease their activity. This will sometimes require bed rest and in most cases can be accomplished at home. An acute herniation usually takes at least 2 weeks of significant rest before the pain substantially eases.

Drug therapy is another important part of the treatment and three categories of pharmacological agents are commonly used: antiinflammatory drugs, analgesics, and muscles relaxants or tranquilizers. Inasmuch as the symptoms of low back pain and sciatica result from an inflammatory reaction as well as mechanical compression, the authors feel that antiinflammatory medication should be taken in conjunction with rest. It should be stressed, however, that no medication can take the place of controlled physical activity. The patient's pain generally will be relieved once the inflammation is brought under control. There may be some numbness or tingling in the involved extremity, but this is usually tolerable.

Analgesic medication is rarely needed if the patient really rests, since the pain is usually adequately controlled by decreased activity.

There is some question as to whether there actually is a muscle relaxant; all drugs that are so designated probably act to some degree as tranquilizers. If one is required, though, methocarbamol and carisoprodol are the ones most frequently used and they can be employed intravenously as well as orally. The use of diazepam (Valium) for this purpose should be discouraged since it is actually a depressant and often will add to the patient's psychological problems.

Eighty percent of those who follow the above regimen will be markedly improved, but it requires patience since frequently at least 6 weeks will have passed before any additional therapy is indicated. Although the noninvasive treatment of a herniated disc can be quite gratifying, it generally takes a significant period of rest and the patient must be aware of the time constraints from the beginning in order to understand the rationale behind the measures employed.

The long-term prognosis for patients with disc herniation is quite good. It has been shown that between 85 and 90% of surgically treated and nonsurgically treated patients were asymptomatic at 4 years. Less than 2% of both groups were symptomatic at 10 years.

Spinal Stenosis

Spinal stenosis can be defined as a narrowing of the spinal canal and the mechanical pressure on the neural structures within will depend upon the degree of narrowing. Every person's spine, however, becomes narrower with age due to osteoarthritis. Not everyone with a narrowed spinal canal, however, will have symptoms.

For those who do suffer, the discomfort can vary from mild annoyance to an inability to walk. The symptom complex is well documented. Patients of either sex, usually not before their fifth decade, will first complain of vague pains, dysesthesias, and paresthesias with ambulation, but will typically have excellent relief of their symptoms when they are sitting or lying supine. The increased lordotic stance assumed when walking, and particularly walking down grades, is most likely the inciting cause. The hyperextension further narrows the spinal canal and increases the symptoms.

With maturation of the syndrome, symptoms may even occur at rest. Muscle weakness, atrophy, and asymmetrical reflex changes may then appear; however, as long as the symptoms are only aggravated dynamically, neurological changes will occur only after the patient is stressed. The following stress tests can be used in an outpatient clinic: after a neurological examination has been performed on the patient, he or she is asked to walk up and down the corridor until symptoms occur or the patient has walked 300 feet. A repeat examination is then done and in many cases the second examination will be positive for a focal neurologic deficit when the first was negative. Plain X-rays are often helpful in visualizing spinal stenosis, particularly degenerative spinal stenosis. One can see intervertebral disc degeneration, decreased interpedicular distance, a decreased sagittal canal diameter, and facet degeneration. If a patient fails conservative treatment and becomes a surgical candidate, the location and degree of neurological compression can be assessed with MRI or CT scan/myelogram.

The majority of patients with spinal stenosis, especially the degenerative and combined variety, can be treated nonsurgically with antiinflammatory medication.

Finally, a lumbosacral corset is often helpful in reminding the patient to avoid excessive motion. Symptoms are usually intermittent and the individual often needs encouragement in getting through the episode without getting depressed. Nonoperative management is preferable as long as the pain is tolerable.

Spondylolisthesis

Spondylolisthesis is a spinal condition where all or part of a vertebra has slipped forward on another. The word is derived from the Greek *spondylos*, meaning "vertebra," and *olisthesis*, meaning "to slip." There are several different types of spondylolisthesis, but the most common is that in which the lesion is in the isthmus or pars interarticularis. If a defect can be identified, but no slipping has occurred, the condition is termed spondylolysis; if one vertebra has slipped forward on another (horizontal translation), it is referred to as spondylolisthesis.

The etiology of the defect in spondylolysis is not clear. Although there may be a hereditary component, the lesion is seldom seen in patients under the age of 5 and is found in 5% of people over the age of 17. The most attractive explanation is that although these children inherit a potential deficiency in the pars, they are not born with any identifiable defect. Between the ages of 5 and 17, however, they become more active and a stress fracture, caused by repetitive hyperextension stresses, can develop into a spondylolysis. It is likely that most of these fractures occur during the period of rapid growth known as the adolescent growth spurt and they are particularly prevalent in gymnasts and football players.

Spondylolisthesis has several characteristic features, but the forward displacement is easily recognized radiographically on the lateral projection (Figs. 7.10 and 7.11). The degree of slip varies from patient to patient and can range from minimal displacement to complete dislocation of the vertebral body. Increased slipping

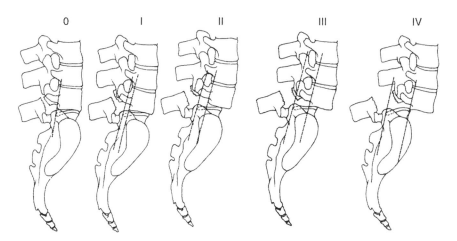

Fig. 7.10 Grading system for spondylolisthesis. (From Borenstein DG, Wiesel SW. *Low Back Pain: Medical Diagnosis and Comprehensive Management*. Philadelphia, PA: Saunders; 1989. Reprinted with permission)

Fig. 7.11 Lateral spot view
of the lumbosacral junction.
A grade I spondylolisthesis is
present with 25% slippage of
the superior vertebral body
(*black arrow*). This view
demonstrates a Type II
spondylolisthesis with a pars
defect (*white arrow*). (From
Borenstein DG, Wiesel SW.
*Low Back Pain: Medical
Diagnosis and
Comprehensive Management.*
Philadelphia, PA: Saunders;
1989. Reprinted with
permission)

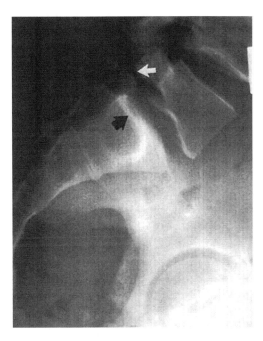

rarely occurs after the age of 20 unless there has been a severe superimposed injury or surgical intervention. The period of most rapid progression coincides with the rapid growth spurt between the ages of 9 and 15.

The most common clinical manifestation of spondylolisthesis is low back pain. Although the cause of this type of back pain in the adult has been studied extensively, its origin is still not clear. There is no clear understanding of how so many patients develop this lesion between the ages of 5 and 17, but still have no back complaints until perhaps age 35, when a sudden twisting or lifting motion will precipitate an acute episode of back and leg pain. Other patients with significant degrees of slipping, however, will go through life with no discomfort.

Although 50% of patients overall normally cannot associate an injury with the onset of the symptoms of those working in industry, almost all report an associated incident. It is possible to sustain an acute fracture of the pars, but it is a very rare occurrence. If the acuity of a pars defect is in question, it can be documented by a bone scan within 3 months of the injury; if the defect is long-standing, the scan will be negative.

There is also frequently a buildup of a fibrocartilaginous mass at the defect and this can cause pain by irritating the nerve root as it exits. It is thus not unusual in spondylolisthesis to have the patient first complain of back pain, but over time have leg pain develop as the most annoying part of the problem.

Once the symptoms begin, the patient usually has constant low-grade back discomfort that is aggravated by activity and relieved by rest. There are some periods during which the pain is more intense than others, but unless the picture is compli-cated by severe leg pain, total incapacitation is rare. The patients are seldom aware of any sensory or motor deficit. At this point, it should be reemphasized that in some people even severe displacement is asymptomatic and gives rise to no disability. It is not uncommon to pick up a previously unrecognized spondylolisthesis on a routine gastrointestinal radiological study of a 50-year-old patient.

The physical findings of this syndrome are fairly characteristic. In the absence of any radicular pain, the patient exhibits no postural scoliosis; but there is usually an exaggeration of the lumbar lordosis and a palpable "stepoff" with a dimple at the side of the abnormality. Occasionally, mild muscle spasm is demonstrable and, in most instances, some local tenderness can be elicited. Although the range of motion is usually complete, some pain can be expected on hyperextension.

Radiographs, particularly the lateral views, confirm the diagnosis. Even the slightest amount of forward slipping of the body of the involved vertebra is readily discernible and the oblique views will disclose the actual defect in the pars.

The nonoperative treatment of the adult with spondylolisthesis is much the same as that used for backache from other causes. When the symptoms are acute, rest is indicated. If leg pain is a significant problem, then antiinflammatory medication can be quite beneficial. Exercises, usually a flexion-extension program, should be started once patients are in remission and they are usually advised to own a corset for use during occasional strenuous activity. If conservative treatment is not successful, an operative approach can be considered and would include a spinal fusion.

Lumbar Spine Algorithm

As with patients with neck pain, the task of the physician when confronted with low back pain patients is to integrate their complaints into an accurate diagnosis and to prescribe appropriate therapy. This problem (universe of low back pain patients) has been formatted into an algorithm (Fig. 7.12), the aim of which is to select the correct diagnostic category and proper treatment avenues for each patient with low back pain. A specific patient may fall outside the limits of the algorithm and require a different approach and the physician must constantly be on the alert for excep-tions. The algorithm can be followed in sequence and is also presented in table form (Table 7.4).

The information necessary to use the algorithm is initially obtained through the history and physical examination. The key points in the history are differentiation of back pain that is mechanical in nature from nonmechanical pain that is present at rest, detecting changes in bowel or bladder function and defining the precise location and quality of the pain. The physical examination must be oriented toward ruling out other medical causes of low back pain, assessing neurologic function, and evaluating for the presence of tension signs.

Following the low back pain algorithm, the first major decision is to make a ruling on the presence or absence of CEC syndrome. Mechanical compression of the cauda

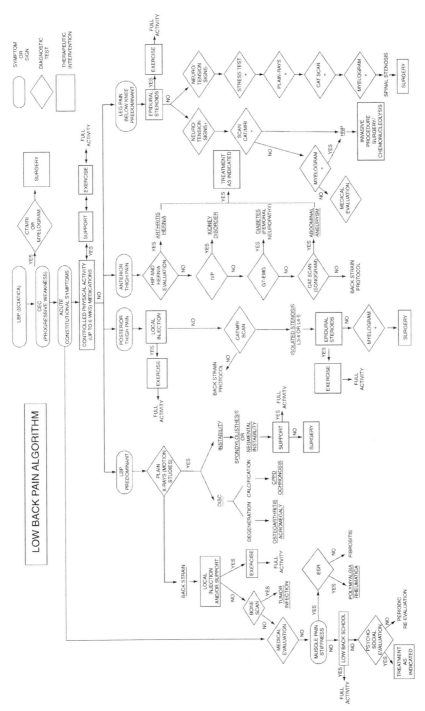

Fig. 7.12 Algorithm for the differential diagnosis of low back pain. (From Boden S, Wiesel SW, Laws E, et al. *The Aging Spine*. Philadelphia, PA: Saunders; 1991. Reprinted with permission)

Table 7.4 Differential diagnosis of low back pain

Evaluation	Back strain	Herniated nucleus pulposus	Spinal stenosis	Spondylo-listhesis/instability	Spondylo-athropathy	Infection	Tumor	Metabolic	Hematologic	Visceral
Predominant pain (arm vs. neck)	Back	Leg (below knee)	Back/leg	Back	Back	Back	Back	Back	Back	Back (buttock, thigh)
Constitutional symptoms					+	+	+	+	+	
Tension sign		+		±						
Neurologic exam		±	± after stress							
Plain X-rays			+	+	+	±	±	+	+	
Lateral motion X-rays				+						
CT/MRI		+	+			+	+			
Myelogram		+	+							
Bone scan					+	+	+	+	+	
ESR					+	+	+	+	+	+
Serum chemistries							+	+	+	+

Ca/P/alk phos calcium, phosphate, and alkaline phosphatase, *CT* computerized tomography, *MRI* magnetic resonance imaging, *CAT* computerized axial tomography, *ESR* erythrocyte sedimentation rate

equina, with truly progressive motor weakness, is the only surgical emergency in lumbar spine disease. This compression from a massive rupture of the L4–L5 disc in the midline is usually due to pressure on the caudal sac, through which pass the nerves to the lower extremities, bowel, and bladder.

The signs and symptoms of CEC are a complex mixture of low back pain, bilateral motor weakness of the lower extremities, bilateral sciatica, saddle anesthesia, and even frank paraplegia with bowel and bladder incontinence or urinary retention. Cauda equina compression can be caused by either bone or soft tissue damage, the latter generally a ruptured or herniated disc in the midline. These patients should undergo an immediate definitive diagnostic test and, if it is positive, emergency surgical decompression. Historically, the myelogram was the study used in this setting; however, the development of the MRI has facilitated the noninvasive diagnosis of CEC. The principal reason for prompt surgical intervention is to arrest the progression of neurologic loss; the chance of actual return of lost neurologic function following surgery is small. Although the incidence of CEC syndrome in the entire back pain population is very low, it is the only event that requires immediate operative intervention; if its diagnosis is missed, the consequences can be devastating.

The remaining patients make up the overwhelming majority. They should be started on a course of conservative (nonoperative) therapy regardless of the diagnosis. At this stage the specific diagnosis, whether a herniated disc or a simple back strain, is not important to the therapy because the entire population is treated the same way. A few of these patients will eventually need an invasive procedure (surgery), but at this point there is no way to predict which individuals will respond to conservative therapy and which will not.

Conservative Treatment

The vast majority of this initial group have nonradiating low back pain, termed lumbago or back strain. The etiology of lumbago is not clear. There are several possibilities, including ligamentous or muscular strain, continuous mechanical stress from poor posture, facet joint irritation, or a small tear in the annulus fibrosis. Patients usually complain of pain in the low back, often localized to a single area. On physical examination they demonstrate a decreased range of lumbar spine motion, tenderness to palpation over the involved area, and paraspinal muscle spasm. Their roentgenographic examinations are usually normal, but if therapy is not successful, films should be obtained to rule out other possible etiological factors. Two exceptions to this rule are patients younger than 15 years of age and patients over age 60; X-rays are important early in the diagnostic process because these patients are more likely to have a diagnosis other than back strain (tumor or infection). Other situations warranting X-rays sooner rather than later include a history of serious trauma, known cancer, unexplained weight loss, and fever.

The early stage of the treatment of low back pain (with and without leg pain) is a waiting game. The passage of time, the use of antiinflammatory medication, and controlled physical activity are the modalities proven safest and most effective. The vast majority of these patients will respond to this approach within the first 10 days, although a small percentage will not. In today's society with its emphasis on quick solutions and high technology, many patients are pushed too rapidly toward more complex (i.e., invasive) management. This quick fix approach has no place in the treatment of low back pain. The physician should treat the patient conservatively and wait up to 6 weeks for a response. As already stated, most of these patients will improve within 10 days; a few will take longer.

Once the patients have achieved approximately 80% relief, they should be mobilized with the help of a lightweight, flexible corset. After they are more comfortable and have increased their activity level, they should begin a program of lumbar exercises and return to their normal lifestyles. The pathway along this section of the algorithm is a two-way street: should regression occur with exacerbation of symptoms, the physician can resort to more stringent conservative measures. The patient may require further bed rest. Most acute low back pain patients will proceed along this pathway, returning to their normal life patterns within 2 months of onset of symptoms.

If the initial conservative treatment regimen fails and 6 weeks have passed, symptomatic patients are sorted into four groups. The first group is comprised of people with low back pain predominating. The second group complains mainly of leg pain, defined as pain radiating below the knee and commonly referred to as sciatica. The third group has posterior thigh pain. The fourth group has anterior thigh pain. Each group follows a separate diagnostic pathway.

Refractory Patients with Low Back Pain

Those patients who continue to complain predominantly of low back pain for 6 weeks should have plain X-rays carefully examined for abnormalities. Spondylolysis with and without spondylolisthesis is the most common structural abnormality to cause significant low back pain. Approximately 5% of the population has this defect, thought to be caused by a combination of genetics and environmental stress. In spite of this defect, most people are able to perform their activities of daily living with little or no discomfort. When symptoms are present, these patients will usually respond to nonoperative measures, including a thorough explanation of the problem, a back support, and exercises. In a small percentage of such cases, conservative treatment fails and a fusion of the involved spinal segments becomes necessary. This is one of the few times primary fusion of the lumbar spine is indicated and it must be stressed that it is a relatively infrequent occurrence.

The vast majority of patients with pain predominantly in the low back will have normal plain X-rays. Before there is any additional workup, a local injection of steroids and Xylocaine may be tried at the point of maximum tenderness. This can be quite successful, and if there is a good response, the patient is begun on exercises with gradual resumption of normal activity. In some instances, if there are no objective findings, such a trigger-point injection can be considered as early as the third week after onset of symptoms.

Should the patient not respond to local injection, other pathology must be seriously considered. A bone scan, along with a general medical evaluation, should be obtained. The bone scan is an excellent tool, often identifying early bone tumors or infections not visible on routine radiographic examinations. It is particularly important to obtain this study in the patient with nonmechanical back pain. If the pain is constant, unremitting and unrelieved by postural adjustments, more often than not the correct diagnosis will be one of an occult neoplasm or metabolic disorder not readily apparent from other testing.

Approximately 3% of cases of apparent low back pain that present at orthopedic clinics are attributable to extraspinal causes. A thorough medical search also frequently reveals problems missed earlier such as posterior penetrating ulcer, pancreatitis, renal disease, or abdominal aneurysm. If these diagnostic studies are positive, the patient should be transferred into a nonorthopedic treatment mode and would no longer be in the therapeutic algorithm.

Those patients who have no abnormality on their bone scans and do not show other medical disease as a cause for their back pain are then referred for another type of therapy—low back education. It is believed that many of these patients are suffering from discogenic pain or facet joint pain syndrome. The low back education concept has as its basis the belief that patients with low back pain, given proper education and understanding of their disease, can often return to a productive and functional life. Ergonomics, the proper and efficient use of the spine in work and recreation, is stressed. Back education need not be an expensive proposition. It can be a one-time classroom session with a review of back problems and a demonstration of exercises with patient participation. This type of educational process has proved to be very effective. It is most important, however, that before patients are referred to this type of program, they be thoroughly screened. One does not want to be in the position of treating a metastatic tumor in a classroom.

If low back education is not successful, the patient should undergo a thorough psychosocial evaluation in an attempt to explain the failure of the previous treatments. This is predicated on the knowledge that a patient's ability is related not only to his or her pathologic anatomy, but also to the patient's perception of pain and stability in relation to the social environment. It is quite common to see a stable patient with a frank herniated disc continue working—regarding the disability as only a minor problem—while a hysterical patient takes to bed at the slightest twinge of low back discomfort.

Drug habituation, depression, alcoholism, and other psychiatric problems are seen frequently in association with back pain. If the evaluation suggests any of these problems, proper measures should be instituted to overcome the disability. There are a surprising number of ambulatory patients addicted to commonly prescribed medications using complaints of back pain as an excuse to obtain these drugs. Oxycodone (Percodan) and diazepam, alone or in combination, are the two most popular offenders. Oxycodone is truly addictive; diazepam is both habituating and depressing. Since the complaint of low back pain may be a common manifestation of depression, it is counterproductive to treat such patients with diazepam.

Approximately 2% of patients who initially present with low back pain will fail treatment and elude any diagnosis. There will be no evidence of any structural problem in the back or criteria for any underlying medical disease or psychiatric disorder. This is a very difficult group to manage. The authors' strategy has been to discontinue narcotics, reassure patients, and periodically reevaluate them. Over time, one-third of these patients will be found to have an underlying medical disease; thus, one cannot abandon this group and discontinue treatment. For the remainder, as much physical activity as possible should be encouraged.

Refractory Patients with Sciatica

The next group of patients consists of those with sciatica, which is pain radiating below the knee. These patients usually experience their symptoms secondary to mechanical pressure and inflammation of the nerve roots that originate in the back and extend down the leg. The etiology of the mechanical pressure can be soft tissue—herniated disc, bone, or a combination of the two.

At this point in the algorithm, the patient has had up to 6 weeks of controlled physical activity and medication, but still has persistent leg pain. The next therapeutic step is an epidural steroid injection, which is performed on an outpatient basis. An epidural injection is worth trying; the chance of success is 40% and morbidity is low, particularly compared with the next treatment step—surgery. The maximum benefit from a single injection is achieved at 2 weeks. The injection may have to be repeated once or twice and four to 6 weeks should pass before its success or failure is judged.

If epidural steroids are effective in alleviating patients' leg pain or sciatica, they are begun on a program of back exercises and encouraged to return promptly to as normal a lifestyle as possible. Should the epidural steroids prove ineffective, and 3 months have passed since the initial injury without relief of pain, some type of invasive treatment should be considered. The patient group is then divided into those with probable herniated discs and those with symptoms secondary to spinal stenosis.

The physician must now carefully reevaluate the patient for a neurologic deficit and for a positive tension sign or SLRT. For those who have either a neurologic deficit or positive tension signs along with continued leg pain, an MRI scan should be obtained. If the MRI scan is clearly positive and correlates with the clinical findings, there is no need for myelography since it is invasive.

As in the cervical spine, there is repeated documentation that for surgery to be effective in treatment of a herniated disc, the surgeon must find unequivocal operative evidence of a nerve root compression. Accordingly, nerve root compression must be firmly substantiated preoperatively, not only by neurologic examination, but also by radiographic data. There is no place for "exploratory" back surgery. Many asymptomatic patients have been found to have abnormal myelograms, EMGs, CT scans, and MRI scans. If the patient has neither a neurologic deficit nor a positive SLRT, then regardless of radiographic findings there is not enough evidence of root compression to proceed with successful surgery. These patients without objective findings are the ones who have poor results and who have given back surgery a bad name.

If there are no objective findings, the physician should avoid surgery and proceed to the psychosocial evaluation. Exceptions should be few and far between. When sympathy for the patient's complaints outweighs the objective evaluation, surgery is fraught with difficulties. For those who meet these specific criteria for lumbar laminectomy, results will be satisfactory: 95% of them can expect a good-to-excellent result.

The second group of patients whose symptoms are based on mechanical pressure on the neural elements are those with spinal stenosis. The diagnosis of spinal stenosis usually can be inferred from the plain X-rays which will demonstrate facet degeneration, disc degeneration, and decreased interpedicular and sagittal canal diameters. A CT scan and/or MRI can confirm the diagnosis (Figs. 7.13 and 7.14). If symptoms are severe, and there is radiographic evidence of spinal stenosis, surgery is appropriate. Age alone is not a deterrent to surgery; many elderly people who are in good health except for a narrow spinal canal will benefit greatly from adequate decompression of the lumbar spine.

Refractory Patients with Anterior Thigh Pain

A small percentage of patients will have pain that radiates from the back into the anterior thigh. This usually is relieved with rest and antiinflammatory medication. If the discomfort persists after 6 weeks of treatment, a workup should be initiated to

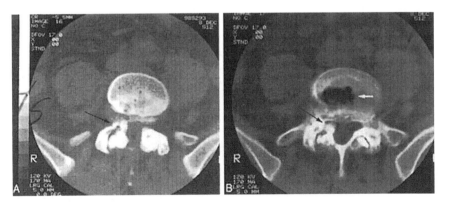

Fig. 7.13 Computerized tomography scan of a 68-year-old man with back pain that is exacerbated with standing. Cross-sectional views demonstrate vacuum phenomenon in intervertebral disc (*white arrow*) and facet hypertrophy (most prominent on the *right*), resulting in canal stenosis at multiple levels (*black arrows*). The patient's symptoms responded to epidural steroid injections. (From Borenstein DG, Boden S, Wiesel SW. *Low Back Pain: Medical Diagnosis and Comprehensive Management.* 2nd ed. Philadelphia, PA: Saunders; 1995. Reprinted with permission)

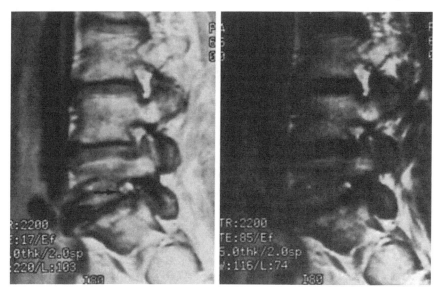

Fig. 7.14 Magnetic resonance imaging of the lumbar spine. Sagittal view of a T2-weighted image demonstrating foraminal narrowing at L5–S1 interspace (*black arrow*) with associated intervertebral disc degeneration. (From Borenstein DG, Boden S, Wiesel SW. *Low Back Pain: Medical Diagnosis and Comprehensive Management*. 2nd ed. Philadelphia, PA: Saunders; 1995. Reprinted with permission)

search for underlying pathology. Although an upper lumbar radiculopathy can cause anterior thigh pain, several other entities must be considered.

A hip problem or hernia can be ruled out with a thorough physical examination. If the hip examination is positive, radiographs should be obtained. An intravenous pyelogram is useful to evaluate the urinary tract, because kidney stones often may present as anterior thigh pain. Peripheral neuropathy, most commonly secondary to diabetes, also can present initially with anterior thigh pain; a glucose tolerance test as well as an EMG will reveal the underlying problem. Finally, a retroperitoneal tumor can cause symptoms by mechanically pressing on the nerves that innervate the anterior thighs. A CT or MRI scan of the retroperitoneal area will eliminate or confirm this possibility.

If any of the entities reviewed above is diagnosed, the patient is treated accordingly. If no physical cause can be found for the anterior thigh pain, the patient is treated for recalcitrant back strain by the method already outlined.

Refractory Patients with Posterior Thigh Pain

This final group of patients will complain of back pain with radiation into the buttocks and posterior thighs. Most of them will be relieved of their symptoms with 6 weeks of conservative therapy. However, if their pain persists after the initial treatment period, they can be considered to have back strain and given a trigger-point injection of steroids and Xylocaine in the area of maximum tenderness.

If the injection is unsuccessful, it is necessary to distinguish between referred and radicular pain.

As noted earlier, referred pain is pain in the mesodermal tissues of the same embryologic origin. The muscles, tendons, and ligaments of the buttocks and posterior thigh have the same embryologic origin as those of the low back. When the low back is injured, the pain may be referred to the posterior thigh, where it is perceived by the patient. Referred pain from irritated soft tissues cannot be cured with a surgical procedure.

Radicular pain is caused by compression of an inflamed nerve root along the anatomic course of the nerve. A herniated disc or spinal stenosis in the high lumbar area can cause radiation or pain into the posterior thigh. An MRI or CT scan and an EMG may be used in this situation to differentiate radicular etiology from referred pain or a peripheral nerve lesion. If the studies are within normal limits, the patient is considered to have back strain and treated according to the algorithm. If a radicular abnormality is found, the patient is diagnosed as having mechanical compression on the neural elements either from a herniated disc or spinal stenosis. Epidural steroids should be tried first; if these do not provide adequate relief, surgery should be contemplated.

This group of patients with unexplained posterior thigh pain is very difficult to treat. The biggest mistake made is the performance of surgery on people thought to have radicular pain who actually have referred pain. Again, referred pain in this setting is not responsive to surgery.

In most instances, the treatment of low back pain is no longer a mystery. The algorithm described here presents a series of easy-to-follow and clearly defined decision-making processes. Use of this algorithm provides patients with the most helpful diagnostic and therapeutic measures at the optimal time. It neither denies them helpful surgery nor subjects them to procedures that are useless technical exercises.

Conservative Treatment Modalities

As the algorithm indicates, all low back pain patients, regardless of diagnosis (except those with CEC syndrome), require an initial period of conservative therapy. At present, there are many modalities available, but few have been scientifically validated because of the difficulty in performing a prospective double-blind study in this field. Each treatment plan in popular use today is surrounded by conflicting claims for its indications and efficacy. The purpose of this section is to discuss the rationale behind the use of some of the more common therapeutic measures.

Bed Rest (Controlled Physical Activity)

Decreased activity has evolved over the years as one of the most important elements in the treatment of low back pain. The degree of rest depends on the severity of the symptoms and can vary from complete bed rest to just a decrease in active exercise.

The amount of rest prescribed varies for each patient; these people should not be mobilized until reasonably comfortable. The type of pathology will determine the duration of rest required. Most patients with acute back strain will need only 2–7 days of bed rest before they can ambulate. However, a patient with an acute herniated disc may require up to 1 week of complete bed rest with another 10 days for gradual mobilization. Complete bed rest for long periods (more than 2 weeks) has a deleterious effect on the body in general and should be closely monitored. As their discomfort eases, the patient should be strongly encouraged to take short walks, but to do as little sitting as possible. Each patient should be followed carefully and not allowed complete mobility until the objective signs, such as a list and/or paravertebral muscle spasm, disappear. The patient's physical activity is tailored to increase movement without incurring a return of symptoms.

The purpose of controlled physical activity is to allow any inflammatory reaction that is present to subside. Bed rest will not result in the disc's return to its original position. However, as the disc herniates, it causes a secondary inflammatory process responsible for the patient's pain; if this reaction can be brought under control, the patient's symptoms will disappear. This relief may or may not be permanent.

Drug Therapy

The judicious use of drug therapy is an important adjunct in the treatment of low back pain. As in the cervical spine, there are three main categories of drugs in common use: antiinflammatories, analgesics, and muscle relaxants.

Antiinflammatory agents are employed because of the belief that inflammation within the affected tissues is a major cause of pain in the low back. This is especially true for those patients with symptoms secondary to a herniated disc.

There are a variety of NSAIDs available. Based on several scientific studies, none of these appear to be superior to the others. Most patients will get significant relief. Again, all antiinflammatory medications are utilized in conjunction with controlled physical activity to relieve pain; they do not replace adequate rest. Occasionally, after an initial recovery, a patient will experience intermittent recurrent attacks or complain of a chronic low backache; in some instances these patients will be helped by a maintenance dose of an antiinflammatory drug.

Analgesic medication is very important during the acute phase of low back pain. The goal is to keep the patient comfortable while in bed. Most of the antiinflammatory agents also have analgesic properties. In more severe cases, patients will respond to 30–60 mg of codeine every 4–6 h. As the pain decreases, nonnarcotic analgesics may be substituted for the more potent drugs.

The biggest mistake seen is treatment with very strong narcotics such as meperidine (Demerol) or oxycodone (Percodan, Tylox) on an outpatient basis. Many of these patients become addicted to the medication. In other cases, patients try to shortcut the controlled physical activity and use analgesic medication instead. This, of course, will not work and when the patient tries to stop the drug, the back pain returns.

Muscle relaxants generally are not recommended for the treatment of low back pain. In most cases, the muscle spasm is secondary to a primary problem such as a herniated disc. If the pain from the ruptured disc can be controlled, the muscle spasm will usually subside.

Occasionally, muscle spasm will be so severe that some type of treatment is required. Carisoprodol (Soma), methocarbamol (Robaxin), or cyclobenzaprine (Flexeril) are the drugs recommended. Diazepam (Valium) should be discouraged since it is actually a physiological depressant and depression is often an integral feature of back pain syndromes. Administering diazepam to depressed patients only increases their problems. If anxiety is prominent and a sedative is needed, phenobarbital will alleviate the symptoms.

In summary, drug therapy for low back pain should be viewed as an adjunct to adequately controlled physical activity. Antiinflammatory medication should be the primary agent employed. Analgesic medication should be used selectively in a controlled environment and not for extended periods. Muscle relaxants are generally not recommended and, if employed, should be carefully monitored.

Trigger-Point Injection

Trigger-point therapy is indicated for nonradiating low back pain when a point of maximal tenderness can be identified. This procedure involves the injection of steroids and Xylocaine at an area of maximal tenderness in the low back. The precise mechanism of action is not clear, but may be related to modulation of peripheral nerve stimulation as it affects the afferent input perceived as pain.

Trigger-point therapy is easy to perform, has a negligible risk, and may help certain patients. Further controlled research is required to delineate the true value of this modality in the treatment of low back pain.

Epidural Steroid Injection

Epidural steroid injections are indicated for severe lumbar radiculopathy, not, in most cases, for nonradiating low back pain. They have generally been viewed as an intermediate form of treatment between conservative and surgical management. It is a more aggressive attempt at pain relief after conservative therapy has failed, yet avoids the disadvantages of surgery. The rationale for this therapy is that lumbar radiculopathy (in the early phase) involves a significant inflammatory component, evoked by chemical or mechanical irritation or an autoimmune response—all of which should be amenable to treatment with corticosteroid drugs in the early stages.

Unfortunately, few studies have systematically and accurately studied the efficacy of this treatment modality. Poorly controlled, nonrandomized studies have yielded controversial results with a range of success rates from 25 to 75%. Another problem is that some studies have attempted to determine the efficacy of epidural steroids compared to epidural saline injection, while others have compared their results to a true placebo.

Despite the lack of optimally designed investigations, upon review of the literature, certain trends seem to be evident. Epidural steroids appear to be more beneficial in acute rather than chronic radiculopathy, especially when no neurologic deficit is present. Improvement may not be noted until 3–6 days after injection and may be only temporary. No neurotoxicity has been reported in humans or animal models; complications stem from the technique of epidural injection and are rare. Suppression of plasma corticosteroid concentration may occur up to 3 weeks following the injection.

The authors maintain that epidural steroids may be helpful in relieving some component of radicular pain in 40% of patients. Until controlled investigations indicate otherwise, this is a treatment worth trying in patients who have failed 6 weeks of conservative management in an effort to avoid a major invasive procedure.

Traction

The application of traction to the lumbar spine is a popular treatment for patients with herniated discs. The theory is that stretching the lumbar spine distracts the vertebrae so that the protruded disc is allowed to return to a more normal anatomic position. In fact, the disc material probably does not change position at all. Scientific evidence indicates that a traction force equal to 60% of body weight is needed just to reduce the intradiscal pressure at the third lumbar vertebra by 25%. Such a force could not practically be applied to a patient. Furthermore, there has never been any proof that disc material returns to its normal position following herniation.

Traction can be applied as gravity lumbar traction, autotraction, and through motorized techniques. None of these methods has been proven to be more effective than the others. While a few studies have shown traction to have a short-lived benefit on sciatica patients, most double-blind studies have not demonstrated any positive effect. In one study, two groups of patients with proven herniated discs (by myelogram) were treated by applying traction apparatuses to each group in the hospital. However, for one group there were weights in the traction bag; for the other, no weights. There was no statistically significant difference between the two groups in terms of relief of symptoms. Traction had no effect on spinal mobility, tension signs, deep tendon reflexes, paresis, or sensory deficit and although it usually was well tolerated, it made some patients worse.

Manipulation

Spinal manipulation is another popular conservative modality in treating low back pain. In the United States, it is somewhat controversial because it is performed mostly by chiropractors. The principle involved is that any malalignment of the spinal structures can be corrected by manipulation; the assumption here is that the malalignment is the etiology of the patient's pain. Unfortunately, there is no scientific proof for or against either the efficacy of this therapy or its pathophysiological foundation.

The authors' experience is that some patients do have short periods of symptomatic relief after manipulation, but must keep returning for repeated sessions to maintain it, substantially increasing the cost of treatment. Some patients, in fact, may be harmed if pathologic bone disease such as a tumor or osteopenia is present when manipulation is performed. At present, it is felt that manipulation is not indicated for the routine treatment of chronic low back pain. There is not adequate scientific evidence to justify its routine use.

Braces and Corsets

External support of the lumbar spine with a corset or brace is indicated for only a short period in the average patient's recovery process, and not every patient requires it. As the acute symptoms subside, a properly fitted corset or brace will aid the patient in regaining mobility sooner. As the recovery progresses, the patient usually should abandon the brace in favor of an exercise program. With continued long-term use of a brace, soft-tissue contractures and muscle atrophy will occur. The young patient should rely on a brace only to hasten ambulation. In theory, strong, flexible lumbar and abdominal muscles function as an excellent internal brace because they are adjacent to the structures (vertebrae) that they are supporting.

Exercises

Some form of exercise is probably the most commonly prescribed therapy for patients recovering from low back pain. There are two regimens commonly advocated: isometric flexion exercises and hyperextension exercises. These programs are purported to reduce the frequency and intensity of low back pain episodes, although there is no scientific evidence to support this contention.

The isometric flexion exercises are the most popular. They are based on the theory that by reducing the lumbar lordosis, back pain is decreased. This goal is achieved by strengthening both the abdominal and lumbar muscles, thereby creating a corset of muscles to support the lumbar spine. Flexion exercises are commonly utilized in patients with spondylolisthesis or spinal stenosis.

Hyperextension exercises are the other form of therapy. They are purported to strengthen the paravertebral muscles. These exercises generally are used after a patient has satisfactorily performed a course of isometric flexion exercises. The goal is to have the paravertebral muscles act as an internal support for the lumbar spine.

The authors believe that an exercise regimen is very important for the rehabilitation of low back patients. This regimen should not be instituted while the patient is experiencing acute pain, but may be started after his symptoms have subsided to the point where no list or paravertebral muscle spasm is present. The number of repetitions is increased gradually; if the patient has any recurrence of acute symptoms, the exercises are stopped. The patient is then closely monitored; when his symptoms again decrease, the exercises can be resumed.

Physical Therapy

There are many other treatment modalities used for low back pain. These include hot packs, cold packs, light massage, ultrasound, transcutaneous electrical nerve stimulation, and diathermy. They are all well tolerated and pleasant. Most patients experience some immediate relief of symptoms, but unfortunately, there is not a long-lasting impact on the disease process. There is no evidence that any of these treatment modalities offers any long-term benefit or even adds to the efficacy of decreased physical activity alone.

Summary and Conclusion

Neck and low back pain affects the majority of adults at some time during the course of their lives. Every physician should have a working knowledge of the common pathologic conditions and be able to differentiate a serious problem from the more common benign types. In both the cervical spine (myelopathy) and the lumbar spine (cauda equina compression), disastrous sequelae such as paralysis or loss of bowel and bladder control can occur if these serious conditions are not recognized in a timely fashion.

To help in the decision-making process, algorithms for both the cervical and lumbar spine were described. This will allow the physician to make the right diagnosis using the indicated diagnostic procedures at the correct time.

Suggested Reading

1. Borenstein DG, Wiesel SW, Boden SD. *Low Back and Neck Pain.* 3rd ed. Philadelphia, PA: WB Saunders; 2004.
2. Frymoyer JW, Wiesel SW. *The Adult & Pediatric Spine.* 3rd ed. Philadelphia, PA: Lippincott Williams & Wilkins; 2004.
3. Wiesel SW, Delahay JN. *Principles of Orthopaedic Medicine and Surgery.* Philadelphia, PA: WB Saunders; 2001.

Chapter 8
The Shoulder

Brent B. Wiesel and Raymond M. Carroll

Introduction

The shoulder joint, as it is commonly called, is not a single joint but a complex arrangement of bones, ligaments, and musculotendinous units that is more aptly called the shoulder girdle. The primary role of the shoulder girdle is to provide a tremendous range of motion for positioning the upper extremity in space. The shoulder girdle also provides power and support for the upper extremity throughout and at the extremes of the range of motion. Many shoulder girdle problems stem from overuse injuries such as pitching a baseball or serving a tennis ball that exploit both the power and range of motion of the shoulder girdle. This chapter will review the anatomy of the shoulder girdle and provide an approach to evaluating and treating common shoulder problems.

Functional Anatomy

The shoulder girdle includes three bones (scapula, clavicle, and proximal humerus) (Fig. 8.1), three joints (glenohumeral, acromioclavicular, and sternoclavicular), an additional articulation (scapulothoracic), and some 17 musculotendinous units. These individual elements function in a synchronous and interdependent manner in order to maximize the power and range of motion of the shoulder girdle. The clavicle is the sole bony link between the upper extremity and the axial skeleton.

The Glenohumeral Joint

The glenohumeral (GH) joint is the articulation of the proximal humeral epiphysis (ball) with the glenoid fossa (socket) of the scapula. This joint contributes to the

B.B. Wiesel (✉)
Shoulder Service, Department of Orthopedic Surgery, Georgetown University Medical Center, Washington, DC 20007, USA

S.W. Wiesel, J.N. Delahay (eds.), *Essentials of Orthopedic Surgery*,
DOI 10.1007/978-1-4419-1389-0_8, © Springer Science+Business Media, LLC 2010

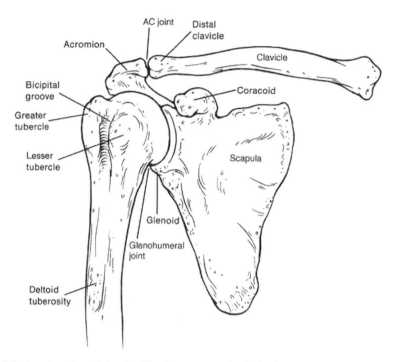

Fig. 8.1 Anterior view of the shoulder demonstrates the skeletal anatomy and two of the four articulations, the glenohumeral and acromioclavicular joints

majority of motion in the shoulder girdle. As only 20–30% of the humeral head is in contact with the glenoid fossa at any point in the shoulder's arc of motion and the radius of curvature of the glenoid is greater than that of the humeral head, there is little inherent bony stability of the GH joint. As a result, the soft tissues surrounding the joint are responsible for maintaining joint stability and congruity while still permitting the tremendous range of motion required of the GH joint. These soft tissue stabilizers include the joint capsule, glenohumeral ligaments, glenoid labrum, long head of the biceps tendon, and the rotator cuff musculature. The burden placed upon these soft tissues leads to the majority of degenerative and traumatic conditions affecting the shoulder girdle.

The Glenohumeral Ligaments

The capsule of the shoulder is a specialized structure that contains distinct thickenings referred to as ligaments (Fig. 8.2). The glenohumeral ligaments are named for their origin from the glenoid rim. This ligamentous complex includes

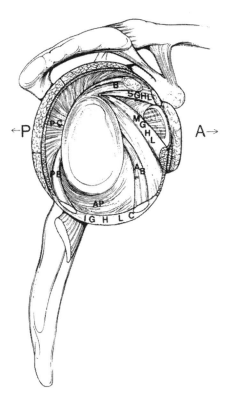

Fig. 8.2 In this cutaway view of the shoulder joint, the humeral head has been removed, allowing visualization of the interior of the normal glenohumeral anatomy. Notice the discrete ligaments that constitute the anterior shoulder capsule, namely the superior (*SGHL*), middle (*MGHL*), and anterior inferior glenohumeral ligaments. In this illustration, the most important anterior restraining structure, the inferior glenohumeral ligament complex (*IGHLC*), is shown to the further subdivided into having anterior (*AB*) and posterior (*PB*) bands and an axillary pouch (*AP*). (From Rockwood CA Jr, Matsen FA III eds. *The Shoulder*. Vol 1. Philadelphia, PA: Saunders; 1990. Reprinted with permission)

the superior glenohumeral ligament (SGHL), the middle glenohumeral ligament (MGHL), and the inferior glenohumeral ligament. These ligaments function as static stabilizers of the glenohumeral joint. The SGHL is the primary restraint to inferior translation and external rotation with the arm in adduction. The MGHL is the primary stabilizer to anterior translation with the arm in 45° of abduction. The inferior glenohumeral ligament complex includes an anterior band (AIGHL), posterior band (PIGHL), and an intervening sling or pouch. The inferior glenohumeral ligament complex becomes taut when the arm is abducted to 90°. In this position, the anterior band resists anterior translation with external rotation, and the posterior band resists posterior translation with internal rotation forces. The sling supports the humeral head.

The Labrum

The labrum is a fibrous structure of variable anatomy that attaches to the rim of the glenoid cartilage through a fibrocartilaginous zone, increasing the depth of the glenoid concavity by 50%. The labrum functions to increase the surface contact area with the humeral head; to act as a static stabilizer through a buttress effect; and to serve as an attachment site for the shoulder capsule, glenohumeral ligaments, and long head of the biceps tendon. The labrum has a variable cross-sectional anatomy, with the superior aspect of the labrum more triangular shaped and well defined and the inferior aspect of the labrum more rounded and less distinct. Common anatomic variations include a sublabral hole (foramen) or an absent labrum in the anterior-superior quadrant of the glenoid. The combination of a cord-like MGHL and absent anterosuperior labrum has been termed a Buford complex. It is important that the surgeon recognize variations in labral anatomy as inappropriate repair of a sublabral foramen or Buford complex will lead to significant postoperative stiffness.

The Rotator Interval

The rotator interval is the triangular region between the superior aspect of the subscapularis tendon and the anterior aspect of the supraspinatus tendon whose base is the coracoid. The rotator interval includes a number of fibrous structures including the coracohumeral ligament (CHL), the SGHL, and the transverse humeral ligament. The coracohumeral ligament is the most significant structure in the rotator interval and is extraarticular. It originates from the lateral base of the coracoid, fanning out to envelope the supraspinatus tendon inserting on the greater tuberosity and the subscapularis tendon inserting on the lesser tuberosity. The CHL is a primary restraint to inferior translation and external rotation in the adducted arm. The transverse humeral ligament forms the apex of the rotator interval and contributes to the superior soft tissue sling that stabilizes the long head of the biceps tendon as it passes through the interval to enter (or exit) the glenohumeral joint.

The Long Head of the Biceps Tendon

The long head of the biceps tendon (LHBT) remains somewhat enigmatic with respect to its function in the shoulder girdle but is nonetheless a potential source of pain and disability. The long head of the biceps enters/exits the glenohumeral joint at the rotator interval by way of the bicipital groove and is an intraarticular structure. The LHBT originates from the superior glenoid tubercle and blends with the fibers of the superior labrum. This intimate relationship of the LHBT with the superior labrum is a significant source of morbidity in the throwing athlete.

Although there is conflicting data, the long head of the biceps is thought to be a humeral head depressor and may contribute to glenohumeral instability. Potentially more relevant is the theory of the "peel-back" mechanism of SLAP (superior labrum anterior posterior) tears. This theory suggests that the LHBT and superior labrum can be torn from the superior glenoid in the late cocking position of a baseball pitch as the LHBT becomes taut and "peels back" the superior labrum off the glenoid rim. Whether or not this theory is correct, SLAP tears can be a significant problem in the throwing athlete. Tendinitis of the LHBT is also a common source of morbidity in the shoulder and is often a component of the impingement syndrome.

The Rotator Cuff

The rotator cuff consists of four muscle-tendon units including the subscapularis, supraspinatus, infraspinatus, and teres minor. These muscles originate on the scapula and insert onto the tuberosities of the proximal humerus. The subscapularis originates on the anterior surface of the scapula and inserts onto the lesser tuberosity. The remaining rotator cuff muscles originate from the posterior surface of the scapula and insert along the greater tuberosity. The roles of the rotator cuff are to keep the humeral head centered in the glenoid fossa throughout the range of shoulder motion and to contribute to the rotation and elevation of the extremity. As such, the rotator cuff is the primary dynamic stabilizer of the glenohumeral joint. Traumatic and overuse injuries to the rotator cuff are the most common problems in the shoulder girdle.

The Subacromial Space

The subacromial space is a potential space beneath the acromion and above the rotator cuff. The subacromial bursa outlines the subacromial space and provides frictionless gliding of the rotator cuff beneath the acromion and coracoacromial arch. Bony osteophytes on the undersurface of the anterior acromion have been postulated to narrow the subacromial space, irritate the subacromial bursa, and contribute to rotator cuff tears.

The Acromioclavicular Joint

The acromioclavicular (AC) joint is a true diarthrodial joint containing a fibrocartilaginous disc. The AC joint helps link the appendicular skeleton with the axial skeleton through the clavicle. Because there is little intrinsic bony stability to the AC joint, a number of ligaments and other soft tissues serve to stabilize this articulation (Fig. 8.3). The superior AC ligament is the most important horizontal stabilizer. The coracoclavicular (CC) ligaments, consisting of the conoid ligament (medial) and the

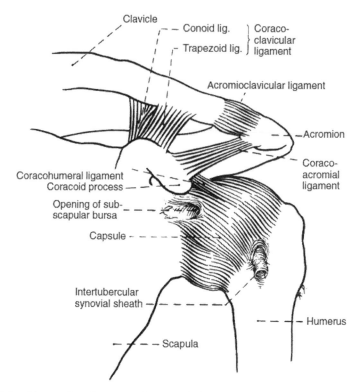

Fig. 8.3 In this anterior view, note the acromioclavicular joint surrounded by the capsule (acromioclavicular ligament), in addition to the supporting coracoclavicular ligaments, the conoid and trapezoid. (From Rockwood CA Jr, Matsen FA III eds. *The Shoulder*. Vol 1. Philadelphia, PA: Saunders; 1990. Reprinted with permission)

trapezoid ligament (lateral), provide the primary restraint to vertical displacement of the clavicle. A significant amount of rotation occurs in the clavicle throughout the arc of elevation of the upper extremity. Approximately 10% of this rotation occurs at the acromioclavicular joint.

The Sternoclavicular Joint

The sternoclavicular (SC) joint is the only bony connection the upper appendicular skeleton has to the axial skeleton and has the least bony stability of any major joint. The majority of clavicular rotation occurs at the sternoclavicular joint, but less than 50% of the bulbous, medial clavicle is in contact with the shallow, sternal articular fossa. Thus, the soft tissues provide stability to the sternoclavicular joint. The ligamentous anatomy of the SC joint includes the intraarticular disk ligament, the costoclavicular ligament, the interclavicular ligament, and the capsular ligament. Of these, the posterior sternoclavicular joint capsule has been shown to be the most important structure for preventing both anterior and posterior displacement of the medial clavicle.

The Scapulothoracic Articulation

The scapulothoracic articulation includes the scapula, posterior thorax, and interposed bursae which provide frictionless motion between the scapula and posterior thorax. The scapulothoracic articulation provides a significant percentage of motion to the shoulder girdle. Specifically, the glenohumeral joint and scapulothoracic articulation function in a synchronous fashion to provide full forward elevation of the upper extremity in a 2:1 ratio. The scapular stabilizer muscles include the trapezius, levator scapulae, rhomboids, latissimus dorsi, and serratus anterior. Dysfunction of scapulothoracic motion, seen clinically as scapular winging, may be a result of nerve injury or muscle dysfunction. Damage to the spinal accessory nerve results in trapezius dysfunction and lateral scapular winging. Long thoracic nerve injury leads to serratus anterior dysfunction and medial scapular winging. Pain and loss of motion in the glenohumeral joint can lead to overuse and fatigue of the scapular stabilizer muscles resulting in scapular winging.

The Brachial Plexus

The brachial plexus is comprised of the ventral rami of cervical roots C5, C6, C7, C8, and ventral thoracic root T1. With the exception of the spinal accessory nerve (XI) which innervates the trapezius, all of the muscles contributing to the function of the shoulder girdle and upper extremity are innervated by nerves originating from the brachial plexus. The brachial plexus includes five nerve roots, three trunks (superior, middle, and inferior), six divisions (three anterior, three posterior), three cords (lateral, medial, and posterior), and six terminal branches (musculocutaneous, ulnar, medial cord branch to median nerve, lateral cord branch to median nerve, axillary, and radial). With the exception of the divisions, nerves originate from each level of the brachial plexus to innervate muscles of the shoulder girdle. Brachial plexus injuries are relatively common with traumatic shoulder girdle injuries such as proximal humerus fractures, glenohumeral dislocations, and fracture/dislocations.

Clinical Examination of the Shoulder Girdle

The history of present illness is critical in the evaluation of shoulder girdle pathology and should be used to develop a reasonable differential diagnosis based on the patient's story and the epidemiology of shoulder pathology. For example, a high school athlete with activity-related shoulder pain is more likely to have instability or labral pathology than a rotator cuff tear. Conversely, a 65-year-old who has shoulder pain with activities of daily living is more likely to have rotator cuff disease than a labral tear or instability. The physical examination is used to narrow the differential diagnosis and make the definitive diagnosis. Most of the time, an accurate diagnosis can be made using only the history and physical examination. Indiscriminate use of imaging studies and additional testing is not recommended. Prior to ordering additional studies, the examiner must have a clear understanding of how the study will contribute to the evaluation and treatment of the patient.

History

Patients with shoulder pathology most often complain of pain, stiffness, instability, and weakness. When pain is the chief complaint, the examiner must characterize the pain, with particular attention to location. Pain from the glenohumeral joint and its surrounding soft tissues typically is localized to the anterosuperior aspect of the shoulder. Localization of the pain to the deltoid insertion in the arm is common in rotator cuff or subacromial pathology. Pain emanating from the neck or to the posterior scapular region is frequently due to cervical spine disease. Pain and crepitation in the periscapular region, however, may be related to scapulothoracic bursitis.

The timing and frequency of shoulder pain must also be given careful consideration. Activity-related pain can provide valuable clues as to the underlying diagnosis. Pain with overhead activities of daily living is common in rotator cuff pathology. Pain with sporting activities such as swimming, throwing, or serving is often related to the labrum or glenohumeral instability. Night pain is often reported with shoulder girdle pathology, especially in the setting of rotator cuff tears. Patients will often report the inability to sleep on the affected side. Rest pain is uncommon but may occur with severe arthropathy or radicular pain from the cervical spine. If rest pain is the predominant complaint, the examiner should consider infection or malignancy as a possible source of pain.

The relationship of pain to injury is important to establish. Pain that begins with a traumatic event such as a fall on an outstretched hand, direct blow to the shoulder, or shoulder dislocation may represent significant damage to the rotator cuff, ligaments, or bony structures. Pain that begins days or weeks after a seemingly innocuous event such as shoveling snow, trimming hedges, or painting may represent tendonitis or early capsulitis. Pain that begins more insidiously or over time is more likely to be related to degenerative lesions of the shoulder girdle such as rotator cuff tears or osteoarthritis.

Complaints of shoulder instability are relatively common. The patient may describe the shoulder "slipping out of place" or "getting stuck" in extreme positions. It is important to establish whether a frank shoulder dislocation was ever documented. True traumatic shoulder dislocations are the result of significant trauma and require a manipulative reduction. Unfortunately, subsequent dislocations may occur with less trauma. Patients who have shoulders which "slip out of place" and "slide back in" on their own are more likely to have multidirectional instability as opposed to traumatic instability.

Weakness or loss of shoulder function is an infrequent complaint. In the absence of pain, a neurologic origin of the deteriorating function should be considered. Insidious onset of pain with deteriorating function may represent a degenerative condition of the shoulder or adhesive capsulitis.

A careful review of systems is important to document as there are a number of disease processes remote from the shoulder girdle that can result in shoulder pain. Cervical spine pathology, cardiac disease, gallbladder disease, and lung disease (pancoast tumor) can present with shoulder pain. A history of cancer is also important to document as metastatic cancer can present with shoulder pain and lesions in the shoulder girdle.

Functional Assessment

In addition to establishing the history of present illness, it is imperative to establish the functional status of the patient. Important patient factors to note include the handedness (right, left, or ambidextrous) of the patient, the vocation of the patient, extracurricular/sporting activities enjoyed by the patient, and, most importantly, the expectations of the patient with regard to his shoulder problem. Understanding the patient's functional demands and expectations allows the clinician to prescribe appropriate treatment regimens and to provide reasonable expectations for functional recovery.

Inspection

The physical examination begins with inspection of the shoulder girdle. The region must be adequately exposed for the examination. The inspection begins with assessment of symmetry between the involved and uninvolved shoulder girdles. Gross deformities such as distal clavicle prominence in an AC separation, prior surgical incisions, skin discoloration, or open wounds are readily appreciated. A more subtle finding is muscle atrophy which may be the result of disuse or injury. Patients with longstanding rotator cuff tears will often have atrophy of the supra- and infraspinatus fossae resulting in prominence of the spine of the scapula. Traumatic injuries can produce subtle deformities. In the setting of an anterior dislocation, the anterior aspect of the shoulder may appear "full" and the posterior aspect may lose its normal contour making the posterior acromion appear more prominent. Inspection should continue through the entire exam as some deformities such as scapular winging may only be revealed during provocative testing.

Palpation

The primary importance of palpation is to localize the source of pain. Palpation of bony prominences and superficial joints yields the most information. In the absence of trauma, palpation includes the SC joint, AC joint, the greater and lesser tuberosities, and the intertubercular or bicipital groove. Tenderness on palpation at any of these sites can be a valuable clue in making a diagnosis. When the presenting complaint is neck or periscapular pain, palpation of the posterior elements of the cervical spine and bony elements of the scapula is warranted. In the setting of trauma, palpation of all bony structures and areas of deformity is critical to localize the zone of injury.

Range of Motion

The evaluation of range of motion is straightforward. The examiner directs the motions and observes for symmetry. The standard motions include forward elevation, external rotation, internal rotation, and abduction. Forward elevation occurs in the plane of the scapula and is a combination of scapulothoracic and glenohumeral motion. Loss of glenohumeral motion can lead to scapulothoracic substitution and scapular winging. External rotation is evaluated with the arms at the side to prevent scapulothoracic contribution to rotation. Internal rotation is evaluated by having the patient place his or her hands as high as possible along the midline of the back. Internal rotation is graded by the approximate vertebral level the patient is able to reach. Assessment of abduction, including internal and external rotation in abduction, is critical for unmasking subtle losses of motion. Throwing athletes often lose some internal rotation in abduction while gaining external rotation in abduction in their throwing arm. There is no net loss of motion, only a resetting of the range of motion relative to the non-throwing shoulder.

When loss of active motion is identified, the examiner must assess the passive range of motion. If there is loss of active and passive motion, there is likely a soft tissue contracture or a physical block to motion (dislocation, loose body, or osteophyte). In the absence of trauma, loss of both active and passive motion usually represents adhesive capsulitis (frozen shoulder) or arthropathy. If there is loss of active motion with preserved passive motion, the examiner must consider tendon (rotator cuff) rupture or, potentially, nerve damage. When examining the rotator cuff muscles, the examiner must appreciate lag signs.

A lag sign can be documented when the patient has a loss of active motion with preservation of passive motion. The examiner positions the shoulder at the end range of full passive motion and instructs the patient to maintain the position. If the patient is unable to maintain the position and the extremity falls away, the patient is considered to have a positive lag sign. The horn blower's sign is the lag sign for the abducted, externally rotated position and is suggestive of a massive rotator cuff tear involving the posterior cuff.

Strength Assessment

The relative strength of muscle groups can be assessed during the physical examination. In order to assess strength, the examiner manually resists the patient's active motion in a defined plane such as abduction, adduction, and internal or external rotation. Asymmetric weakness on the involved side can provide additional diagnostic information. Weakness or paralysis of the scapular stabilizer muscles can be assessed by having the patient perform pushups against a wall. Scapular winging can be elicited using this technique.

Neurologic Examination

In the absence of trauma or brachial plexopathies, most neurologic lesions about the shoulder involve a peripheral nerve. Common peripheral neuropathies in the shoulder girdle include the suprascapular, spinal accessory, and long thoracic nerves. Although these conditions can be painful, many patients report dysfunction or cosmetic deformity as the presenting complaint. These lesions are appreciated during the inspection, range of motion and strength testing of the shoulder girdle. Suprascapular neuropathy can occur at the level of the suprascapular notch or proximal and involve both the supra- and infraspinatus tendons resulting in prominence of the scapular spine and weakness of forward elevation and external rotation. Suprascapular nerve lesions at the level of the spinoglenoid notch involve only the infraspinatus muscle resulting in atrophy of the infraspinatus fossa and weakness of external rotation. Spinal accessory nerve injury is often iatrogenic from a posterior cervical node biopsy or a radical neck dissection for malignancy. Injury to the spinal accessory nerve (cranial nerve XI) results in trapezius dysfunction and lateral scapular winging. Long thoracic nerve injury is thought to be secondary to traction or contusion and affects the serratus anterior muscle resulting in medial scapular winging. Medial or lateral refers to the direction toward which the inferior border of the scapula is directed. Nerve lesions in the shoulder girdle should be further evaluated with electromyography (EMG) and nerve conduction testing. The majority of these nerve lesions (except iatrogenic laceration) recover without surgical intervention.

Special Tests and Signs

There are a variety of special tests or maneuvers that have been described to evaluate individual structures or reveal specific pathology. A few of these tests and signs are reviewed below.

Rotator Cuff

The most commonly used tests attempt to recreate the pain that occurs with rotator cuff impingement under the coracoacromial (CA) arch by rotating the greater tuberosity under the acromion. The painful arc sign occurs when the patient experiences pain while elevating the upper extremity from 70 to 120°. The Neer impingement sign is positive when shoulder pain is reproduced as the upper extremity is passively elevated in the scapular plane with the scapula stabilized (Fig. 8.4). Hawkins's impingement sign is tested by passively internally rotating the humerus when the arm is at 90° of forward flexion with the elbow flexed. A positive test is defined as shoulder pain with this maneuver. The drop arm test is performed by placing the upper extremity at shoulder level (90°) in the scapular plane with the thumb pointing downward. The test is considered positive when the patient is unable to maintain the extremity in this position and is indicative of superior rotator cuff pathology.

Fig. 8.4 Impingement of the rotator cuff is demonstrated by passively elevating the shoulder against the fixed scapula. Pain suggests the possibility of mechanical compression of the rotator cuff against the anterior inferior acromion, a process known as impingement. (From DeLee JC, Drez D Jr. *Orthopaedic Sports Medicine: Principles and Practice.* Vol 1. Philadelphia, PA: Saunders; 1994. Reprinted with permission)

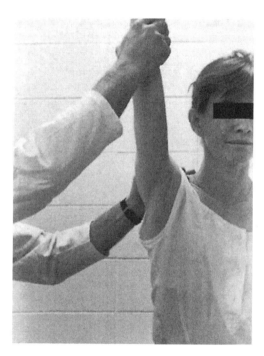

Two tests have been described to evaluate the subscapularis. The lift-off test is performed by having the patient place his or her hands behind the back with the arm internally rotated and the elbow flexed. The patient is then asked to lift the hands off the back without extending the elbows. If the patient is unable to perform the lift-off, the test is considered positive and indicative of subscapularis insufficiency. For patients who are unable to reach behind their back, the belly press test can be used to evaluate the subscapularis. The belly press test is performed by having the patient place his or her hands on the abdomen and, while pressing the hands to the abdomen, bringing the elbows anterior to the coronal plane of the body. Inability to perform the belly press maneuver is a positive test.

Biceps Tendon (Long Head and Superior Labrum)

Speed's test is used to evaluate the long head of the biceps tendon. The test is performed by having the patient maintain forward elevation of the upper extremity at shoulder height against resistance with the elbow extended and the forearm supinated. The test is considered positive when pain is produced in the area of the bicipital groove with the maneuver.

The active-compression test, or O'Brien's test, is used to evaluate the superior labral-biceps tendon complex. The test is performed in two steps. The upper extremity is brought to shoulder height in forward flexion with the forearm fully pronated (thumb down) and adducted approximately 15°. The patient resists the examiner's downward pressure from this position. If this maneuver elicits pain in the shoulder, the test is repeated with the forearm supinated. If the pain is reduced or absent with the second maneuver, the test is considered positive. A positive test indicates that the biceps tendon-superior labral complex is torn or detached from the superior glenoid.

Shoulder Instability

A number of tests have been described to evaluate shoulder instability. All of the following tests can be performed with the patient supine on the examining table. The apprehension test is performed with the shoulder abducted to 90° and externally rotated to 90° in the coronal plane of the body. From this position, the examiner continues to externally rotate the shoulder. If the patient experiences apprehension (fear of the shoulder dislocating), the test is considered positive. If the patient has a positive apprehension test, the examiner can reduce the subluxated humeral head by applying a posterior directed force against the proximal humerus, thereby reducing the humeral head. If the apprehension is relieved, the relocation test is positive. The examiner can then release the proximal humerus. If apprehension recurs with release of the posterior directed force, the release test is positive.

The load-and-shift test is used to assess the direction and degree of shoulder laxity. The examiner uses one hand to apply a longitudinal load to the humerus directed toward the glenohumeral joint. This hand is located at the elbow with the elbow flexed. The other hand is used to apply a perpendicular force to the proximal humeral shaft in an attempt to shift (subluxate or dislocate) the humeral head relative to the glenoid. The test is performed while maintaining the upper extremity in the coronal plane of the body. The degree of abduction/rotation and the direction of the applied force can be varied to evaluate the various glenohumeral ligaments. The test is graded by the examiner who determines through tactile sense whether the humeral head translates to the glenoid rim (1+); over the glenoid rim but spontaneously reduces (2+); or over the rim requiring manual reduction (3+).

Imaging Studies and Other Diagnostic Tests

The use of routine imaging studies and tests to evaluate the shoulder girdle for diagnostic purposes is not recommended. At the conclusion of the history and physical examination, the examiner should have a reasonable diagnosis. Additional tests or studies are used to answer specific questions. If the clinical diagnosis is frozen shoulder but the examiner is concerned that the patient has glenohumeral arthritis, it is reasonable to order radiographs to rule out osteoarthritis since the natural history and treatment of osteoarthritis and adhesive capsulitis are dissimilar. If the clinical diagnosis is rotator cuff impingement or tendonitis, there is no reason to obtain further studies initially as they will not change the recommended course of treatment.

Radiographs

The standard shoulder series includes an anteroposterior (AP) X-ray in the plane of the scapula; a Y-outlet view; and an axillary view. This series of X-rays is mandatory in the evaluation of shoulder girdle trauma. Unfortunately, the axillary view is often not obtained, yet it is the most sensitive for documenting shoulder dislocations. AP views with the humerus internally and externally rotated may be used to critically evaluate greater tuberosity fractures or calcific tendonitis. The scapula is approximately 45° oblique to the coronal plane of the body; therefore, in order to obtain a true AP view of the glenohumeral joint, the X-ray beam must be obliquely oriented to the coronal plane of the body (Fig. 8.5). The AP view is useful for evaluating the clavicle, AC joint, glenohumeral joint space, glenoid, scapular body, proximal humeral shaft, surgical neck, and greater tuberosity. The Y-outlet view is useful for evaluating the scapular spine, scapular body, coracoid, shape of the acromion, and spur formation in the CA ligament. The axillary view is critical in evaluating glenohumeral joint congruence. Anterior or posterior dislocations are best seen on the axillary view.

Magnetic Resonance Imaging

The magnetic resonance imaging (MRI) scan is commonly employed to evaluate the soft tissues of the shoulder girdle and is considered is the gold standard for evaluating the rotator cuff tendons. Subacromial fluid, tendon inflammation, and rotator cuff tears are all visible with MR imaging. MRI scans can be performed with an arthrogram (intraarticular contrast dye) to better delineate intraarticular structures such as labral tears and articular-sided partial rotator cuff tears. Standard MRI views of the shoulder include coronal oblique, sagittal oblique, and axial cuts. The coronal and sagittal views are termed oblique because they are obtained in the plane of the scapula which is oblique to the coronal and sagittal planes of the body. Although the MRI scan is a powerful tool in the evaluation of shoulder problems, it is a very sensitive test. Positive findings, therefore, may correlate poorly with a patient's clinical presentation. For example, MRI scans obtained on patients with normal, pain-free shoulders have documented a greater than 50% incidence of rotator cuff tears in

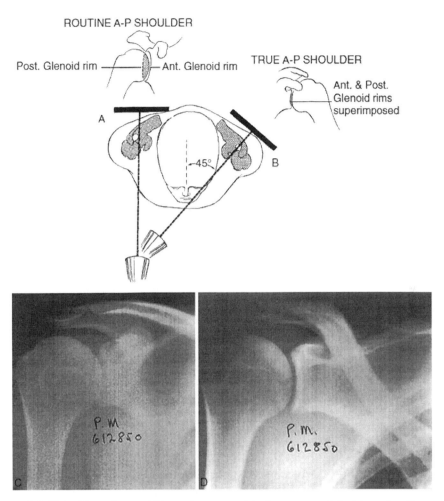

Fig. 8.5 These illustrations and X-rays demonstrated the importance of obtaining a "true" anterioposterior (AP) perspective of the glenohumeral joint. In X-ray (**a**), note that the AP view is actually one of the thorax, yielding an X-ray which shows overlap of the glenohumeral joint. When the beam is angled, however, as in (**b**), a "true" AP view of the glenohumeral joint is obtained. Note the differences in appearance in these views in (**c**) (AP view of the thorax) and (**d**) (true AP view of the glenohumeral joint) (From Rockwood CA Jr, Matsen FA III eds. *The Shoulder*. Vol 1. Philadelphia, PA: Saunders; 1990. Reprinted with permission)

patients over the age of 60. It is therefore important to treat the patient and not the MRI scan.

Computerized Tomography

Computerized tomography (CT) scans are useful in the evaluation of bone abnormalities. In the setting of complex or comminuted shoulder girdle fractures,

CT scanning with or without image reconstruction is a powerful tool for clinical decision making and/or preoperative planning. CT scans are also valuable in assessing bone deficiencies such as glenoid wear prior to shoulder arthroplasty.

Electrodiagnostic Testing

Electromyography (EMG) and nerve conduction velocity (NCV) testing are commonly used to evaluate neurologic lesions of the shoulder girdle. EMG testing involves placing small needle electrodes into the muscles to record resting potentials and firing patterns. NCV testing is used to document the speed with which an impulse is conducted along a peripheral nerve. Abnormalities such as a conduction block may indicate severe nerve injury. Electrodiagnostic testing is useful in documenting both the presence and recovery of peripheral nerve lesions.

Evaluation and Treatment of Common Shoulder Problems

The majority of common shoulder girdle problems result from degenerative changes, overuse, or traumatic injury. Atraumatic shoulder pain is common and includes rotator cuff disease, arthropathy, adhesive capsulitis, calcific tendinitis, and multidirectional instability. Most atraumatic shoulder pain is initially treated with activity modification, anti-inflammatory medication and physical therapy. Treatment regimens may vary depending on the specific diagnosis. Calcific tendinitis, for example, responds well to subacromial corticosteroid injections. The physical therapy prescription may also vary depending on the diagnosis. Patients with adhesive capsulitis require stretching exercises, in contrast to patients with rotator cuff tendonitis who are treated with rotator cuff strengthening exercises. Surgical treatment in the atraumatic population is generally reserved for those patients who fail to respond to nonoperative treatment regimens. A basic algorithm for the evaluation of atraumatic shoulder pain is provided in Fig. 8.6.

Traumatic injuries to the shoulder girdle are common and include both soft tissue and bony injury. Treatment is individualized based on the age of the patient, functional status of the patient, and the severity of the injury. Depending on the injury, nonoperative or operative treatment may be appropriate. Common traumatic injuries to the shoulder girdle include shoulder dislocations, AC joint injuries, clavicle fractures, and proximal humerus fractures and are reviewed in the skeletal trauma chapter. Contrary to popular belief, traumatic rotator cuff tears are relatively uncommon.

Rotator Cuff Disease

Degenerative and overuse injuries of the rotator cuff (RC) are common sources of shoulder pain and disability. Anterosuperior shoulder pain emanating from the

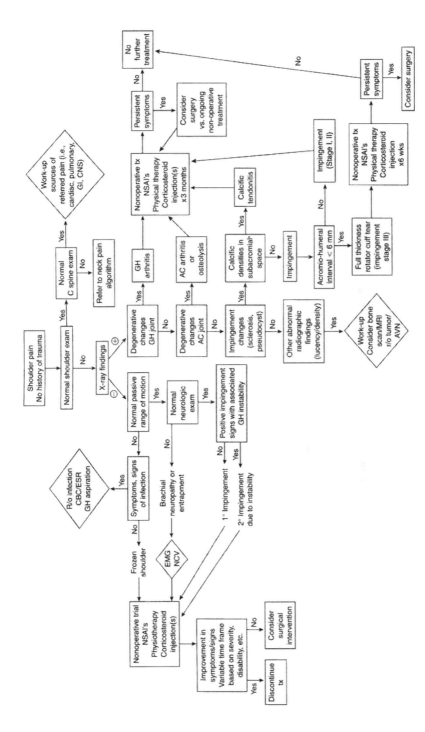

Fig. 8.6 Algorithmic approach to the diagnosis and treatment of atraumatic shoulder pain

rotator cuff under the coracoacromial arch has historically been called impingement syndrome. Impingement syndrome encompasses a spectrum of pathology in the subacromial region including subacromial bursitis, RC tendinopathy, partial-thickness RC tears, and full-thickness RC tears. Partial and full-thickness tears of the rotator cuff become more prevalent with increasing age. It is unusual for patients under the age of 40 years to present with rotator cuff tears in the absence of significant trauma. Conversely, older patients may present with massive rotator cuff tears after an innocuous event. There are two main theories which attempt to explain such degenerative cuff tears. The external impingement model suggests an extrinsic cause of rotator cuff tears such as abrasion of the anterosuperior cuff under the acromion and coracoacromial arch. The intrinsic model suggests that a relatively poor blood supply to the critical zone of the rotator cuff in combination with high stresses across the cuff leads to RC tears. The true pathophysiology likely results from a combination of these models.

History

The chief complaint is usually anterosuperior shoulder pain which often radiates to the lateral deltoid region. The pain is typically worse with overhead activities and at night. The patient may recall a minor traumatic event, or the pain may have started insidiously.

Examination

Inspection of the shoulder girdle usually reveals symmetry, but patients with degenerative cuff tears may present with atrophy of the supra- or infraspinatus fossae. The patient typically has discrete tenderness at the cuff insertion on the greater tuberosity. The active range of motion is generally normal; however, some patients with large RC tears may exhibit loss of active motion with preservation of passive motion. In this setting, the clinician may be able to document lag signs. Strength testing may reveal weakness of the supraspinatus or infraspinatus tendons. Special tests include the Neer and Hawkins's impingement signs. If the patient has concomitant biceps tendon pathology, there may be tenderness at the bicipital groove and Speed's test may be positive. Tenderness over the AC joint may indicate that the AC joint is contributing to the painful condition. A cross-body adduction test recreating pain at the AC joint is considered confirmatory.

Differential Diagnosis

The differential diagnosis varies with the age of the patient. In older patients, the differential diagnosis includes arthritis, cervical spine pathology, metastatic disease, and visceral pathology such as cardiac disease. In younger patients, instability and labral pathology should be considered. In any age group, the differential diagnosis includes adhesive capsulitis, calcific tendinitis, and a variety of other less common shoulder problems (avascular necrosis, scapulothoracic dysfunction, and infection).

Radiographic Evaluation and Magnetic Resonance Imaging

The AP radiograph may reveal sclerosis and cyst formation of the greater tuberosity. The Y-outlet view shows the acromial morphology with potential narrowing of the subacromial space. In patients with longstanding RC tears, there may be superior migration of the humeral head and the distance between the humerus and acromion on the AP view may be narrowed. The axillary view illustrates the joint space and may reveal an os acromiale. An MRI scan is useful for a number of reasons. Confirmation of rotator cuff disease (and exclusion of other etiologies) is reassuring, but not necessary. The MRI scan is extremely useful for assessing the RC tendons and muscle bellies (Fig. 8.7). The presence, size, and chronicity of an RC tear directly impacts patient care (surgical options), recovery, and, ultimately, prognosis.

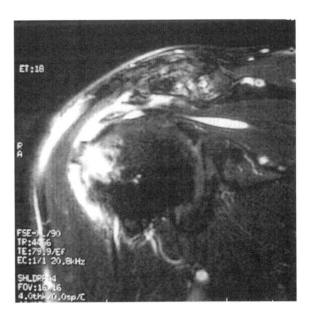

Fig. 8.7 A tear of the supraspinatus tendon with fluid in the gap is easily appreciated in this coronal oblique magnetic resonance imaging (MRI) scan of the glenohumeral joint

Initial Treatment

The goal of treatment is to return the patient to pain-free activity. Initially, treatment consists of education, rest, and activity modifications. If the pain is significant, an oral anti-inflammatory medication can be prescribed. Once the painful period subsides, the patient may benefit from a course of physical therapy to strengthen the rotator cuff and scapular stabilizers. Radiographs are generally obtained in patients who fail initial therapy. A subacromial corticosteroid injection can be considered in a patient who fails to respond to the initial treatment over 1–2 months. Additional physical therapy can also be helpful. Patients who fail to respond to nonoperative management over 3–6 months may benefit from surgical treatment. Most surgeons will obtain an MRI scan prior to surgical treatment.

Surgical Treatment

In the absence of a rotator cuff tear, most surgeons recommend a subacromial decompression performed either openly or arthroscopically. This involves removing the inflamed subacromial bursa, releasing the coracoacromial ligament and shaving the undersurface of the acromion (acromioplasty) to create more room in the subacromial space for the rotator cuff. Patients who have reparable RC tears are treated with primary repair, and most surgeons will perform an acromioplasty although several studies suggest this may be unnecessary. RC repairs can be done both openly and arthroscopically (Fig. 8.8). While technically more challenging, arthroscopic rotator cuff repair is quickly becoming the standard of care as it allows for better

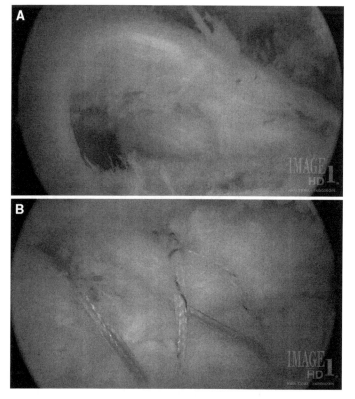

Fig. 8.8 (**a**) Arthroscopic photography of a right shoulder with a full-thickness tear of the supraspinatus tendon. (**b**) Arthroscopic photography following arthroscopic repair of the tear with suture anchors

visualization of the tear pattern and a more anatomic repair. The initial results of arthroscopic repair were inferior to open repair but improved arthroscopic skills and technology have led to equivalent or superior outcomes in more recent studies.

Care should be taken to preserve the CA ligament in patients with large tears and multiple tendon tears to prevent superior migration of the humeral head if the repair fails. There are a variety of options for patients with irreparable tears, including arthroscopic debridement, partial tendon repair, and tendon transfers. Patients with irreparable RC tears and arthropathy may be candidates for a hemiarthroplasty or reverse shoulder arthroplasty. If biceps tendon pathology is found at the time of surgery, either tenodesis or tenotomy can be performed. Patients who are noted to have AC joint arthropathy and pain prior to surgery may benefit from a distal clavicle resection. Recovery from RC surgery can take anywhere from 4 to 6 months. The goal of early (4–6 weeks) postoperative physical therapy is recovery of passive shoulder motion. Restoration of strength and function is the goal of subsequent postoperative therapy. Failure of the patient to adhere to postoperative physical therapy can result in a poor outcome.

Osteoarthritis

Degenerative arthritis, or osteoarthritis (OA), occurs in the glenohumeral joint but is less common than in the hip or knee joints. Osteoarthritis of the glenohumeral joint has the same pathophysiology as in other joints with progressive articular cartilage destruction.

History

Patients with early osteoarthritis may have a clinical syndrome that is virtually indistinguishable from impingement syndrome. In patients with advanced osteoarthritis, pain is more likely to be chronic, occur at rest, and be resistant to standard analgesics and anti-inflammatory medications. In addition, loss of shoulder motion is a common complaint.

Examination

Patients with early osteoarthritis may examine similarly to those with impingement syndrome. In more advanced OA, generalized disuse atrophy of the shoulder girdle may be noticeable and there is often significant crepitus of the glenohumeral joint. In general, active motion is decreased in all planes, but loss of external rotation with the arm at the side is often the most dramatic. Passive motion is similarly decreased and there is often a significant amount of pain associated with passive stretching of the joint capsule near the end ranges of motion.

Differential Diagnosis

Adhesive capsulitis and inflammatory arthropathy can have similar presentations. The examiner must have a high index of suspicion for locked posterior shoulder dislocations in older patients who are poor historians as a result of dementia or stroke.

Radiographs

A standard shoulder series is recommended. Joint space narrowing, subchondral sclerosis, osteophytes, and subchondral cyst formation are classic findings in osteoarthritis and are best seen on the AP and axillary view (Fig. 8.9). In the glenohumeral joint, inferior humeral osteophytes predominate. Often, eccentric posterior glenoid wear is present. MRI scans are generally not used in the evaluation of OA. A CT scan to assess the glenoid for eccentric wear or bone loss is common during preoperative evaluation for shoulder arthroplasty.

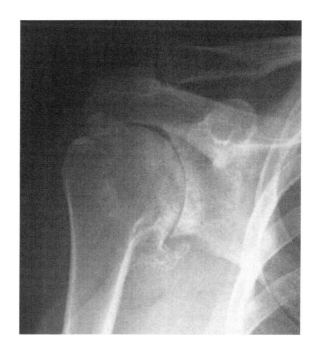

Fig. 8.9 All of the classic findings of osteoarthritis are present in this true AP X-ray of the glenohumeral joint, including joint space narrowing, subchondral sclerosis, osteophyte formation, and subchondral cyst formation

Treatment

Initial treatment for OA includes education, rest, activity modification, and anti-inflammatory medications. Physical therapy for stretching and maintenance of motion is an important component of nonoperative treatment. Intraarticular corticosteroid injections provide inconsistent and incomplete pain relief in this setting. With advanced disease, some patients require narcotic analgesia for pain relief. When nonoperative management is no longer able to control the patient's pain, surgical management is a reasonable option. In select patients with concentric wear with or without some joint space preservation and reasonable motion may benefit from arthroscopic debridement. The goal of debridement is pain relief and postponement of prosthetic joint arthroplasty.

In the setting of painful, end-stage OA, prosthetic joint replacement with either a hemiarthroplasty or a total shoulder arthroplasty (TSA) is recommended (Fig. 8.10). Hemiarthroplasty involves resection of the humeral head and replacement with a metallic sphere attached to an intramedullary stem. For a TSA, a plastic glenoid component is cemented onto the patient's glenoid in addition to replacement of the humeral head. Slight improvement with respect to motion and pain relief has been demonstrated with TSA relative to hemiarthroplasty. TSA introduces the risk of glenoid-sided prosthetic loosening and wear which may require revision surgery; however, hemiarthroplasty can fail as a result of inadequate pain relief. The surgery is performed via the deltopectoral interval and the subscapularis muscle must be detached in order to access the joint. The muscle is repaired following placement of the implant but the repair must be protected during the early phase (first 6 weeks) of postoperative rehabilitation.

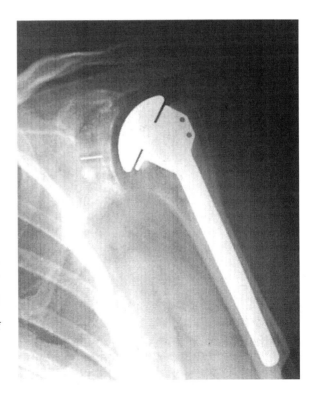

Fig. 8.10 A total shoulder arthroplasty is demonstrated in this true AP X-ray of the glenohumeral joint. The metallic humeral component is cemented into the proximal humerus. The pegged glenoid component is cemented into the glenoid and is represented by the reproduction of the joint space. The central peg of the polyethylene glenoid component is identified by the horizontal radioopaque marker

Miscellaneous Arthropathy

A variety of other disease processes can lead to glenohumeral joint destruction. Inflammatory arthropathy, such as rheumatoid arthritis, can lead to joint destruction as a result of synovial disease. While the clinical presentation may be similar to osteoarthritis with pain and loss of motion, there are some important differences. In particular, rheumatoid arthritis can result in rotator cuff deficiency and incompetence. In these patients, total shoulder arthroplasty is contraindicated, since glenoid loosening in the setting of rotator cuff deficiency is a common problem. If arthroplasty is required in the setting of significant destruction of the rotator cuff, then hemiarthroplasty is the procedure of choice. Progressive bony destruction of the humeral head and glenoid can result from rheumatoid arthritis, making prosthetic arthroplasty difficult, if not impossible. Avascular necrosis can occur as a result of trauma, corticosteroid use, alcoholism, and other less common etiologies. Avascular necrosis of the humeral head can lead to pain and loss of motion in the glenohumeral joint. Hemiarthroplasty is an option for patients with humeral head collapse and chronic pain. Total shoulder arthroplasty is indicated when secondary destruction of the glenoid is present. Charcot or neuropathic arthropathy is typically a painless condition that results in severe joint destruction. Charcot arthropathy in the glenohumeral joint is commonly related to a cervical spine syrinx. There are no reliable surgical options for Charcot arthropathy.

Adhesive Capsulitis

Adhesive capsulitis, or frozen shoulder, is a painful condition in which the synovial lining of the glenohumeral joint is inflamed. Adhesive capsulitis is a clinical diagnosis in which examination reveals an equal loss of active and passive motion. Primary adhesive capsulitis is idiopathic meaning that no trigger can be identified. It occurs in middle-aged persons and is associated with diabetes and thyroid dysfunction. Secondary adhesive capsulitis implies that a trigger or cause of the disease process can be identified. Trauma, surgery, and concomitant shoulder girdle pathology may result in secondary adhesive capsulitis.

History

The patient reports an insidious onset of shoulder pain and progressive decreased range of motion. Pain often occurs during rotational movements such as reaching behind the back, putting on a coat, or fastening a bra. Often the patient may recall a minor event that precipitated the condition. It is important to obtain a past medical and surgical history to identify possible risk factors. Insulin-dependent diabetes is a strong risk factor for adhesive capsulitis.

Examination

In the absence of prior trauma or surgery to the shoulder girdle, the inspection and palpation portions of the exam are usually unremarkable. Active motion can be extremely limited in all planes of motion, and the passive motion is similarly restricted. The patient often experiences pain at the end range of motion (active or passive).

Differential Diagnosis

Early adhesive capsulitis can mimic impingement. Subtle losses of internal and external rotation in abduction may be the only clues to differentiate between the two diagnoses. Unrecognized trauma (locked posterior shoulder dislocations) and glenohumeral joint arthropathy can mimic adhesive capsulitis but these entities can be easily excluded with standard radiographs.

Radiographs

A standard shoulder series is useful in excluding other diagnoses; however, there are no radiographic findings for adhesive capsulitis. Further studies are generally not indicated unless additional pathology is suspected.

Treatment

Once the diagnosis is made, education of the patient is paramount. In general, the treatment of adhesive capsulitis is twofold: treatment of the synovial inflammation and restoration of motion. Anti-inflammatory medications can be used, but a corticosteroid injection into the glenohumeral joint space is more efficient and effective for treating the synovial inflammation. The patient must start a stretching program to regain motion in all planes. Initially, supervised physical therapy is helpful, but the patient must independently perform a battery of home stretching exercises daily. A gradual restoration of motion is the anticipated course although this can often take 12–18 months. In patients who fail to show any response to nonoperative treatment after 3–6 months, surgery may be a reasonable option. Historically, patients with diabetes have a higher failure rate of nonoperative treatment compared to patients without risk factors. Additionally, patients with secondary adhesive capsulitis from trauma or prior shoulder surgery often fail to respond fully to nonoperative treatment. Manipulation of the shoulder under anesthesia was once the preferred treatment and continues to be a reasonable option. However, proximal humerus fractures can occur with manipulations under anesthesia, and osteoporosis is a risk factor for this complication. Arthroscopic capsular release is a more invasive, yet more anatomic, procedure. The surgery involves releasing the shoulder capsule under direct vision with a combination bitters and electrofrequency devices. The axillary nerve is at particular risk during release of inferior capsule. Aggressive physical therapy with active-assisted and active range of motion is mandatory to maintain the postoperative range of motion and should be started on the day or surgery. Shoulder strengthening and resistance therapy is instituted only after restoration of full, active shoulder motion.

Calcific Tendinitis

Calcific tendinitis of the rotator cuff is a painful condition of the shoulder girdle and is a common clinical problem (Fig. 8.11). The etiology of calcific tendinitis is a matter of debate. The pathogenesis of calcifying tendinitis includes various stages of tendon degeneration, calcium deposition, and calcium resorption. In the formative phase of calcium deposition, there may be little or no pain. Typically the resorptive phase is more painful and clinically relevant.

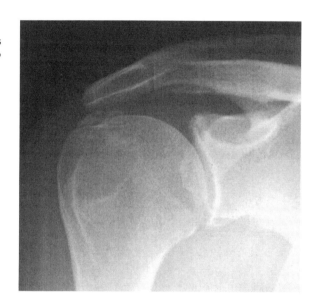

Fig. 8.11 A calcium deposit is present in the supraspinatus tendon immediately medial to its attachment site on the greater tuberosity in this true AP X-ray of the glenohumeral joint

History

In the resorptive phase, the patient may present with an acute onset of severe shoulder pain. In the formative phase, the patient may present with more chronic symptoms that mimic impingement syndrome.

Examination

Acute bursitis in the resorptive phase may lead to fullness of the anterosuperior shoulder, but otherwise the inspection is typically unremarkable. Typically there is tenderness at the rotator cuff insertion corresponding to the calcium deposition. There may be a loss of active motion secondary to pain, but passive motion, although painful, is generally preserved. Impingement signs are often positive.

Differential Diagnosis

The differential diagnosis includes rotator cuff disease and adhesive capsulitis. Referred pain from cardiac origin or other visceral organs and radicular pain from the cervical spine should be considered.

Radiographs

The appearance of calcific tendonitis on radiographs varies depending on the phase of the disease. In the formative phase, the calcium deposit is usually well circumscribed and easily identified. In the resorptive phase, the deposit may appear fluffy and less well defined. In addition to the standard shoulder series, internal and external rotational AP views can be helpful for identifying more subtle deposits. Additional studies are not usually indicated.

Treatment

Treatment generally involves pain management. Noninvasive treatment options include anti-inflammatory medications and extra-corporeal shock wave therapy. More invasive options include corticosteroid injections and lavage therapy. Surgical treatment is a last resort and involves arthroscopic debridement of the calcium deposit.

Multidirectional Instability

Shoulder instability is a complex problem with a spectrum of pathology ranging from atraumatic multidirectional shoulder instability to traumatic, unidirectional shoulder dislocations. Multidirectional instability (MDI) generally refers to shoulder pain and disability caused by excessive laxity of the static shoulder stabilizers (capsule and glenohumeral ligaments).

History

In the overhead athlete (pitchers, swimmers, and volleyball players), MDI can present with activity-related pain, scapular winging, and occasionally neurologic symptoms down the arm. Other patients may present with shoulder subluxations and dislocations that may easily reduce on their own but are a significant source of disability and distress to the patient.

Examination

Scapular winging may be noticeable on inspection during range of motion and strength testing. The active and passive ranges of motion are often excessive compared to the average shoulder. Additionally, the patient may exhibit generalized ligamentous laxity at other joints. The sulcus sign (hollowing of the subacromial region with downward traction on the arm) may be noticeable and indicative of shoulder laxity. Provocative shoulder testing such as the apprehension test may produce pain rather than apprehension. Other patients may have true apprehension. Load-and-shift testing often reveals subluxation or dislocation in multiple directions.

Differential Diagnosis

The differential diagnosis includes rotator cuff disease, labral pathology, and peripheral nerve injury in the setting of scapular winging.

Radiographs

The standard radiographs are typically unremarkable although bony abnormalities such as glenoid hypoplasia can be identified. Patients who have had previous traumatic anterior shoulder dislocation may have a posterosuperior impression fracture of the humeral head (Hill-Sachs lesion) or a bony deficiency of the anteroinferior glenoid rim (bony Bankart lesion). An MRI arthrogram can be useful to exclude labral injury (Bankart lesion) and document the patulous capsule.

Treatment

The mainstay of treatment for MDI is rehabilitation. Physical therapy is focused on strengthening the dynamic stabilizers of the shoulder girdle, including the rotator cuff and scapular stabilizers. More specialized therapy can be prescribed for athletes and is based on their specific sport and needs. Patients who fail rehabilitation may be candidates for surgical treatment. In most cases, rehabilitation should be continued for at least 6–12 months. Surgical treatment involves decreasing the volume of the shoulder joint by surgically altering the capsule (capsulorraphy). Surgery may be performed by arthroscopic or open methods. Arthroscopic methods tend to preserve motion better and may be preferable in athletes who would not tolerate minor losses of motion. Open surgical treatments historically have had lower rates of recurrent instability. Criticisms of open procedures such as the inferior capsular shift include loss of motion and potential subscapularis deficiency.

Summary

The shoulder is a complex structure that provides tremendous versatility and power to the upper extremity. The majority of painful shoulder girdle conditions are readily diagnosed with a thorough history and physical examination. Successful treatment of shoulder girdle problems is often accomplished by following a relatively simple algorithm of rest, activity modification, nonsteroidal anti-inflammatory drug therapy, and physical therapy. More invasive treatment options, such as arthroscopic and open surgery, are highly effective in appropriately selected patients.

Suggested Reading

1. Galatz LM ed. *Orthopaedic Knowledge Update: Shoulder and Elbow.* 3rd ed. Rosemont, IL: American Academy of Orthopaedic Surgeons; 2008.
2. Iannotti JP, Williams GR Jr. *Disorders of the Shoulder: Diagnosis & Management.* 2nd ed. Philadelphia, PA: Lippincott Williams & Wilkins; 2007.

Chapter 9
The Elbow

Scott G. Edwards and Brent B. Wiesel

Introduction

In looking at the arm as a whole, the tremendous range of motion of the shoulder can be thought of as positioning the hand on the outer surface of a sphere. It is the flexion, extension, pronation, and supination of the elbow and forearm that allow positioning of the hand within that sphere, thus creating the ability to function throughout a huge volume of space surrounding a person. When elbow and forearm function are compromised by pain, injury, or loss of motion, significant disability can result. The goals of this chapter are to present the elbow's functional anatomy, describe how to evaluate this region, and present an approach to diagnosis and treatment of common elbow problems.

Functional Anatomy

Skeletal

The elbow contains two distinct types of joints which allow hinge-type motion in the flexion–extension plane, and rotatory motion in the pronation–supination plane. Its bony anatomy starts several centimeters proximal to the joint itself, as the humeral shaft divides and flares into medial and lateral columns which end in condyles (Fig. 9.1). The lateral condyle consists of the lateral epicondyle and the capitellum, a hemispherical structure that articulates with the proximal surface of the radial head. The medial column develops a broad outcropping called the medial epicondyle; laterally it is bridged to the capitellum by the trochlea, a spool-shaped articular segment that engages the proximal ulna with a high degree of congruity and constraint. The trochlea has a 300° arc of cartilage when viewed in the sagittal plane,

S.G. Edwards (✉)
Division of Hand and Elbow Surgery, Center for Hand and Elbow Specialists, Department of Orthopedic Surgery, Georgetown University Medical Center, Washington, DC 20007, USA
e-mail: sge1@gunet.georgetown.edu

S.W. Wiesel, J.N. Delahay (eds.), *Essentials of Orthopedic Surgery*,
DOI 10.1007/978-1-4419-1389-0_9, © Springer Science+Business Media, LLC 2010

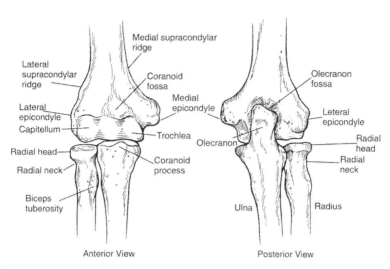

Fig. 9.1 Anterior and posterior views of the elbow joint demonstrate the three articulations, including the ulno-trochlear joint, the radiocapitellar joint, and the proximal radioulnar joint

allowing for the tremendous flexion–extension arc of the elbow while maintaining stability. The humeral columns and condyles create two fossae on the volar and dorsal aspects of the distal humerus. They are, respectively, called the coronoid and olecranon fossa; they allow for the coronoid and olecranon processes of the ulna to recess below the surface level of the humerus in extremes of flexion and extension.

The proximal ulna has a deep sigmoid notch, framed by the olecranon and coronoid processes, which cradles the trochlea. Radially, it has a lesser sigmoid notch, which articulates with the periphery of the radial head. Distally, it narrows to the tubular bone of the ulnar shaft. The radial head has a cup-shaped proximal surface articulating with the capitellum; its sides are covered with a 240° arc of articular cartilage, which interfaces with the lesser sigmoid notch and allows nearly 180° of pronation and supination. Distally, a prominent tuberosity is present on the radius for the attachment of the biceps.

Unlike the shoulder, whose stability is dependent on surrounding soft tissues, the elbow is a highly congruent joint with significant inherent stability. It is further supplemented by two important ligament complexes medially and laterally. The medial ulnar collateral ligament has three segments; the most important for stability is the anterior bundle (Fig. 9.2). The lateral complex consists of the lateral ulnar collateral ligament, which originates on the lateral epicondyle and inserts on the ulna; the annular ligament, which surrounds and stabilizes the radial head; and the radial collateral ligament, which extends from the lateral epicondyle to the annular ligament.

Anteriorly and posteriorly the elbow joint is lined by a single-cell layer of synovium, which in turn is covered by a relatively thick fibrous capsule. In the olecranon and coronoid fossa, a fatty layer of tissue is present between the synovium and the capsule. This layer is of significance in radiographic evaluation of elbow

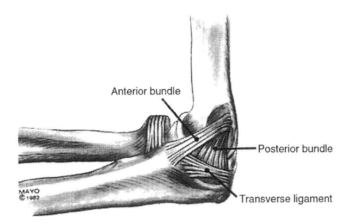

Fig. 9.2 A medial view of the elbow demonstrating the three bundles or bands of the medial collateral ligament. The anterior band is most important in elbow stability. (From Morrey BF ed. *The Elbow and Its Disorders*. 2nd ed. Philadelphia, PA: Saunders; 1993. Reprinted with permission from the Mayo Foundation for Medical Education and Research. All rights reserved)

trauma, in which intra-articular (intra-capsular) effusion (fluid) or hemarthrosis (bleeding into the joint) causes capsular distension and displacement of these fat pads either anterior or posterior to their usual position (Fig. 9.3). Identification of

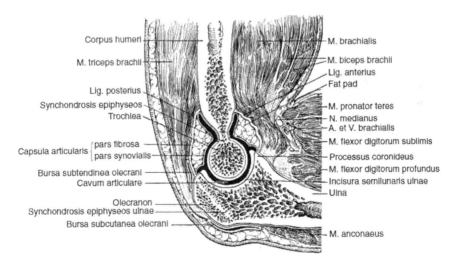

Fig. 9.3 Sagittal illustration of the elbow joint demonstrates the normal skeletal and soft tissue anatomy. Note the presence of fat pads both anteriorly and posteriorly, directly outside the joint capsule. Intra-articular swelling can lead to displacement out of the olecranon (posterior) or coronoid (anterior) fossae, leading to the appearance of "positive fat pad sign(s)" on lateral X-rays. (From Morrey BF ed. *The Elbow and Its Disorders*. 2nd ed. Philadelphia, PA: Saunders; 1993. Reprinted with permission from the Mayo Foundation for Medical Education and Research. All rights reserved)

these usually absent fat pads (particularly the posterior fat pad which is usually deeply contained within the olecranon fossa) suggests joint injury or fracture.

Muscles

The muscles surrounding the elbow can be divided into four separate groups on the basis of location and function. The two groups that originate in the upper arm include the elbow flexor and extensor compartments. The flexor compartment is on the anterior surface and consists of the brachialis, which inserts on the coronoid process, and the biceps, which inserts primarily on the radial tuberosity to provide both flexion and supination. The brachioradialis, which arises from the lateral aspect of the distal humerus and inserts on the radial styloid, also participates in flexion of the elbow. The extensor compartment of the elbow consists of the triceps, which inserts on the olecranon process to provide a powerful extension moment.

The two forearm muscle groups originating around the elbow include the wrist and finger extensors and the flexor-pronator mass. The extensor compartment muscles arise from the lateral epicondyle and include the extensor carpi radialis longus and brevis, which insert on the index and middle metacarpal, respectively, the extensor digitorum and extensor digiti mini, which extend the fingers, and the extensor carpi ulnaris. Deep to these muscles lies the supinator muscle which originates on the proximal ulna and inserts on the proximal radius. It assists the biceps with supination of the forearm. In addition, there is a muscle called the anconeus. This relatively small triangular structure originates on the lateral epicondyle and inserts on the lateral aspect of the olecranon. It is thought to assist with elbow extension and lateral stability of the elbow. The flexor-pronator mass takes its origin from the medial epicondyle, the medial ulna, and the interosseous membrane. It consists of the muscles that flex the fingers and wrist as well as the pronator teres.

Neurovascular

In contrast to the deeper-seated neurovascular structures of other extremities, those about the elbow are both tightly concentrated and superficial, making them uniquely vulnerable to both direct and indirect injuries. Injuries or symptoms due to nerve involvement around the elbow make familiarization with normal neurovascular anatomy crucial.

Musculocutaneous Nerve

Continuing from the lateral cord of the brachial plexus and composed of fibers from the C5–C8 nerve roots, this nerve travels through (and innervates) the biceps and brachialis. It terminates as the lateral antebrachial cutaneous nerve of the forearm which is vulnerable to injury during anterior approaches to the elbow, especially during distal biceps repair.

Median Nerve

Arising from C5–T1 nerve roots, combined from the upper and lower cords, the median nerve travels along anterior to the brachialis muscle, enters the antecubital fossa, then passes medial to the biceps tendon and the brachial artery. It then passes through the pronator teres and gives off the anterior interosseous branch, which supplies motor innervation to the flexor pollicis longus, the index and middle flexor digitorum profundus, and the pronator quadratus. The remainder continues distally in the forearm under the flexor digitorum sublimis. Distally the median nerve provides motor and sensory innervation to part of the radial aspect of the hand.

Radial Nerve

Originating from C6–8 nerve roots, the radial nerve is a continuation of the posterior cord and travels in the radial groove of the humerus. It innervates the triceps, brachioradialis, and extensor carpi radialis longus and brevis muscles. In the antecubital fossa the nerve divides into a deep motor branch (posterior interosseous nerve) and a superficial sensory branch. The superficial branch continues underneath the brachioradialis to provide sensation to the dorsum of the radial aspect of the wrist and hand.

Ulnar Nerve

Derived from roots C8 and T1, the ulnar nerve continues from the medial cord of the brachial plexus along the arm until passing posteriorly through the intermuscular septum at the level of the mid-humerus. It then travels through the cubital tunnel, where pathologic compression, traction, or irritation can occur. In the forearm, the ulnar nerve innervates the flexor carpi ulnaris and the ulnar half of the flexor digitorum profundus. Distally, it continues to provide motor function to many of the intrinsic hand muscles and sensation to the skin of the ulnar wrist and hand.

Brachial Artery

The brachial artery lies anterior to the medial aspect of the brachialis muscle, entering the antecubital space medial to the biceps tendon and lateral to the median nerve. At the level of the radial head, it divides into its terminal branches, the ulnar and radial arteries.

Evaluation of Elbow Problems

The evaluation of elbow problems relies on a thorough history, physical, and radiographic examination, supplemented by other pertinent tests when indicated.

History

Elbow problems can be divided into two major categories: (1) acute traumatic injuries and (2) atraumatic problems which tend to be more chronic in nature. In the situation of acute trauma, a detailed history of the event must be obtained. The mechanism of injury including the position of the arm, initial treatment, and subsequent symptoms are all very important in guiding further evaluation and management. It is also important to elicit a history of any prior injury or underlying symptoms in the elbow and forearm.

For non-acute elbow conditions, the most common complaint is pain, although stiffness or other mechanical symptoms such as locking, catching, or instability may accompany or become the primary problem. The examiner must try to define the complaint as completely and accurately as possible and identify the onset of the symptoms, including the time frame before the examination and whether it was acute or insidious. The exact location of the symptoms and any zone to which they radiate is important. As is the nature of the pain, Is it burning or radiating (nerve), or is it an aching related only to activity (tendinitis)? Does it hurt at rest or at night (tumor, infection)? Is it associated with any other symptoms, such as neck pain (referred pathology from the cervical spine) or wrist pain (distal radioulnar joint problem)?

The relationship of the patient's activity to the symptoms must be established. For example, in a throwing athlete, when during the pitch or throw does the pain occur? Medial elbow pain when the arm is in the "cocking position" suggests medial collateral ligament pathology, whereas medial pain during follow-through suggests involvement of the flexor-pronator group or impingement in the posterior ulna-humeral joint.

The examiner should determine what treatments, such as cortisone injections, physical therapy, anti-inflammatories, the patient has had and if any of them have been effective. The specifics of any pervious surgery is also important.

The elbow is commonly involved (and sometimes one of the first joints affected) in inflammatory arthritides, so it is important to elicit a history of other joint complaints, known arthritis, and family history. Is there a history of skin problems (lupus, dermatitis, psoriasis) or gastrointestinal problems (colitis)? Have there been any systemic symptoms of illness (malaise, fevers)?

Numbness, tingling, and weakness may be obvious clues to neurologic involvement, but sometimes nerve entrapment syndromes present with pain only. In addition to inquiring about tingling or numbness, ask about weakness or loss of dexterity.

Perhaps the most important part of the history is determining how the symptoms interfere with function. This directs the treatment more than any other factor. For example, inability to flex the elbow completely is well tolerated by most patients, because an arc of motion of 30–130° is generally relied upon for most activities of daily living. But in patients with rheumatoid arthritis, in whom shoulder motion is also compromised, elbow restriction may interfere with their ability to feed or clean themselves.

Physical Examination

The examination of the elbow begins with inspection, palpation, range of motion assessment, and evaluation for strength and neurovascular integrity. These maneuvers are then followed by special tests designed to evaluate specific conditions, based on a differential diagnosis from the history and initial tests. A thorough physical exam should also include a directed evaluation of the shoulder, wrist and hand, and, when relevant, the cervical spine.

Inspection begins with careful observation of elbow use as soon as one begins interaction with the patient. Does the patient extend the elbow to shake hands with the examiner? Are there obvious adaptive maneuvers that the patient uses to avoid pain or compensate for functional loss? A more formal visual exam is then performed to look for the presence of swelling, ecchymosis, atrophy, asymmetry, or masses. One should evaluate the "carrying angle" formed between the longitudinal axis of the humerus and the forearm which is normally 10–15°.

With the elbow flexed 90°, note that the normal bony prominences (medial and lateral epicondyles and the olecranon) form an equilateral triangle. In dislocations, this normal relationship is distorted. Look for evidence of joint swelling laterally by inspection of the soft tissue triangle bordered by the radial head, olecranon tip, and lateral epicondyle.

Palpate for tenderness, soft tissue integrity, and crepitus. Include the anterior, medial, lateral, and posterior structures in an organized systematic fashion. Be specific in trying to identify the exact area of tenderness. For example, lateral epicondylitis (lateral tennis elbow) causes focal tenderness over the lateral epicondyle. Tenderness more distally in the proximal forearm may instead suggest posterior interosseous nerve entrapment. Medial elbow pain may reflect medial epicondylitis (medial tennis elbow) if tender directly over the epicondyle. When more distal, it may be due to medial ulnar collateral ligament (MCL) insufficiency. Palpate posteriorly over the olecranon fossa. Notice the presence of any bursae over the olecranon tip, occasionally containing fluid, palpable fibrous fragments, or both (olecranon bursitis). Palpate over the antecubital fossa for any defect in the biceps tendon attachment (distal biceps tendon rupture).

Check both active and passive motion, noting any difference between them. If passive motion is greater than active motion, consider pain, muscle, or nerve injury as possible causes. Patients tend to splint their elbow at 80–90° following trauma because the joint capsule accommodates the maximum amount of fluid in this position. In the absence of trauma, pain on passive elbow motion suggests infection.

Note the location and timing of pain during motion. Discomfort at terminal extension is common in posterior olecranon impingement secondary to osteophytes in patients with ulnohumeral arthritis. Crepitus over the radiocapitellar joint during pronation/supination may indicate synovial or chondral pathology, degenerative changes, or radial head fracture.

The extent of neurologic evaluation depends on the patient's symptoms, but be familiar with sensory, motor, and reflex exam. Check for sensation to light touch in the distribution of the specific peripheral nerves. For the ulnar nerve, check the ulnar border of the little finger. For the median, use the radial border of the index finger. Check radial sensory function over dorsal thumb–index web space. The specific nerve roots have overlapping innervation, but in general, the lateral aspect of the deltoid is the C5 dermatome, the dorsal first web space is C6, the middle finger tip is C7, and the ulnar aspect of the forearm and arm is T1.

Strength testing depends on familiarity with the innervation of the various muscle groups. Elbow flexion relies on C5, whereas wrist extension is mainly C6. Elbow extension is from C7, which also provides finger extension and wrist flexion. Reflex testing is performed for the biceps (C5), brachioradialis (C6), and triceps (C7).

Vascular assessment includes palpation of the radial and ulnar arteries at the wrist, and the brachial artery in the antecubital fossa.

Additional specific physical examination tests may be useful depending on the condition suspected. When considering medial epicondylitis, check for pain on wrist flexion or forearm pronation against resistance. Medial collateral ligament sprain or attenuation is determined by applying a valgus stress to the 15–30° flexed elbow, looking to reproduce pain or joint opening. Lateral epicondylitis can be assessed by eliciting pain with wrist extension or grip, whereas radial tunnel syndrome is implied by pain with resisted middle finger extension or forearm supination.

The Tinel's sign is useful in assessment of nerve problems. Gently tapping over a nerve in the vicinity of suspected entrapment or pathology reproduces the symptoms, causing numbness, tingling, or pain in the nerve's distribution. During flexion and extension, the ulnar nerve may be "unstable" and can be felt subluxating or completely dislocating out of its groove posterior to the medial epicondyle in the cubital tunnel.

Radiographic Evaluation

Anteroposterior (AP) and lateral X-rays are the minimum views necessary to evaluate the elbow joint. Following trauma, additional views are sometimes helpful, including oblique and radial head views. Beyond this, the following special radiographic tests can be helpful.

Stress X-Rays

Stress views may be helpful in evaluating the patient with a suspected tear of the medial collateral ligament. This is achieved through manual stress, during which the clinician applies a valgus stress to the elbow in an effort to open up the medial side. A difference in medial gapping of more than 2 mm between the affected and normal elbow is usually significant.

Computed Tomography/Magnetic Resonance Imaging Examination

Computed tomography (CT) scans are effective in preoperative planning of complex elbow trauma, assessment of bony and joint deformity, and occasionally for evaluation of loose bodies of the elbow.

Magnetic resonance imaging (MRI) provides superior soft tissue imaging and allows visualization of marrow and vascularity changes in bone. Its current use about the elbow includes imaging occult fractures, tumors, infections, synovitis or other causes of joint effusion, and osteochondritis dissecans. It is occasionally useful in evaluating ligament disruptions, but it is usually unnecessary in evaluating medial or lateral epicondylitis and rarely helpful in nerve entrapment syndromes.

Technetium-99 Bone Scan

Technetium-99 injected intravenously is taken up in areas of increased vascularity. Although it is very sensitive, this test is not very specific, because increased blood flow can occur due to fracture, infection, tumor, or arthritis. In patients with heterotopic ossification, serial bone scans may help determine when the process has become quiescent enough to permit safe bone mass excision.

Electrodiagnostic Tests

Electromyography (EMG) and nerve conduction velocity (NCV) testing have definite indications in the patient with suspected nerve entrapment or injury. Such testing may indicate the site of the compression or injury. However, failure to demonstrate specific neurologic findings by electrodiagnostic testing does not rule out their presence. This is commonly the problem in working up the patient with early ulnar nerve symptoms, or the patient with suspected radial tunnel syndrome, in whom such tests are commonly negative.

Arthroscopy

The techniques and procedures for arthroscopy of the elbow have developed more slowly than in other joints such as the knee, shoulder, or wrist. Because of the very tight concentration of nerves and blood vessels in the area, the depth of the joint capsule under the musculature, and the tight articular constraint, the procedure is technically difficult and involves more risk than arthroscopy at most other joints. Although it provides a minimally invasive means with which to visually inspect and, when necessary, palpate the intra-articular structures, it is rarely used for diagnostic purposes alone.

Treatment of Elbow Problems

Treatment of elbow problems is algorithmic, dividing conditions into either traumatic or atraumatic cause (Figs. 9.4 and 9.5). One general principle of treatment in the elbow is to minimize the length of immobilization. The elbow has a high propensity for developing contractures with immobilization, especially after fractures or dislocations. The resultant loss of motion can be disabling, and treatment for it can be prolonged and difficult. When necessary, splinting is usually done with the elbow in 90° of flexion and neutral pronation to allow for maximal capsular volume and maintenance of the most useful arc of function.

With any significant elbow trauma, after appropriate initial treatment, one should carefully follow the patient's neurovascular exam, as the multiple confined fascial compartments of the forearm leave patients vulnerable to compartment syndrome or other severe compromise.

Nonoperative Treatment

Rehabilitation

Rehabilitation, through either a patient self-guided program or formal occupational or physical therapy, plays an important role in the treatment of elbow problems. The goals should include (1) reduction of pain and inflammation, (2) restoration of motion, (3) rebuilding strength, and (4) return to normal function and activity. These goals should be carefully monitored by the treating physician until the patient is discharged or alternative management is instituted.

Inflammation and pain are treated acutely with rest, ice, compression, and elevation (RICE). Later treatment includes activity modification, analgesics, nonsteroidal anti-inflammatories, and local modalities, including ice, heat, electrical stimulation, and ultrasound. Occasionally corticosteroid injection or systemic therapy is warranted.

Restoration of motion is done through careful stretching exercises. Elbow stiffness is best treated by prevention. Do not immobilize or use a sling any longer than absolutely necessary. Motion loss is usually in extension (inability to completely straighten the elbow) and takes much longer to regain than to lose. Once lost, motion return is best achieved through active exercise by the patient, rather than passive stretching by the therapist. A unique characteristic of the elbow is its propensity to develop heterotopic ossification (HO), bone formation within the soft tissues. This is particularly common anteriorly because of the presence of the brachialis

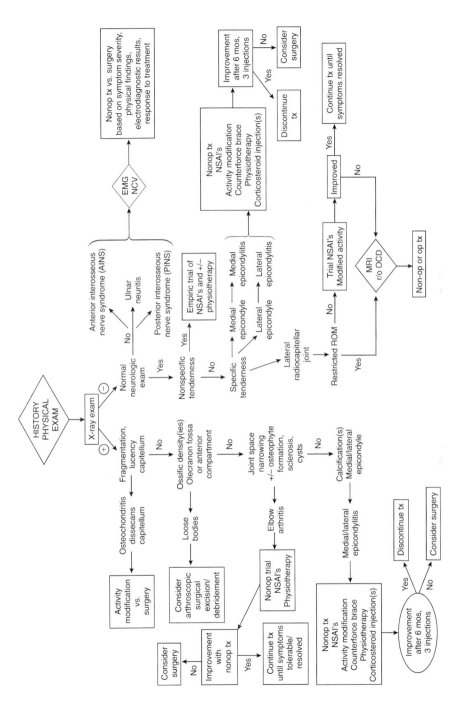

Fig. 9.4 Algorithmic approach to the diagnosis and treatment of atraumatic elbow pain

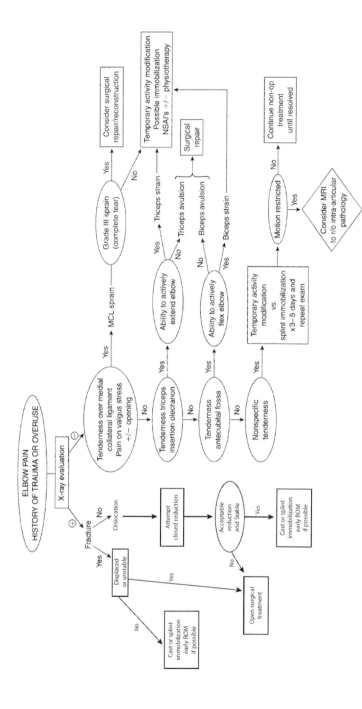

Fig. 9.5 Algorithmic approach to the diagnosis and treatment of traumatic elbow pain

muscle immediately anterior to the elbow capsule. The risk of ossification is increased with passive stretching, and for this reason, aggressive passive motion is discouraged. Specially designed splints which exert a dynamic force across the elbow are sometimes effective in restoring motion.

Corticosteroid Injections

The use of corticosteroids about the elbow facilitates treatment of a number of conditions, including medial and lateral epicondylitis, olecranon bursitis, and, less commonly, inflammatory or degenerative arthritis.

Because corticosteroid injections can lead to tendon damage, dermal de-pigmentation, and infection, they should not be used arbitrarily or excessively. Generally, their use is reserved for conditions which fail initial activity modification, anti-inflammatories, and therapy. The exact timing and number of injections is controversial, but in general, no more than three injections should be given over a 6-month time period.

Some authors have argued against using corticosteroids for conditions such as epicondylitis, arguing that the disease does not involve inflammation. Despite this, most orthopedic surgeons feel they are a useful treatment adjunct at this time.

Operative Treatment

Surgery for the elbow is reserved for patients in whom nonoperative management has failed or is inappropriate, such as traumatic injuries requiring rigid fixation and early mobilization. Surgery can be performed via open or arthroscopic methods. Elbow arthroscopy should only be done by surgeons who are comfortable with the surrounding anatomy, and even then should be approached cautiously. Therapeutically it has been used effectively for removal of loose bodies, synovectomy, debridement of the capsule and extensor carpi radialis brevis (ECRB) origin for lateral epicondylitis, radial head resection, release of contracture, and excision of osteophytes, and osteochondral debridement (osteochondritis dissecans, arthritis). Relative contraindications include severe contracture, previous ulnar nerve transposition, significant bone or joint distortion, and prior open elbow surgery.

Evaluation and Treatment of Common Elbow Problems

The following discussion highlights selected examples of common elbow problems.

Trauma

Fractures

Fractures around the elbow at the distal humerus, radial head and neck, and proximal ulna are fairly common. They occur through a wide variety of mechanisms, and one must be vigilant for associated soft tissue injuries. The treatment goals are complete healing of the fracture with pain-free motion and good function. Treatment options include casting, traction, percutaneous pin fixation, rigid internal fixation, resection, and replacement arthroplasty. Stable, non-displaced injuries such as simple radial head fractures can be treated with a brief period (1–2 weeks) of splinting followed by gentle range of motion. Most other fractures, however, require operative management with rigid internal fixation (Fig. 9.6) and early motion to avoid stiffness, non-union, and other complications. Severely comminuted, intra-articular fractures of the distal humerus in elderly or rheumatoid patients are sometimes best treated with a total elbow arthroplasty.

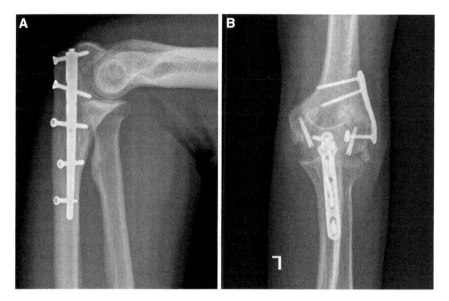

Fig. 9.6 (**a**) Proximal ulna fracture treated with a rigid intramedullary nail. (**b**) Supracondylar humerus fracture treated with plates and screws

Dislocations

Elbow dislocations are second only to those of the shoulder in frequency for major joints. They usually occur after a fall on an outstretched hand. By far the most common type is posteriolateral, in which the radius and ulna dislocate posteriorly and laterally relative to the humerus. Associated injuries are common, such as radial head and neck fractures (5–10%), avulsion fractures from the medial or lateral epicondyle (12%), and fractures of the coronoid process (10%).

Upon physical examination, there is visible deformity, with loss of the normal bony equilateral triangle, significant swelling, and loss of motion. A careful neurologic exam is mandated; the ulnar nerve is the most commonly injured nerve. Significant swelling anteriorly can lead to compartment syndrome of the forearm.

An AP and lateral X-ray are sufficient to make the diagnosis. The radial head should line up with the capitellum on both views. Failure to do so suggests residual subluxation. Special tests are rarely necessary. In the patient with median nerve injuries, one must consider arterial injury because of the median nerve's proximity to the brachial artery. If there is any question, arteriography is appropriate.

Initial neurovascular and radiographic assessment is followed by prompt reduction under sedation. Reduction is effected through manual forearm traction and brachial countertraction. The elbow is assessed for stability following reduction. If it is stable throughout the range of motion, application of a splint and sling, followed by early range of motion exercises, is indicated. If the elbow starts to sublux or dislocate, immobilization at 90° is appropriate for a longer period, but usually no more than 3 weeks to minimize the risk of permanent stiffness. Rarely, the elbow will remain unstable, even at 90° of flexion, in which case acute surgical repair of the lateral and possible medial collateral ligaments is indicated.

Ligamentous Injuries

Ligamentous injuries causing chronic elbow instability can be difficult to diagnose and treat. Anterior or posterior instabilities are usually due to displaced olecranon or coronoid fractures or, more rarely, anterior capsule and brachialis disruptions. Addressing the source of pathology usually leads to a stable elbow. Other types include varus, valgus, and posterolateral rotatory instabilities. They can all result from a single traumatic event such as a dislocation, but they can also come from repetitive stresses or iatrogenic injuries from excessive removal of epicondyles for ulnar nerve decompression or treatment of epicondylitis.

Patients with posterolateral rotatory instability have a spectrum of injury starting with disruption of the lateral ulnar collateral ligament and progressing to posterior capsule and even medial collateral ligament injury. They usually present with lateral elbow pain and often a mild flexion contracture. They have clicking and recurrent symptoms of popping or subluxation of the elbow. Varus stress test and elbow pivot shift test help make the diagnoses. X-rays are usually negative although stress views can be helpful. Treatment involves reconstruction of the lateral ligamentous structures; this often requires a tendon graft.

Injuries to the medial ulnar collateral ligament (MCL) cause valgus instability. It ranges from the Grade I sprains with microscopic hemorrhage causing chronic pain to complete Grade III disruption and true instability to valgus stress. The problem is particularly common in throwing athletes. Patients have a sense of "giving way" of the medial elbow. They have medial elbow pain and tenderness, especially with throwing. Pain typically occurs when the arm is in the "late cocking position" of throwing, that is, with the shoulder maximally abducted and externally rotated. Occasionally the patient has sudden onset of symptoms with one particular event such as in javelin throwing, but more commonly, prodromal symptoms precede the "final event" when the ligament completely tears.

Physical examination shows focal tenderness over the MCL or its coronoid insertion. On valgus stress there may be pain, tenderness, or the subtle sensation of medial joint opening. Look for signs of ulnar nerve irritability, which commonly accompanies MCL pathology. X-rays may show ossification or the "spur" sign at the ulnar insertion of the ligament.

The most difficult differential diagnosis is that of medial epicondylitis. Valgus stress may cause pain in this condition as well because of stress on the medial epicondylar tendinous origin. However, in the isolated MCL sprain, forearm pronation or wrist flexion against resistance (common in epicondylitis) should not cause pain.

Special stress X-rays may be helpful to document subtle instability. By flexing the elbow 30°, thereby unlocking the olecranon from its fossa, either gravity or manual force can apply a valgus stress. Any opening is likely of some significance, although it is appropriate to compare with the other side. When positive, these stress views are confirmatory. When negative however, they do not exclude MCL insufficiency.

In almost all Grade I and II injuries, symptomatic treatment, including rest, ice, compression, and strengthening, allows return to activity. Grade III tears, especially in throwing athletes, often require surgical reconstruction, in which a tendon graft is used to reconstruct the MCL.

Tendon Ruptures

Ruptures of the distal biceps tendon are common injuries. They nearly always occur in muscular men aged 30–60 years. They can occur as partial tears at the insertion or the musculotendinous junction, but they are most commonly complete insertional detachments from the biceps tuberosity of the radius. They almost always occur during a heavy eccentric load to the biceps, and patients usually feel a "pop" and sharp pain in the antecubital space at the time. Patients are tender anteriorly and have weakness with elbow flexion and supination. If the diagnosis is unclear, an MRI can be helpful, but it is rarely needed.

Complete ruptures should be surgically reattached with 10–14 days to prevent future weakness which is more dramatic in supination than flexion. Surgery involves finding the ruptured tendon via an incision over the anticubital fossa and then reattaching it to the biceps tuberosity. This can be done using bone tunnels placed via a second incision over the posterior lateral elbow (two incision technique) or with suture anchors or an Endobutton[TM] (Smith & Nephew, Memphis, Tennessee) placed from the anterior incision (one incision technique). In chronic presentations, patients can be treated with graft reconstructions or just observed if their functional losses are tolerated.

Triceps tendon ruptures are more uncommon. Patients again present after an eccentric load. A defect in the triceps is often palpable, and elbow extension is weak. These injuries should be treated with surgical reattachment of the tendon to the olecranon process.

Atraumatic and Overuse Injuries of the Elbow

Lateral and Medial Epicondylitis

In skeletally mature adults, strains to the medial and lateral epicondyle can result in epicondylitis and are the most common elbow pathology seen in clinical practice. These conditions can also result from a single, particularly strenuous action, or with any repetitive stress such as sports (especially racket sports, golf, and baseball), carrying heavy bags, or even typing or cleaning activities. The tendon origin is thought to undergo microtears, degeneration, replacement with abnormal scar and granulation tissue (called angiofibroblastic hyperplasia due to its microscopic appearance) within the extensor carpi radialis brevis (ECRB) on the lateral side or the flexor carpi radialis (FCR) and pronator teres (PT) muscles on the medial side.

Lateral epicondylitis is popularly known as tennis elbow, despite the fact that only 5% of patients play tennis. Conversely, nearly 50% of tennis players will develop the condition during their sports careers. Medial epicondylitis is often called golfer's elbow.

Patients complain of pain on activity over the medial or lateral epicondyles of the elbow, often with some radiation into the forearm. The key physical exam finding is focal tenderness over the epicondyle or the muscles just anterior to it. Resisted wrist extension and grip reproduce symptoms in lateral epicondylitis, and wrist flexion and forearm pronation against resistance reproduce the symptoms in medial epicondylitis. X-rays are usually normal.

On the lateral side, the differential diagnosis includes radial tunnel syndrome (which coexists in 5% of patients), varus or posterolateral rotatory instability, or radiocapitellar arthrosis. On the medial side, the main diagnoses to also consider are ulnar nerve compression and medial collateral ligament injury.

Treatment is almost always conservative, emphasizing rest, ice, avoidance of provocative activities, and nonsteroidal anti-inflammatory drugs (NSAIDs). In addition, modalities such as ice, heat, or contrast therapy are helpful. Identification and correction of faulty technique, use of a counterforce brace, and a structured physical therapy (PT) program can be helpful. Cortisone injections are used in those unresponsive to early conservative management or those presenting with severe symptoms.

Surgery is required for less than 10% of patients who develop epicondylitis. It may be indicated in patients who fail an appropriate conservative trial, usually considered at least 6 months' duration, and up to three injections of cortisone. Successful surgery involves identification and debridement of the pathologic tissue, usually located within the substance of the flexor carpi radialis and pronator teres on the medial side or the extensor carpi radialis brevis on the lateral side. For lateral epicondylitis, some surgeons are now advocating an arthroscopic technique in which the lateral joint capsule and the ECRB origin are debrided from the joint surface outward, without opening the superficial skin or musculature. The reported advantage of this technique is a faster return to work following surgery although it is associated with risk of neurovascular injury that accompanies arthroscopy.

Ulnar Nerve Compression (Cubital Tunnel Syndrome)

Patients with cubital tunnel syndrome present with complaints of numbness and tingling in the distribution of the ulnar nerve. They often have elbow pain with or without radiation; it is usually worse with sleep or long periods of elbow flexion. The patient may feel clumsy or weak in grasping or throwing; he or she may note actual "snapping" in cases in which the ulnar nerve is unstable.

The position of the ulnar nerve at the elbow renders it susceptible to both compression and direct trauma. There are five major sites of compression of the ulnar nerve in the region: the arcade of Struthers (a fascial band 5–10 cm proximal to the medial epicondyle), the medial intermuscular septum, the groove behind the medial epicondyle, the ligament of Osborne [a fascial band between the humeral and ulnar heads of the flexor carpi ulnaris or flexor carpi ulnaris (FCU) muscle], and the exit of the nerve from the FCU. Extremes of elbow flexion can cause tethering of the ulnar nerve around the medial epicondyle and compression. Up to 16% of patients are further predisposed to symptoms by having "instability," with either subluxation or frank dislocation out of the groove.

In early disease, there is usually no sensory or motor deficit, although Tinel's sign over the cubital tunnel may be positive. It is important to check for nerve instability by flexing and extending elbow while feeling the ulnar nerve. As the compression progresses, patients can lose sensation over the ulnar border of the ring finger and all of the small finger. Weakness to finger abduction and eventually intrinsic atrophy can develop. A positive Froment's test, in which the thumb collapses into IP joint flexion and is weak with key pinch, is an important diagnostic sign. X-rays are almost always negative. Electrodiagnostic tests are often negative in early disease, but can show slowing of conduction velocity specifically at the elbow.

It is important to rule out other similarly presenting compressive neuropathies such as thoracic outlet or ulnar tunnel syndrome, as well as medial epicondylitis.

Treatment is initially nonoperative, with rest, ice, NSAIDs, night-time extension splinting, or occasional cast immobilization for 2–3 weeks. For patients with continued symptoms or significant deinervation on nerve conduction study/electromyography (NCS/EMG), surgery involves decompression and possibly anterior transposition of the ulnar nerve (Fig. 9.7).

Little Leaguer's Elbow

In the skeletally immature athlete, injury to the medial epicondylar apophyseal structures is known as little leaguer's elbow because of its high incidence in young baseball players. Repetitive stresses to the vulnerable epicondylar origin of the flexor-pronator group and MCL, during both acceleration and follow-through phases of throwing, result in abnormalities in secondary ossification and physeal plate structures. These children present with medial elbow pain, diminished throwing effectiveness, and decreased throwing distance.

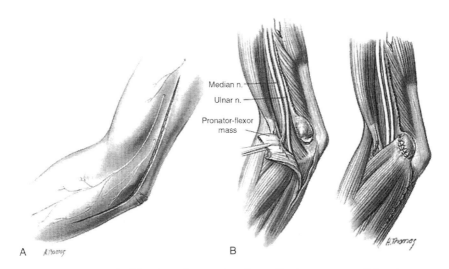

Fig. 9.7 (**a**) A medial incision is made over the elbow, allowing exposure of the ulnar nerve proximal, through and distal to the cubital tunnel through which it travels. (**b**) The ulnar nerve is transposed sub-muscularly underneath the flexor-pronator muscle mass, after which the muscle origin is reattached to the medial epicondyle. (From Morrey BF ed. *The Elbow and Its Disorders*. 2nd ed. Philadelphia, PA: Saunders; 1993. Reprinted with permission from the Mayo Foundation for Medical Education and Research. All rights reserved)

On examination there is focal tenderness over the medial epicondyle and pain on attempting active wrist flexion or forearm pronation, especially against resistance. X-ray findings vary and include apophyseal fragmentation, irregularity or enlargement, abnormality of the physis, or avulsion of the medial epicondyle. Stress views are useful; even an innocent appearing minimally displaced fracture may be unstable.

Fortunately, treatment is rarely operative and includes rest, ice, and gradual return to activity as pain resolves. Restricting the number of innings pitched in Little League has led to a reduction in the incidence of elbow complaints. Surgery is reserved for those with displaced or unstable avulsion injuries or symptomatic non-unions.

Osteochondritis Dissecans (Panners' Disease)

This condition is particularly common among adolescent throwing and gymnastic athletes. It has been described as the leading cause of permanent disability in the young throwing athlete. The most common symptom is that of activity-related lateral elbow pain. There may be associated swelling, limitation of motion, and catching or locking episodes.

In throwing, enormous valgus stresses are imparted to the elbow joint. Absorbed primarily by the medial collateral ligament, the second line of defense is the radiocapitellar buttress, which is subjected to significant compression and shear. This also occurs in gymnastics, particularly during vaulting, balance beam, uneven parallel bars, and floor exercises. In skeletally immature individuals, such repetitive stresses lead to damage of the capitaller cartilage and subchondral bone and possibly are a result of avascular necrosis (AVN).

There is a classification system based on articular involvement. Type I lesions have no articular involvement. In Types II and III, there is articular involvement. In Type II, there is formation of an osteochondral fragment without separation, and in Type III there is separation with loose body formation.

On physical exam, there is often a restriction in motion, especially extension, crepitus on supination/pronation, and tenderness over the radiocapitellar joint. X-rays are initially often normal, although there may be lucency or irregular ossification of the capitellum. In later stages, there may be a crescent sign, fragmentation, or loose body formation. MRI or CT with arthrogram is probably the best method of establishing the diagnosis and assessing the degree of articular involvement. MRI is also useful in assessing subchondral involvement and the extent and status of healing of the lesion.

Treatment depends on clinical and radiographic findings. Nonoperative treatment for Type I includes rest, ice, NSAIDs, extension splinting, and physical therapy with modalities. Because the healing process is slow, the area must be protected against overzealous activity (i.e., hard throwing or weight-bearing) for a long time.

Treatment of Type II and III (articular involvement) lesions is initially nonoperative but operative treatment is frequently required. Typically, this involves arthroscopically removing loose bodies, curetting, and/or drilling the lesion's base. Return to throwing or gymnastics after surgery is highly variable.

Arthritis

Arthritis of the elbow is much less common than that of the hip or knee. The three major types are primary osteoarthritis, post-traumatic arthritis, and inflammatory. In patients with inflammatory (especially rheumatoid) arthritis, 20–50% have elbow involvement. It can lead to severe loss of arm function due to pain, instability, or loss of motion, especially when there is concomitant shoulder and hand involvement. In some cases rheumatoid disease first presents in the elbow. These patients require appropriate lab tests for evaluation of systemic arthritis including erythrocyte sedimentation rate (ESR), anti-nuclear antibody (ANA) test, rheumatoid factor (RF) test, and complete blood count (CBC). Additional rheumatologic tests should be determined in consultation with a rheumatologist. The differential diagnosis includes septic arthritis, gout or other crystalline arthropathy, or osteoarthritis. Aspiration for cell count with differential, gram stain, and crystal examination of the joint fluid is very helpful. X-ray changes are variable, ranging from periarticular osteopenia in early disease to subchondral erosions, destructive appearing joint collapse, and ultimately bony ankylosis as the disease progresses.

Treatment of the rheumatoid elbow varies with the stage of presentation. Early in the course, anti-inflammatory and anti-rheumatoid medication, analgesics, and activity modification may be sufficient. Initial goals are to decrease pain and inflammation, maintain motion, and avoid further destructive changes. Later, efforts to relieve pain and improve function may rely on surgical treatment such as arthroscopic or open synovectomy with or without radial head resection. In end-stage disease, a total elbow replacement may be the only option.

Summary and Conclusions

The elbow is the critical link between the highly mobile shoulder joint and the precisely coordinated wrist/hand complex. Conditions which interfere with the elbow's normal motion can significantly compromise a patient's ability to feed, dress, and clean himself or herself. In the athlete, compromise in function often precludes the ability to participate. Fortunately, most conditions affecting the elbow do not result in significant limitations. The majority elbow problems can be readily diagnosed with a thorough history, physical, and basic radiographic examination. An algorithmic approach to treatment facilitates resolution of most problems of the elbow.

Suggested Reading

1. Morrey BF ed. *The Elbow and Its Disorders.* 3rd ed. Philadelphia, PA: WB Saunders; 2000.
2. Galatz LM ed. *Orthopaedic Knowledge Update: Shoulder and Elbow.* 3rd ed. Rosemont, IL: American Academy of Orthopaedic Surgeons; 2008.

Chapter 10
The Hand

Scott G. Edwards

Introduction

The human hand is one of the most important interfaces of a person's body with the outside world. It allows us to touch, feel, manipulate, and modify our environment. Its cortical representation in the brain is nearly as large as the rest of the musculoskeletal system combined. Loss of hand function can have devastating effects on a person's ability to work or perform activities of daily living. Unfortunately, because of its constant use and its position at the forefront of human activity, it is frequently affected by trauma and other disease processes. Nearly all physicians will see patients with hand problems, so some familiarity with these processes and the basic hand evaluation is very important.

History

As in all fields of medicine, the history begins by carefully determining the patient's chief complaint, followed by a detailed history of the present illness. It is also very important to obtain supplemental information important to hand function, such as hand dominance, and the patient's specific use patterns for his or her hands such as their occupation, sports involvement, and other hobbies.

The history of present illness is tailored to the patient's chief complaint and does require some background understanding of various pathologic processes in the hand and upper extremity. In patients with congenital hand differences or birth-related injuries, one must obtain a careful understanding of the gestational and birth history. One must inquire about gestational diabetes, preeclampsia, and other maternal and fetal health problems including exposure to teratogens. The presence of consanguinity or a family history of similar anomalies should also be determined. The physician

S.G. Edwards (✉)
Division of Hand and Elbow Surgery, Center for Hand and Elbow Specialists, Department of Orthopedic Surgery, Georgetown University Medical Center, Washington, DC 20007, USA
e-mail: sge1@gunet.georgetown.edu

S.W. Wiesel, J.N. Delahay (eds.), *Essentials of Orthopedic Surgery*,
DOI 10.1007/978-1-4419-1389-0_10, © Springer Science+Business Media, LLC 2010

should also see if improvement in the condition has occurred and determine some of the parental goals and expectations of outcome.

In nontraumatic situations, it is important to have the patient focus as closely as possible on the exact site of the problem and to try to analyze the history of onset, the progression, and interventions. An understanding of what helps relieve symptoms and what aggravates them can be very important in determining treatment. In patients who attribute their problems to repetitive activities, it is further important to understand the length of time it takes before symptoms begin, how long the patient had been doing this activity before this problem developed, and whether symptoms are now present when the patient is not involved in these activities.

When a traumatic injury is present, the exact nature of the injury and the surrounding circumstances under which they occurred should be carefully noted and documented. This includes such information as the environment in which this occurred, whether it was clean or dirty, and whether the patient perceives that the injury was due to another person's fault, their own error, or an unavoidable circumstance. Many of these patients later become involved in worker's compensation or other medicolegal litigation. By carefully determining and recording the events that occurred, the treating physician can give the most accurate representation of the injury and avoid later difficulties in trying to reconstruct events from memory.

Many times these patients will present late after having been treated elsewhere or avoiding treatment altogether. In these stages, it is very important to note the evolution of the patient's problems, what treatments have occurred, and what the current functional losses are.

The remainder of the patient's medical history is also quite important. A good understanding of the patient's diseases including the presence of diabetes, hypothyroidism, heart disease, or other problems can help determine contributing factors to a hand problem. Previous surgical history, including complications of anesthetics, is also very important in the treatment process. Medications and allergies have obvious implications in the treatment. Social history should include the patient's occupation and hobbies as well as tobacco, alcohol, and illicit drug use. Family history and review of systems that include questions about the patient's psychiatric history help complete a thorough evaluation of the patient's history.

Physical Examination

In the physical examination of the hand and upper extremity, one must often start proximally at the neck or shoulder, especially for nerve and tendon problems. One begins the evaluation with observation of the upper extremity looking for atrophy, deformity, or any other lesions with comparison to the opposite side. Palpation of the area of the chief complaint should be performed next. In this section, one should make every effort to localize the patient's pain or other complaints as anatomically as possible to help define the diagnosis. An understanding of the surface anatomy is critical to this. For example, one must know that the scaphoid waist underlies the anatomical snuff box, or that the A-1 pulley of the flexor tendon sheath is at the level of the metacarpophalangeal joint. Next, one should determine both the active and passive range of motion of the elbow, wrist, and hand. This should be recorded carefully for later comparison testing.

Injuries that involve open wounds of the hand and upper extremity should rarely, if ever, be probed or explored on the initial evaluation. Examination of the distal hand function can usually determine what structures are injured. Vascular function can be determined by evaluating capillary refill or performing a Doppler ultrasound evaluation of pulses distal to the laceration. Flexor and extensor tendon function can almost always be determined by evaluation of active range of motion. Nerve function can be assessed by performing motor and sensory examination as well. In evaluating the sensory function, it is often helpful to obtain some quantifiably measured data such as two-point discrimination or Semmes-Weinstein monofilament threshold testing. For young children, assessment of wrinkling after immersion under water or the presence or absence of sweating can be helpful, as they are functions of the autonomic nervous system and cease as soon as a peripheral nerve is cut.

Specialized testing for specific injuries or problems can help confirm a diagnosis, and they will be addressed under the sections describing those specific disease processes.

Imaging

Imaging of the hand and upper extremity typically starts with plain radiographic evaluation. The standard views used in the hand and wrist include AP, lateral, and oblique views, and all physicians who will ever evaluate the hand should have some familiarity with the basic radiographic anatomy of the carpal, metacarpal, and phalangeal bones in these views. In particular, one should recognize the overall alignment and arcs that are present to avoid missing a dislocation in an emergency room setting. There are many additional special views such as a carpal tunnel, a Brewerton, and scaphoid views that help profile specific injury patterns.

Advanced imaging modalities are used for disease or injury processes that are more difficult to define. Bone scans can be very useful for helping define infection, reflex sympathetic dystrophy, and occult fractures. Computed tomography (CT) scans are helpful for better understanding bony lesions and defining tumors. Magnetic resonance imaging (MRI) is typically the imaging modality of choice for soft tissue lesions. It is also becoming more frequently used for occult fractures. When accompanied by an arthrogram, it can be very helpful in diagnosing ligamentous injuries of the wrist. Ultrasound is rapidly becoming a very useful imaging technique as well, especially to define soft tissue lesions, bony abnormalities, and ligamentous injuries. It can be particularly helpful in differentiating between rupture or scarring of a tendon repair and for visualizing foreign bodies that are not radiopaque. It allows for a dynamic study in which tendons or other soft tissue structures can be evaluated while they are moving. It is an extremely cost-effective imaging modality, but, unfortunately, at this time it is still very operator dependent.

Arthroscopy

Arthroscopy has become an important treatment modality particularly for the wrist. In some situations, such as chondral injuries, some ligament tears, and capsular tears, it is the best way to make a diagnosis as well. As the technology and experience level increases in these techniques, arthroscopy may become an important diagnostic and treatment method for the metacarpophalangeal and other small joints.

Pathophysiology

Hand problems can be grouped into seven major categories of disease: congenital, developmental/idiopathic, inflammatory/infectious, traumatic, metabolic, vascular, and neoplastic. There is tremendous overlap between these divisions and a given disease process may actually have roots in more than one category. However, keeping these major categories in mind and eliminating the ones that do not fit a patient's complaint can help narrow down one's differential diagnosis and arrive at the proper diagnosis and treatment protocol. The remainder of this section reviews the most common disease entities within each category.

Congenital Hand Differences

In the human embryo, the upper extremity begins to develop as a limb bud at 4 weeks after fertilization when a segment of mesoderm outgrows and protrudes into the overlying ectoderm. A small segment of ectoderm then condenses and forms the apical ectodermal ridge which guides further longitudinal growth of the limb. A second area named the "zone of polarizing activity" forms in the posterior margin of the limb bud and controls radial and ulnar growth and differentiation. A third area in the dorsal ectoderm helps control formation of volar and dorsal characteristics of the limb. From weeks 4–8 after fertilization, this small outgrowth of mesoderm becomes a fully differentiated upper extremity with separated joints and digits. It is during this time that most congenital upper extremity anomalies originate.

Failure of Formation of Parts (Arrest of Development)

Failures of formation of parts come in two varieties: transverse and longitudinal. Transverse failures are due to injuries to the apical ectodermal ridge. They result in complete congenital amputation distal to the site of injury. This can vary from loss of fingertips to complete absence of the arm. The most common presentation is a congenital below-elbow amputation at the level of the proximal third of the forearm; it is treated by fitting a passive mitten when the child is old enough to sit, then a prosthesis a few years later.

Longitudinal failures of formation involve loss of only part of the distal segment. They can be divided into radial (preaxial), central, and ulnar (postaxial). The most common of these are the radial-sided deficiencies such as congenital absence of the thumb or radial clubhand (Fig. 10.1a). These problems are often associated with visceral and bone marrow abnormalities and abnormalities such as Holt-Oram (cardiac septal defects), thrombocytopenia absent radius (TAR), and (vertebral, anal, cardiac, tracheoesophageal, renal, and limb abnormalities (VACTRL). These patients should all undergo evaluation by the appropriate pediatric subspecialists. Central defects are much less common and mainly involve the cleft hand. Ulnar-sided deficiencies include ulnar clubhand and its variations. These are often associated with other orthopedic anomalies. A very uncommon form of longitudinal growth arrest

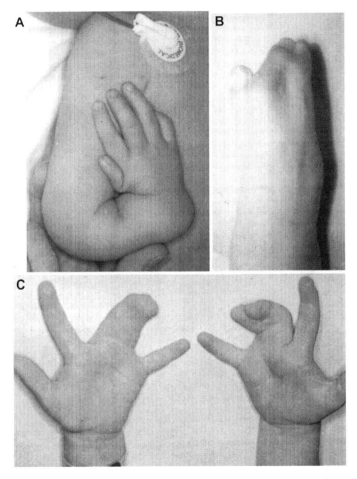

Fig. 10.1 Congenital malformations. (**a**) Radial clubhand produced by longitudinal absence of radius. (**b**) Failure of formation of parts combined with failure of separation. (**c**) Simple syndactyly of middle and ring fingers

involves the intrasegmental losses such as phocomelia, in which a relatively normal hand is attached to either the trunk or a very short segment of arm.

Failure of Differentiation (Separation of Parts)

Failure of differentiation occurs when the normal programmed cell death between tissues fails to occur, and bones, joints, or individual digits fail to form. The most common manifestation of this is syndactyly, in which individual digits are still linked together either by webs of skin or sometimes continued fusion of the bones (Fig. 10.1c). These often require surgical separation when the patient reaches the appropriate age. Other fairly common failures of separation include congenital lunotriquetral coalition. This rarely causes any problems and is often an incidental finding. Synostosis, particularly of the proximal radius and ulna, which restricts pronation and supination, and symphalangism in which there is congenital fusion of the proximal interphalangeal (PIP) joint are other manifestations that can be more problematic.

Duplication

Duplication or polydactyly is another fairly common congenital hand difference. This can range in scope from a simple skin tag attached to the small finger to a complete mirror hand. The very small skin tags formed on the ulnar aspect of the hand can sometimes be treated with suture ligation in the nursery, but more complex polydactylies require formal surgical resection and reconstruction. This is particularly true when a joint is involved as this may require osteotomy to allow the joint surfaces to maintain normal congruity and ligament reconstruction to reestablish stability. Often, the individual duplicated segments are not equal in size to a normal part and function may not be completely normal after reconstruction. Many of the thumb reconstructions, in particular, require later secondary operations to fine-tune the result or to make adjustments for growth-induced deformities (Fig. 10.2a).

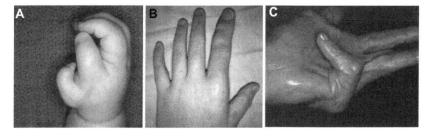

Fig. 10.2 Congenital and developmental anomalies. (**a**) Duplication of thumb. (**b**) Gigantism of index finger with enlarged soft tissues as well as skeleton. (**c**) Dupuytren's contracture. Bands extending from proximal palm into middle segment of finger have caused near 90° contractures of MCP and PIP joints with dimpling and shortening of skin

Other Congenital Anomalies

The remaining categories of congenital hand differences are less common. Overgrowth is a condition that can affect either an entire limb or an individual digit or section of the upper extremity (Fig. 10.2b). When this is encountered, the physician should look for an underlying cause such as a vascular malformation or neurofibromatosis. The problem can be exceedingly difficult to treat, and when debulking procedures fail, this can often require ray amputation of affected digits.

Undergrowth or hypoplasia also shows a wide spectrum of problems including such minor differences as brachymetacarpia (short metacarpals), or to involve significant hypoplasias of the entire upper extremity. It is sometimes associated with other syndromic conditions such as Poland syndrome (pectus excavatum and other chest wall abnormalities, hypoplasia of the hand, syndactyly, and other associated abnormalities). The treatment is very patient specific, and often supportive care is all that is needed.

Congenital constriction band syndrome is a process in which the underlying cause is not fully understood. It is thought that amniotic bands form across segments of the extremities causing deep constriction rings, amputations, or fusions of distal parts. In some rare instances, surgery very soon after birth is required to prevent neurovascular compromise, but most cases can be treated in a delayed fashion. Treatment often involves excision of the deep constriction band and multiple Z-plasties for reconstruction. In some situations, a separation of distal syndactyly of the digits can be required.

The final category of congenital hand differences involves generalized skeletal abnormalities. These are disease processes such as enchondromatosis, multiple hereditary exostoses, and chondroplasia. Frequently, no hand surgery is required. One should just monitor the patient's symptoms closely and make sure follow-up is done by the appropriate specialists if the symptoms get worse.

Developmental or Acquired Disease

Arthritides

Arthritis of the hand and wrist is a fairly common problem, and as it becomes progressively more severe, patients can experience marked limitation in hand use due to pain or loss of function.

Nearly all types of arthritis will eventually affect the hand, but osteoarthritis is by far the most common form that develops. The distal interphalangeal (DIP) joints of the fingers and interphalangeal (IP) joints of the thumbs are the usual sites where this first develops, and patients often notice painless nodules early on in the disease process. Mucous cysts can result at these joints. The PIP joints also become involved and can develop significant angular deformity. The thumb carpometacarpal (CMC) joint, also known as the basilar joint or trapeziometacarpal joint, is a common site of early involvement; it can be extremely painful and cause debilitating loss of pinch and grasp function. In the carpus itself, the scaphotrapeziotrapezoid (STT) joint also has fairly high rates of involvement and is often accompanied by thumb CMC arthritis.

The diagnosis can often be made by the patient's description of symptoms alone. Physical examination often shows a deformity and nodule formation. Thumb CMC arthritis can further be diagnosed by a positive thumb CMC grind test. The thumb metacarpal is carefully grasped between the examiner's thumb and index finger. The remainder of the wrist is stabilized with the other hand and an axial load and circumduction force is applied to the thumb metacarpal. This usually results in severe pain for patients who have arthritis of this joint. Plain radiographs confirm the diagnosis in nearly all cases and advanced imaging is rarely, if ever, needed. Classic radiographic findings are joint space narrowing, subchondral sclerosis, subchondral cyst formation, and osteophyte formation.

Treatment is usually directed by the patient's level of symptoms and the radiographic staging. For moderate pain and earlier radiographic stages, simple rest and antiinflammatories can often help tremendously. Splinting is often a very usual adjunct, particularly for the thumb CMC joint and for the STT joint. Corticosteroid injections can also give tremendous pain relief, again, particularly at the thumb CMC joint and the STT joint. If patients have significant mucous cysts at the DIP joint causing pain, skin breakdown, or nail deformities, surgical treatment with resection of the mucous cysts and the underlying osteophytes is indicated. More severe PIP and DIP joint involvement causing unremitting pain or deformity is usually treated by a fusion. Joint replacement arthroplasties are available for very limited indications. Isolated STT joint arthritis is usually treated with fusion. Arthritis of the CMC joint can be treated with arthrodesis or arthroplasty using trapezial resection and ligament reconstruction. Some surgeons prefer implant arthroplasties, but they have had problems with stability and wear.

Posttraumatic arthritis is another very common form of arthritis. It is due to a ligament, cartilage, or bone injury resulting in increased wear of the joint surface and eventual loss of the cartilage space and arthritis formation. One of the most frequently seen forms is the scapholunate advanced collapse pattern or SLAC wrist. The underlying problem here is a rupture of the scapholunate interosseous ligament that goes untreated. The scaphoid eventually assumes a flexed posture and rotates within the scaphoid fossa of the radius, the lunate goes into a hyperextended position, and arthritis develops. This first starts in the radial styloid region and extends to the entire scaphoid fossa and then to the scaphocapitate interval and eventually around the entire wrist. Treatment options depend upon the stage and include symptomatic treatment initially followed by scaphoid excision and capitate–hamate–triquetral and lunate fusion, or proximal row carpectomy and total wrist fusion for more advanced states.

Rheumatoid arthritis has extensive involvement in the hand and wrist (Fig. 10.3). This disease is a systemic problem, and in the hand nearly all tissues can be involved including bone, joint, tendon, and vascular tissues. The distal radioulnar joint is frequently involved with erosions into the ulnar head eventually causing instability which allows the ulnar head to abrade the overlying extensor tendons and cause rupture; this is called a Vaughn-Jackson lesion. The remainder of the carpus can develop extensive erosion, frequently causing volar and ulnar subluxation of the carpus on the radius and a radial deviation deformity of the wrist. The thumb CMC joint often erodes and dislocates, pushing the thumb into an adduction deformity. The metacarpophalangeal (MP) joint of the thumb is also frequently involved. The MP joints of the remaining digits usually drift into an ulnar deviation deformity, further compromising hand function. The PIP joints develop severe synovitis that can lead to either a boutonnière or swan-neck deformity. The DIP joints are usually spared. In the early phases of the disease, treatment is focused on medical management. Accompanying therapy and splinting can be useful adjuncts for maintaining strength

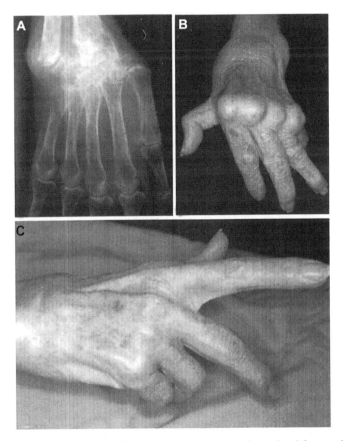

Fig. 10.3 Rheumatoid arthritis. (**a**) Severe erosive destruction of carpal and forearm bones with dislocation of distal radioulnar joint and moderate osteoporosis of all bones. (**b**) Clinical picture of advanced rheumatoid changes with tenosynovitis at wrist, dislocations of MCP joints of fingers resulting in ulnar drift, and typical deformities of the thumb. (**c**) Rupture of extensors of ulnar three digits as a result of tenosynovitis at wrist with dislocation of distal radioulnar joint. (**d**) Results of surgery with relocation of MCP joints of fingers by prosthetic insertion, fusion of thumb joints, and synovectomy of wrist joint and extensor tendons

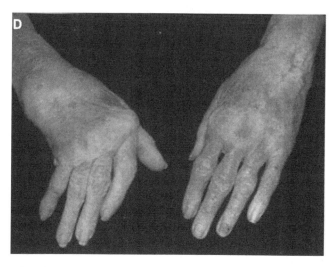

Fig. 10.3 (continued)

and slowing the progress of deformity. As the disease progresses, the individual problems that develop must be addressed. Persistent tenosynovitis is treated with surgical tenosynovectomy, which is often performed in conjunction with resection of any potential sharp bony protrusions that may erode tendons, resection of the ulnar head or bony osteophytes at Lister's tubercle or the scaphoid are also often performed. Rheumatoid destruction of the wrist itself is usually addressed with a fusion. Several types of wrist replacements are available, including Silastic implants and metal and plastic options as well. The thumb CMC joint is usually addressed with a nonimplant arthroplasty, with trapeziectomy and ligament reconstruction. The MP joint of the thumb is usually fused when necessary and MP joints of the other digits are either fused or replaced with Silastic or other implant arthroplasties. Fusions and replacements are available for the PIP joints and DIP joints. Many other treatments and surgical options are available. Needless to say, these procedures need to be done by an experienced hand surgeon who can follow the many problems that these patients will develop over time.

Nerve Compression Syndromes

Compressive neuropathies of the upper extremity are common problems which cause significant disability and pain in many patients. Carpal tunnel syndrome is by far the most common of these problems. Unfortunately, this condition has gotten so much attention that people are often labeled with this disease as soon as they present with any hand problems and the diagnosis can often be faulty. Carpal tunnel syndrome is due to compression of the median nerve at the wrist underneath the transverse carpal ligament. The hallmark symptoms include numbness, tingling, and paresthesias in a median nerve distribution (the thumb, index, middle and radial half of the ring finger), loss of dexterity in the hand, and discomfort, particularly with wrist flexion or at sleep. In more advanced stages, patients may develop weakness of the hand and dropping of objects, pain radiating to the elbow or even the shoulder, or atrophy of the thenar musculature.

The underlying cause of carpal tunnel syndrome is unknown in most patients. Patients with metabolic diseases such as hypothyroidism, diabetes, and renal failure are at much higher risk for developing this disease. The relationship of repetitive motion tasks, especially keyboarding, with carpal tunnel syndrome is very controversial, and hand surgeons still debate the causal role of such activities.

Physical examination findings include a positive Tinel's sign, in which tapping over the median nerve at the wrist crease elicits paresthesias in a median nerve distribution. A positive Phalen's sign occurs when symptoms are reproduced by holding maximal flexion of the wrist for a minute or less. The carpal tunnel compression test is positive if pressure directly over the carpal tunnel applied by the examiner elicits symptoms within 30 s or less. Thumb abduction strength should be tested, and a sensory evaluation should be documented. When patients have an atypical presentation or physical examination, an electromyograph (EMG) and nerve conduction study as well as X-rays can be very helpful for sorting out other diseases or making sure that a more proximal nerve compression process is not present.

Carpal tunnel syndrome can be treated initially by bracing and oral antiinflammatory medications. If this does not help, a corticosteroid injection into the carpal tunnel will give temporary relief in nearly 80% of patients with true disease. Finally, when conservative measures have failed and the patient has had persistent symptoms for over 3–6 months, a surgical release is indicated. This can be done through one of many open techniques or through an endoscopic technique. Overall results are excellent through both methods.

Cubital tunnel syndrome, or compression of the ulnar nerve at the elbow, is the second-most common compressive neuropathy. Patients present with numbness and tingling in the small finger and the ulnar half of the ring finger and frequently complain of elbow pain. Symptoms are often worse at night or after long periods in which the elbow has been flexed. Physical examination findings include a positive Tinel's sign over the ulnar nerve and behind the medial epicondyle, a positive elbow flexion test in which full flexion of the elbow for more than 30s reproduces symptoms, and in some cases, subluxation of the ulnar nerve out of the retrocondylar groove when flexing the elbow. Distally, one can often find decreased sensation in an ulnar nerve distribution. In advanced cases, weakness to finger abduction or even intrinsic atrophy can be present. Froment's test, in which the patient is required to pinch a card between the thumb and index finger, is positive when the patient either cannot strongly pinch the card or collapses into a flexed IP joint position and hyperextended MP joint position of the thumb. The main differential diagnosis includes cervical radiculopathy, thoracic outlet syndrome (i.e., brachial plexus compression in the region from the scalenes to the clavicle), and ulnar nerve compression at the wrist. An EMG and nerve conduction study can be helpful to differentiate between these sites, but it is often negative even in moderately advanced stages of cubital tunnel syndrome. Treatment usually starts with extension splinting, activity modification, and antiinflammatories. If symptoms do not resolve in 3–6 months or if patients develop significant atrophy, an anterior transposition of the ulnar nerve or a medial epicondylectomy is often indicated.

Tendon Compression Syndromes

Stenosing tenosynovitis is the name given to conditions in which tendon segments with a synovial sheath become compressed by the overlying ligamentous or retinacular structures. Patients initially present with pain and eventually develop problems with gliding motion and sometimes even develop frank catching or triggering of the tendon as it passes through its retinacular housing. These problems are frequently associated with diabetes and renal failure. They are sometimes felt to be due to overuse. Most of the time, however, the underlying cause is unknown. The most common of these tendon disorders is trigger finger, in which the flexor tendons are entrapped underneath the A-1 pulley of the flexor tendon sheath. Patients will often end up with locking of the finger in flexion requiring a prying open of the digit with a palpable and sometimes visible pop as the finger fully extends. Initial treatment with a corticosteroid injection has very high success rates. If symptoms recur or do not go away, a surgical release of the A-1 pulley is indicated.

Another very common stenosing tenosynovitis is de Quervain's tenosynovitis, in which the abductor pollicis longus and extensor pollicis brevis tendons become constricted under the extensor retinaculum at the first dorsal compartment of the wrist. This is especially common in mothers with newborn children. Hallmark physical findings are significant tenderness over the first dorsal compartment at the radial styloid and a positive Finkelstein's test, in which the thumb and wrist are forcibly maneuvered into ulnar deviation eliciting severe pain over the first dorsal compartment. Treatment options include nonsteroidal antiinflammatory medications, corticosteroid injections, bracing (which must include the thumb and wrist), and eventually surgical release of the first dorsal compartment. Other less common tendon compressions around the wrist include tendinitis of the flexor carpi radialis (FCR) tendon, extensor carpi ulnaris (ECU) tendon, and extensor carpi radialis brevis (ECRB) and extensor carpi radialis longus (ECRL) tendons (intersection syndrome). Treatment of these conditions proceeds in a similar fashion to that of de Quervain's tenosynovitis.

Dupuytren's Contracture

This disease involves changes in the palmar fascia in which normal fibroblast cells become transformed into myofibroblasts and thicken and contract, turning the normal fascial bands anchoring the fat of the palm into thickened, contractile cords which pull the digits into flexion contractures and cause web space narrowing (Fig. 10.2c). Over time, the contractures can become so severe that patients cannot place their hands in their pockets or put on a glove. The disease is particularly common in older men of Celtic and Scandinavian origins, suggesting a hereditary component to the process. The usual presentation starts as a painless nodule in the palm. Over time it will often progress into a cord along the digit, pulling the MP or PIP joint into a flexion contracture. Therapy, splinting, and other modalities have shown no effect on the progression of the disease. The mainstay of treatment at this time is surgical with excision of the cords, but this does not halt the disease process. There is still a 10% per year risk of recurrence of the disease in a digit that has had cords removed. Clostridial collagenase enzyme injection is another way to rupture the cord and relieve the contracture; it has shown good promise in early trials, and it may eventually become the treatment of choice for these problems.

Kienböck's Disease

This rare condition is due to osteonecrosis of the lunate bone. Over time, collapse of the carpus may occur resulting in severe pain and loss of wrist function. It most commonly occurs in the second, third, and fourth decades of life. It is seen some-what more often in patients with repetitive loading type activities such as gymnastics or football. X-rays often make the diagnosis, and the patients have a tendency to be ulnar-negative, i.e., the radius is longer than the ulna. In situations where the X-rays do not show the disease but it is still suspected, one should obtain an MRI which will definitively make or rule out the diagnosis. Treatment options include immo-bilization and rest for the earliest phases, drilling and vessel implantation and bone grafting, joint leveling procedures, intracarpal fusions, proximal row carpectomies, and, for the most advanced stages, a total wrist fusion.

Inflammation and Infection

Although the hand is relatively resistant to infection as a result of its excellent blood supply, its frequent exposure to trauma, particularly lacerations, open fractures, puncture wounds, foreign body penetration, and paronychial or cuticle injuries, leads to fairly high incidences of infection overall. A paronychia is an infection that affects the soft tissues overlying the proximal nail fold or the lateral edges of the nail (Fig. 10.4a). It is usually caused by *Staphylococcus* and presents as a red, swollen, painful abscess overlying the nail fold. If it is diagnosed at an early enough stage, warm water soaks and oral antibiotics can cure it. In more advanced stages, surgical drainage is required.

A felon is a more involved infection that invades into the pulp of the fingertip. Patients present with a very swollen, tense, and painful finger pulp (Fig. 10.4b–d). It is very important to drain this as soon as possible and release all of the septa between the skin of the pulp and the bone, thereby completely decompressing the infec-tion. If this is not performed, the infection can spread to the bone or to the tendon sheath.

Purulent or septic flexor tenosynovitis is an extremely serious infection that can result in loss of the finger if not treated aggressively. Four classic findings for this

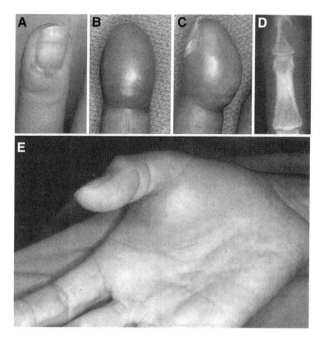

Fig. 10.4 Infections of the hand. (**a**) Paronychia with collection of pus beneath eponychium and base of nail. (**b–d**) Felon with marked distention of pulp of finger, impending necrosis of skin on palmar surface, and dissolution of bone of distal phalanx. (**e**) Thenar space abscess

are called Kanavel's signs. They include fusiform swelling of the digit, severe tenderness over the flexor tendon sheath, semiflexed posture of the digit, and severe pain to passive extension of the digit. This problem should be surgically drained as soon as possible and subsequently treated with several weeks of antibiotics and soaks. If left untreated, it can spread into the palmar bursa and enter the thenar space, the palmar space, or even the carpal tunnel, causing a more severe and widespread infection.

Human bite infections can cause extensive damage before treatment has begun. The injury often occurs in a fight in which the patient's metacarpal head strikes a tooth and seeds the MP joint and the metacarpal head with several different bacteria. These wounds should be debrided aggressively and allowed to heal by secondary intent or a delayed primary closure. The antibiotic selected should cover *Eikenella corrodens*. Dog and cat bite wounds can also cause significant hand infections including septic flexor tenosynovitis and septic arthritis. Appropriate debridement should be performed when necessary and antibiotic coverage should include drugs that will eradicate *Pasteurella multocida*. Infections to the hand and wrist from fungi, mycobacteria, and other atypical flora are relatively rare, but should be kept in mind. A history of exposure to soil, birds, or seawater is particularly important to check. These infections often require extensive debridement and long periods of antibiotic therapy.

Trauma

As mentioned earlier in the chapter, the hand is subject to high rates of trauma, ranging from very minor accidents to devastating injuries to the hand and wrist. It is important for all physicians to have a basic approach to dealing with trauma of the hand and to know when to urgently involve a hand surgeon with these problems.

Lacerations

Lacerations and puncture injuries to the hand can show obvious and extensive injury in some situations, but many of the more subtle small lacerations can also mask significant deep injury. In general, these wounds should not be probed in an emergency room or office setting; all the necessary information can be gleaned by distal evaluation of the affected digit or hand. A careful assessment of nerve, vessel, tendon, ligament, and bone function should be assessed and plain X-rays should also be taken to ensure that no fracture or residual foreign body is present. Appropriate tetanus and antibiotic coverage should be instituted. If the decision is made to take a wound to the operating room right away, the wound can just be loosely dressed and splinted to await passage to surgery. If the external wound is minor, but the patient needs a tendon or other repair, a loose closure can be performed in the emergency room. Splinting is usually initiated and the patient can follow up with the hand surgeon on an elective basis. Minor lacerations that are clean and do not have deep tissue involvement should be definitively closed and dressed in the emergency room. It is important to note here that whenever nerve, tendon, or other significant structural involvement is present, the hand surgeon who will eventually and definitively treat the patient should be contacted so that appropriate care and follow-up can be arranged and the patient does not fall through the cracks or lose an opportunity for timely care. Nerve and flexor tendon injuries in particular need to be addressed within a week or two to avoid permanent loss of function.

Fractures and Dislocations

Fractures and dislocations of the hand and wrist can occur through a variety of mechanisms including falls on an outstretched wrist or hand, crush injuries, or direct blows. Appropriate X-rays can usually make the diagnosis, but for some of the carpal injuries in particular, bone scans and MRIs are needed to confirm the problem. Assessment of the fracture should also include whether it is open or if there is associated soft tissue injury involving the nerves, tendons, or vessels. Fractures of the phalanges can involve a variety from simple tuft fractures to extensive intraarticular fractures with comminution. The fractures must be assessed for stability, angular deformity, rotational malalignment, and shortening. If these factors are all found to be acceptable, the fracture can be treated closed with 3–4 weeks of immobilization or protected early range of motion until healing occurs. If these factors are not acceptable in the fracture pattern, surgical management should be initiated. The most commonly used fixation techniques involve K-wire or plate-and-screw

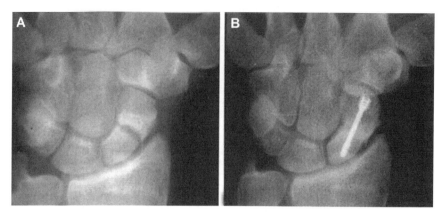

Fig. 10.5 Fracture with nonunion of carpal scaphoid. (**a**) Established nonunion with sclerosis and cyst formation 6 months after untreated "wrist sprain." (**b**) Operative treatment with screw resulted in union

fixation. This is especially important for intraarticular fractures that are displaced in order to restore adequate range of motion.

The vast majority of metacarpal fractures can be treated nonoperatively. Exceptions to this include fractures with rotational malalignment, excessive angular deformity, or intraarticular displacement—especially of the thumb or small metacarpal bases. Fractures of the thumb metacarpal base often occur in a pattern in which the ulnar segment of the base stays attached to the trapezium and index metacarpal through the volar oblique ligament. The remainder of the metacarpal shaft subluxates radially. This pattern is called a Bennett's fracture and often requires fixation. Boxer's fractures are small metacarpal neck fractures that are extremely common. If no rotational deformity is present, up to 70° of apex dorsal angulation can be treated nonoperatively in most cases. Index and middle metacarpal neck fractures are more problematic as their metacarpal bases are quite stiffly attached to the carpus and less compensation can occur.

Carpal bone fractures occur frequently as well. The most commonly injured wrist bone is the scaphoid (Fig. 10.5). When patients are tender over the anatomical snuff box or the scaphoid tubercle, one should maintain a high index of suspicion for this fracture. If initial X-rays are negative, advanced imaging techniques such as bone scan or MRI should be obtained, or the patient should be immobilized for 3 weeks and repeat radiographic views should be considered. Scaphoid fractures have high rates of complications due to the poor vascularity of this bone; nonunions and avascular necrosis of the proximal pole can occur, especially when treatment is delayed or missed. Another common carpal fracture is the dorsal triquetral avulsion injury which often occurs after a fall on an outstretched wrist. This is best seen on lateral radiographic views in which a small fleck of bone is noted dorsal to the triquetral region. Immobilization in a cast or brace for 3–4 weeks usually results in a very good outcome.

Dislocations of the interphalangeal joints are quite common and can usually be reduced using closed techniques. It is important to initiate early range of motion soon after to avoid excessive stiffness. It is particularly important to do brief periods of extension splinting once the joint is stable enough to prevent flexion contractures from developing. At the MP joints, dislocations can result in irreducible situations in which the volar plate becomes incarcerated between the articular surfaces. This requires surgical treatment, but, again, nearly always has excellent stability once reduction is obtained. Here, too, it is very important to initiate range of motion exercises soon after surgical treatment to avoid stiffness afterward. Injuries to the collateral ligaments of the PIP and MP joints are common. This is especially true at the thumb. An injury to the thumb MP joint ulnar collateral ligament is often called a "gamekeeper's" or "skier's" thumb and is a frequent athletic injury. Patients who have tenderness over the ligament but good stability should be immobilized for 3–4 weeks and then range of motion should be initiated. If the patient has more than 45° of opening to radially directed stress or more than 50% subluxation of the joint on stress views or has a palpable Stener's lesion (a completely ruptured ulnar collateral ligament that is incarcerated in the adductor pollicis muscle), surgical repair of the ligament is indicated. It is also important to note that sprains and strains of the PIP joints can result in very long periods of swelling and stiffness of the joint and some patients lead to some permanent thickening of the collateral ligaments.

Severe and Complex Upper Extremity Injuries

Amputations of portions of the upper limb, especially the fingers, are very common especially in industrial and agricultural environments. Modern microvascular surgical techniques allow reimplantation of the amputated parts in many situations. The severed part should be wrapped in a gauze dressing soaked in sterile saline and placed in a container or sealed plastic bag that can be immersed in ice and transported to a treating facility. The part should never be placed directly on ice, and dry ice should never be used. An experienced hand or reimplantation surgeon should be consulted right away to assess whether the part is a good candidate for reattachment. Typical indications at this time include any part that is large enough in a child, the thumb at any level that can be reattached, multiple digits, or an amputation through the midpalm or proximal. Severe contamination, crush injury, avulsion, or broad areas of vascular damage are contraindications to reimplantation of the part.

Extensive mangling injuries must be treated by an experienced hand surgeon as soon as possible. Initial care rendered often determines the final outcome and, therefore, must be carefully planned with a long-term treatment plan and an outcome firmly in mind. Inadequate debridement, primary closure, improper splinting, nominal or poor understanding of the injury all too often result in more significant disability than needed.

Crush injuries and high-energy trauma should always be carefully evaluated for the development of compartment syndrome. The early symptoms may be very subtle. The history may be vague, for example, an intoxicated patient sleeping on an arm for a long period of time (and the damage may take a long time to develop). Iatrogenic causes include cast or dressings that are too tight or extravasation injuries. One should maintain a high degree of suspicion for this problem and observe for the five P's: pain out of *p*roportion to the injury, severe pain with *p*assive stretch, later *p*aresthesias, *p*allor, and *p*ulselessness. The condition occurs from increased pressure in the forearm or hand muscle compartments preventing flow through the venules and capillaries and preventing perfusion of the soft tissues of the compartment. Compartment pressures can be measured, but determining the threshold pressure at which to release the compartments is not always easy.

When this diagnosis is confirmed, it constitutes a surgical emergency. It is imperative to take the patient to the operating room and release the compartments as soon as possible to prevent necrosis of the muscle and other tissues, resulting in severe patterns of function loss, such as a Volkmann's contracture.

Thermal, chemical, or electrical injuries cause soft tissue problems of varying depth. The skin is the initial point of contact and may show first-degree (redness), second-degree (blistering), or third-degree (full-thickness or charring) injuries, particularly with burns. Early care of the second-degree injury can minimize the chance of an infection converting it to a third-degree injury. Early referral to a hand therapist for exercise and splinting may avoid extensive late contractures. Third-degree burns should be treated by early surgical excision of the eschar and skin grafting. Chemical injuries should be treated in a facility that has experience in managing these conditions as specific antidotes can be used to neutralize many chemicals and minimize damage.

Cold injury varies from minor frostbite to extensive freezing of tissues and peripheral parts. The initial treatment should involve rapid rewarming of the area of frostbite followed by observation to see what survives. Early amputation is not necessary in the absence of infection. Electrical burns can be quite deceptive as to the extent in damage and require repeated evaluation.

Other Injuries

Mallet finger may occur from rupture of the terminal extensor tendon often with trivial injury. Fracture of the dorsal lip of the distal phalanx may be seen on X-ray in some cases. Full passive extension is present, but active extension is not. Treatment usually involves splinting in full extension for 6 or more weeks.

Boutonnière deformities occur from disruption of the central slip of the extensor tendon over the PIP joint by blunt trauma or laceration. Over time, the lateral bands slip progressively volar to the axis of rotation of the PIP joint, especially if the triangular band is disrupted. The patient develops a flexion deformity at the PIP joint and compensatory hyperextension at the DIP joint. When diagnosed early, this can be treated with closed extension splinting of the PIP joint. After prolonged presence of deformity, surgical treatment can be required.

Metabolic Disease

Many metabolic illnesses such as diabetes, hyperthyroidism, hyperparathyroidism, and renal failure can be underlying causes to hand problems such as carpal tunnel syndrome. One should be careful to check a patient's medical history and make sure these underlying problems are adequately treated prior to initiating any surgical intervention.

Gout is a common metabolic illness in which uric acid forms crystals and accumulates in joints or soft tissues. Although it is most common in the first MTP joint of the foot, it can occur in the joints and soft tissues of the hand. Often, it presents as a warm, tender, swollen, erythematous region and can mimic infection. Aspiration of a joint and visualization of negatively birefringent crystals under polarized light microscopy evaluation of the fluid confirm the diagnosis. The condition of severe tophaceous gout in the hands, which can cause extensive destruction of tendons or joints, is fairly uncommon due to improvements in medical management of this disease, but it still can be seen. Treatment options include rest, immobilization, antiinflammatory medications, corticosteroids, and other antigout medications. Surgery can sometimes be indicated for erosive tophi.

Calcium pyrophosphate dihydrate deposition disease is another metabolic problem in which crystals accumulate in joints and around tendons. This, too, can cause redness, swelling, and warmth over a joint and, again, aspiration and visualization of crystals in the fluid can be diagnostic for the problem. Treatment includes corticosteroid injections, nonsteroidal antiinflammatories, prednisone or colchicine for acute flareups, and surgery in severe cases.

Vascular

Arterial occlusions and small vessel disease in the hand can cause severe problems with pain and occasionally necrosis of the fingers. Although uncommon, ulnar artery occlusions, which usually occur at the level of the hamate hook, can cause significant ulnar nerve symptoms as well as diminished flow to the digits. When this occurs after a repetitive trauma situation, it is called hypothenar hammer syndrome, and it is seen in manual laborers who use their hypothenar eminence as a hammer on the objects they are working with. A diagnosis for this can be made at times with ultrasound, but usually requires an angiogram. The treatment involves decompression of the nerve and artery, and reconstruction or ligation of the thrombosed segment of the artery. Thrombosis of digital arteries is sometimes seen in patients with atherosclerotic disease proximally, but it is quite uncommon.

Vascular deficiencies secondary to other underlying diseases can be a significant problem in the hand, particularly in diabetes and scleroderma. Many of these patients go on to require amputations of digits, but in earlier stages of scleroderma, a digital sympathectomy or removal of the vascular adventitia can decrease the amount of spasm that occurs and limit the damage done to the digits.

Patients who have severe loss of flow to the hands can also develop gangrene of the digits. This is particularly common in patients who go into systemic vascular shock and require vasopressors, which restrict flow to the extremities. Once again, many of these patients develop gangrene of the digits and require formal amputations at a later point in time.

True aneurysms of the wrist and hand are relatively uncommon. They usually occur in the ulnar artery. They cause symptoms very similar to hypothenar hammer syndrome and can be treated the same way. Pseudoaneurysms are more common and can occur anywhere in the hand and are the result of trauma to an artery. They are usually treated by ligating or reconstructing the artery involved.

Neoplasms

Skin Cancer

Skin cancers (squamous cell and basal cell carcinomas and melanoma) are relatively common, especially in the elderly or those with predisposing factors. These factors include prolonged exposure to the sun in farmers and other outdoor workers, and excessive exposure to X-rays, arsenicals, or other chemicals (Fig. 10.6a). Squamous and basal cell carcinomas can usually be cured by wide excision if they have not already metastasized. Melanomas are much more unpredictable in their behavior and need to be addressed quickly (Fig. 10.6b).

Other Soft Tissue Masses

Benign soft tissue masses are very common in the hand and wrist. They can arise in any of the tissues making up the hand including nerves, vessels, fat, and fascia. The most common "tumors" of the hand arise from the synovium and include ganglions, mucous cysts, and giant cell tumors of the tendon sheath. Ganglia occur in four locations: on the dorsum of the wrist, on the volar aspect of the wrist adjacent to the radial artery, in the flexor tendon sheath at the base of the finger, and over the dorsum of the DIP joint (mucous cyst), usually associated with osteoarthritis and osteophyte formation of the joint. A ganglion on the dorsum of the wrist or over the flexor tendon sheath can be aspirated, although rates of recurrence are fairly high. Aspiration of a volar wrist ganglion should be approached cautiously, if at all, due to the proximity of the radial artery. Surgical resection is a more definitive option, with only 5–10% recurrence rates when done correctly. Arthroscopic resection is now available for dorsal wrist ganglia. Giant cell tumors of the tendon sheath are solid lesions arising from the synovium of the tendon sheath or from the finger joints. Simple excision is usually curative, although occasional recurrences are seen.

Other common benign soft tissue masses include foreign body granulomas, epidermal inclusion cysts, arteriovenous malformations and hemangiomas, neurilemmoma, and glomus tumors.

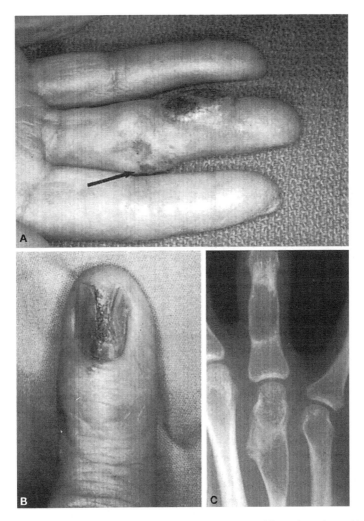

Fig. 10.6 Neoplasms of the hand. (**a**) Squamous cell carcinoma of finger in patient with 30-year history of holding children being radiographed. Note atrophic skin changes (*arrow*) from the radiation exposure. (**b**) Subungual melanoma with splitting of the nail from involvement of nail bed. (**c**) Enchondroma of proximal phalanx with expansion of the diaphysis. Note the enchondroma of the metacarpal with callus from a healed pathologic fracture

Malignant soft tissue tumors in the hand are very rare outside of skin cancers. The most common ones are epithelioid sarcomas, synovial cell sarcomas, and malignant fibrous histiocytoma. Delay in diagnosis is a common problem to these tumors. Limb salvage surgery is the treatment of choice whenever possible.

Tumors of Bone

Benign tumors of the hand bones are often diagnosed incidentally on radiographic examination for trauma. The most common is the enchondroma (Fig. 10.6c). Treatment is not required unless pathologic fracture through the lesion has occurred or is impending. Simple curettage, with or without bone grafting, often suffices. Osteochondromas, fibrous dysplasia, and giant cell tumor of bone can also present in the small hand bones and may require surgery for diagnosis or treatment. Malignant tumors of the hand skeleton are very rare. Partial or total hand amputation may be required along with adjuvant radiation therapy or chemotherapy. Metastatic tumors of the hand seldom occur as isolated metastases, but are not uncommon during widespread metastatic disease, especially from lung or breast lesions.

Management Protocols

As one can see, a broad variety of complex problems can affect the hand and wrist. It is, therefore, important to have in mind a standardized approach to patients with these problems to help arrive at the correct diagnosis and management options. The physician should start with a careful and detailed history of the chief complaint. With a differential diagnosis in mind, the physician should perform a directed, but thorough physical examination. Plain radiographs are usually, but not always, indicated. Algorithms have been developed beyond this to help streamline a patient's care and avoid missing important diagnoses. Although the algorithms are overall quite complete, one should be wary of unusual presentations or diagnoses that are not included. These rare occurrences may require further evaluation or consultation by a hand specialist. The algorithms divide patients into groups with or without a specific history of injury (Figs. 10.7 and 10.8).

Nearly all patients with a specific injury should be X-rayed. If the initial radiographs show a fracture, dislocation, or carpal instability pattern, appropriate operative or nonoperative treatment should be initiated. When X-rays are negative, a soft tissue injury may have occurred or an occult fracture may be present. When a specific soft tissue injury is noted, appropriate treatment should be initiated. If none is found and the patient's symptoms cannot be explained, either further imaging should be performed or splinting or casting for a period of time followed by reevaluation should be considered.

Figure 10.8 deals with patients who have had no specific history of trauma or injury. Unless patients have a very classic history and physical examination for a soft tissue process, plain X-rays should be taken. If they are positive for arthritis, tumor, or occult bony injury, appropriate operative or nonoperative management should be undertaken. If they are negative, further evaluation and/or indicated treatment should be initiated according to the algorithm.

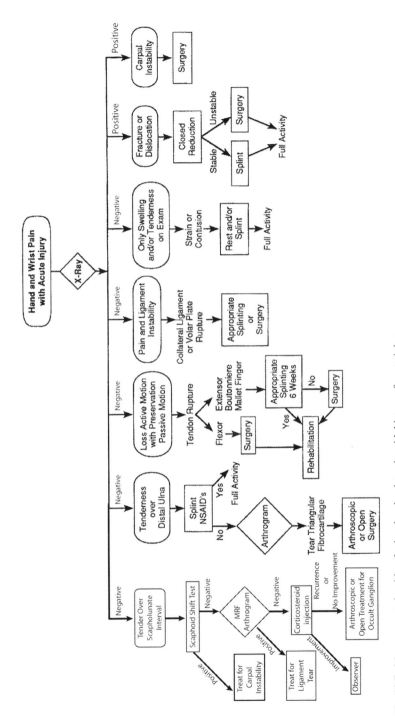

Fig. 10.7 Management algorithm for hand and wrist pain with history of acute injury

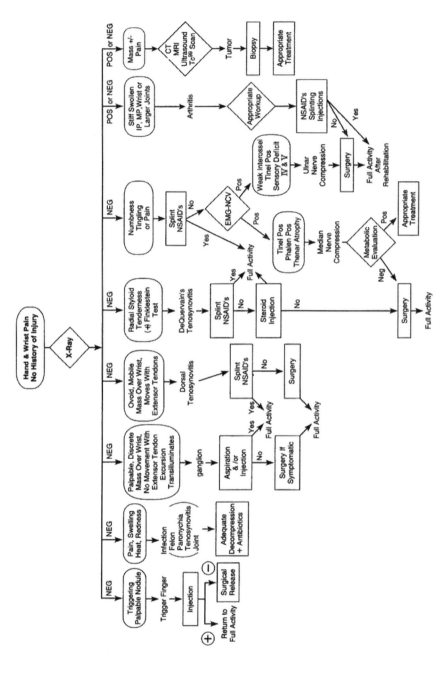

Fig. 10.8 Management algorithm for hand and wrist pain with no history of injury

Suggested Reading

1. Green DP, Hotchkiss RN, Peterson WC eds. *Green's Operative Hand Surgery*. New York, NY: Churchill Livingston; 1999.
2. Seiler JG III ed. *Essentials of Hand Surgery*. Philadelphia, PA: Lippincott Williams & Wilkins; 2002.
3. Trumbull TE ed. *Hand Surgery Update 3*. Rosemont, IL: American Society for Surgery of the Hand; 2003.

Chapter 11
The Hip and Femur

Brian G. Evans and Mark W. Zawadsky

The primary function of the lower extremities is locomotion. Any alteration of the function of the lower extremities will result in an alteration in the ability to walk and run. The hip is the most proximal joint in the lower extremity. Alteration in the hip due to disease will significantly affect the biomechanics of gait and place abnormal stress on the joints above and below the hip, which can lead to pain in areas such as the lumbar spine and the knee.

This chapter will briefly review the anatomy of the hip and its relationship to normal and pathologic gait. The important history and physical examination findings of hip pathology will be discussed. Diseases affecting the hip will be reviewed and treatment outlined. Surgical management of end-stage disease of the hip will commonly be treated by one of several options and these will be reviewed. The indications and outcome for each treatment option will also be reviewed.

Anatomy

Development

The hip joint is a ball and socket joint with the round femoral head articulating within the matching acetabular socket. The acetabulum is formed from the confluence of three bones: the ischium, ilium, and pubis. In skeletally immature patients, these three bones are joined in the medial acetabulum by the triradiate cartilage, which is a growth plate for the acetabulum. There is also appositional growth from the edges of the acetabulum and pelvis resulting in increased depth of the acetabulum and size of the pelvis. Normal development of the acetabulum requires the femoral head to articulate with the acetabular cartilage. The acetabular socket will

B.G. Evans (✉)
Department of Orthopedic Surgery, Georgetown University Medical Center, Washington, DC 20007, USA
e-mail: evansb1@gunet.georgetown.edu

S.W. Wiesel, J.N. Delahay (eds.), *Essentials of Orthopedic Surgery*,
DOI 10.1007/978-1-4419-1389-0_11, © Springer Science+Business Media, LLC 2010

not develop normally if the femoral head is chronically dislocated or subluxed out of the acetabular fossa. This often results in a shallow and malformed acetabulum and is termed developmental dysplasia of the hip (DDH). The severity of this condition is determined by the degree of subluxation of the femoral head. If DDH is identified at birth or soon thereafter, the hip can be reduced with either casting or surgery. This treatment can allow the hip to grow and develop almost normally. If the hip is left subluxed or dislocated, the acetabulum will be shallow and predispose the patient to develop osteoarthritis as an adult. This is reviewed in greater detail in the chapter on pediatric orthopedic conditions.

Osteology and Musculature

The innominate bone consists of the ilium, ischium, and pubis, which are joined in the area of the acetabulum (Fig. 11.1). The ilium is a large flat bone providing broad surfaces for muscular attachment. The ischium extends posteriorly and forms the posterior aspect of the acetabulum. The ischium joins the ilium superiorly and the pubis inferiorly through the inferior pubic ramus. The ischium also serves as the origin of the hamstring and short external rotator muscles of the hip. The pubis consists of the superior pubic ramus, inferior pubic ramus, and the pubic symphysis.

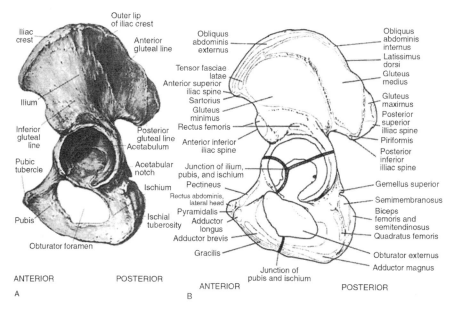

Fig. 11.1 (**a**) Lateral aspect of left hip bone. (**b**) Attachments and epiphyseal lines are shown (From Williams PL, Warwick R. Gray's Anatomy, 36th ed. Churchill Livingstone, New York, NY; 1980:378–379. Reprinted with permission. From Steinberg M, ed. *The Hip and Its Disorders*. Philadelphia, PA, WB Saunders; 1991:32. Reprinted by permission)

The superior pubic ramus joins the pubic symphysis with the ilium and the inferior pubic ramus connects the pubic symphysis with the ischium. The pubis serves as the site of insertion of the musculature of the abdominal wall, as well as the site of origin for the adductor muscles of the thigh.

The acetabulum is formed at the junction of the ilium, ischium, and pubis. The ilium forms the superior dome of the acetabulum. The ischium forms the posterior acetabulum and the pubis the anterior acetabulum. The lateral opening of the acetabulum forms a circular horseshoe with the open end directed inferiorly. The medial base of the acetabulum contains a depression called the acetabular fovea. This is filled with a fatty tissue called the pulvinar and the ligamentum teres. The ligamentum teres is a ligament that extends from the acetabular fovea and the fovea of the femoral head. The artery of the ligamentum teres is a branch of the obturator artery and supplies approximately 10–20% of the bone of the femoral head.

The fovea of the femur is a depression on the femoral head, which serves as the site of attachment of the ligamentum teres. Attached to the rim of the horseshoe is a fibro-cartilaginous labrum, which is similar to the meniscus in the knee. This serves to improve stability and to cushion the femoral neck when the femur is rotated and impinges upon the acetabular rim at the extremes of motion. The hip joint capsule is a dense fibrous structure extending from the base of the intertrochanteric region of the femur to the acetabular rim. Thickenings within the capsule are the iliofemoral and pubofemoral ligaments anteriorly and the ischiofemoral ligament posteriorly. These ligaments as well as the ligamentum teres and the labrum augment the stability of the hip joint.

The femoral head is essentially spherical in geometry (Figs. 11.2 and 11.3). The spherical portion of the femoral head is covered by articular cartilage. The sphere

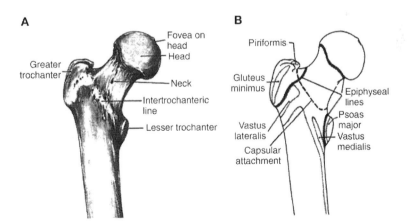

Fig. 11.2 (**a**) Anterior aspect of proximal right femur. (**b**) Attachments and epiphyseal lines (From Williams PL, Warwick R. *Gray's Anatomy*, 36th ed. Churchill Livingstone, New York, NY; 1980:392–393. Reprinted with permission. From Steinberg M, ed. *The Hip and Its Disorders.* Philadelphia, PA, WB Saunders;1991:28. Reprinted by permission)

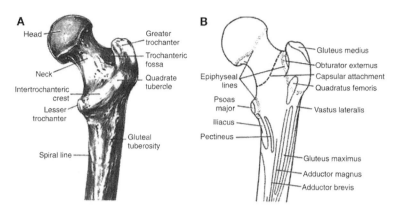

Fig. 11.3 (**a**) Posterior aspect of proximal right femur. (**b**) Attachments and epiphyseal lines (From Williams PL, Warwick R. *Gray's Anatomy*, 36th ed. Churchill Livingstone, New York, NY; 1980:394. Reprinted with permission. From Steinberg, M ed. *The Hip and Its Disorders*. Philadelphia, PA, WB Saunders; 1991:28. Reprinted by permission)

Fig. 11.4 Average rotary, or torsion, angle of the femur. It may be anteverted (A) or retroverted (R). (From Steinberg M, ed. *The Hip and Its Disorders*. Philadelphia, PA, WB Saunders; 1991:29. Reprinted with permission)

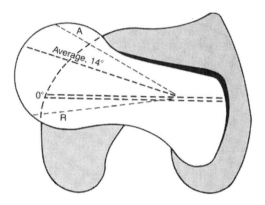

is altered in two areas, laterally where the femoral neck begins and medially at the fovea of the femoral head. The femoral neck joins the femur at approximately 125° angle. The neck is also rotated anteriorly 12–14° relative to the axis represented by the posterior femoral condyles (Fig. 11.4). The femoral neck flares laterally to join the proximal femur in between the greater and lesser trochanters. The greater trochanter, a large osseous prominence at the proximal lateral aspect of the femur, serves as the site of attachment of the abductor musculature. Between the greater and lesser trochanters is an osseous ridge, which serves as the site of attachment of the short external rotators. The lesser trochanter is the site of attachment of the iliopsosas tendon. This leaves the pelvis over the anterior column and superior pubic ramus and then travels over the anterior femoral neck to insert on the lesser trochanter, which lies on the posterior inferior aspect of the intertrochanteric ridge. Within the proximal femur and femoral neck is a large and dense trabeculation known as the calcar. The calcar provides increased strength to the proximal femur. Frequently the proximal postero-medial femur from the base of the femoral neck including the lesser trochanter is also referred to as the calcar. If the medial calcar region of the proximal femur is a separate fragment of a proximal femur fracture, the fracture is usually very unstable.

The muscles of the hip form several distinct groups. The anterior muscles are the hip flexors. These consist of the iliopsosas and rectus femorus and sartorius muscles. The femoral nerve innervates the rectus and sartorius muscles. Motor branches from spinal roots L2, L3, and L4 innervate the iliopsosas. The lateral group consists of the abductors, the gluteus medius, minimus, and tensor fascia lata. These muscles are essential for normal gait. They stabilize the pelvis in single limb stance phase of normal gait. The anterior one-third of the gluteus medius muscle is also the principle internal rotator of the hip. The superior gluteal nerve innervates the gluteus medius, minimus, and tensor fascia lata. Surgical dissection that extends greater than 5 cm proximal to the greater trochanter can disrupt the nerve and will result in a limp.

The posterior muscles are in two layers. The superficial layer consists of the gluteus maximus, the primary extensor of the hip, which is innervated by the inferior gluteal nerve. The deep layer consists of the short external rotators of the hip, the piriformis, superior gemellus, obturator internus, inferior gemellus, obturator externus and the quadratus femoris, and the gluteus minimus and medius. These muscles externally rotate the femur and provide abduction. Small branches from the sacral plexus innervate the short external rotators. The medial muscle group consists of the pectineus, adductor brevis, longus, and magnus, and the gracilis. The adductors and gracilis are supplied by the obturator nerve, with the posterior portion of the adductor magnus also receiving innervation from the tibial division of the sciatic nerve. The femoral nerve innervates the pectineus.

The sciatic nerve crosses the hip joint posteriorly. It exits the pelvis through the superior sciatic notch, under the piriformis muscle, and lies superficial to the short external rotators. The nerve has two distinct divisions within the single nerve sheath, the tibial and peroneal divisions. The peroneal division is more susceptible to injury, compared to the tibial division, at all levels along the course of the sciatic nerve. The increased susceptibility is due to the more lateral location and a more tenuous blood supply of the peroneal division within the sciatic nerve sheath. Therefore, a partial injury to the sciatic nerve, such as can occur with a stretch injury during total hip replacement surgery, will commonly result in a foot drop, clinically similar to the deficits seen in an isolated injury to the common peroneal nerve injury at the level of the fibular neck. One anatomic point with important clinical relevance is that the peroneal division of the sciatic nerve has only one motor branch in the posterior thigh supplying the short head of the biceps. Determining if the short head of the biceps is normally innervated can assist in determining the level of peroneal nerve injury clinically (i.e., the hip or knee).

Vascular Anatomy of the Proximal Femur and Femoral Head

The medial and lateral femoral circumflex vessels in conjunction with the artery of the ligamentum teres provide the vascular supply to proximal femur and femoral head (Fig. 11.5). The medial femoral circumflex artery extends posteriorly and ascends proximally deep to the quadratus femorus muscle. At the level of the hip it joins an arterial ring at the base of the femoral neck. The lateral femoral circumflex artery extends anteriorly and gives off an ascending branch, which also joins the arterial ring at the base of the femoral neck. This vascular ring gives rise to a group of vessels which run in the retinacular tissue inside the capsule to enter the femoral head at the base of the articular surface. These vessels provide 80–90% of the blood supply to the femoral head. The artery of the ligamentum teres, a branch of the obturator artery, travels within the ligamentum teres and supplies only 10–20% of the blood supply to the femoral head.

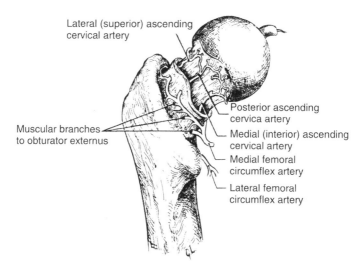

Fig. 11.5 Arterial supply to the head and neck of the posterior aspect of the left proximal femur. Note the extracapsular arterial ring on the surface of the capsule, the ascending cervical arteries on the neck of the femur, and the intra-articular sub-synovial arterial ring at the articular cartilage margin (From Steinberg, M ed. *The Hip and Its Disorders*. Philadelphia, PA, WB Saunders; 1991:19. Reprinted with permission)

Biomechanics

The joint reaction force is the sum of all forces that cross a joint. This includes components from gravity, body weight, and muscle forces acting upon the joint. In two-legged stance with both feet on the ground and static conditions, a joint reaction force of approximately 1.3–1.5 times body weight will cross each hip joint.

However, in single limb stance this force will increase to 2.5–3 times body weight across the hip joint. The primary contribution to the increase is the force generated by the abductor muscles to maintain balance and to keep the pelvis level. If the system is in motion, such as with walking, the joint reaction forces can be as high as 4 times body weight.

Several studies have measured the actual joint reaction forces during rehabilitation using an implanted-instrumented prosthesis. The greatest joint reaction force was noted when the patients arose from a low chair or during stair climbing. However, even non-weight-bearing activities, such as getting onto a bedpan, were found to have a joint reaction force of 1.5–1.8 times body weight. The lowest joint reaction forces with ambulation were recorded when patients used touch-down weight-bearing. Touch-down weight-bearing allows the patient to rest the foot on the ground to balance the weight of the leg, but not to step down or weight-bear on the involved lower extremity.

Gait

As mentioned previously, the principle function of the lower extremities is ambulation. In gait analysis, a gait cycle examines one leg, beginning with heel strike and continues until the next heel strike of the same leg. Gait can be divided into two principle phases: stance and swing. The stance phase is defined as that portion of the gait cycle when the foot is in contact with the ground. The swing phase is therefore the portion of each step when the foot is not in contact with the ground. The stance phase makes up 60% of each step, with the remainder being made up by the swing phase. Therefore, in 20% of the gait cycle, both feet are in contact with the ground. Normal gait requires a stable pelvis, which is provided by the hip abductor muscles. Normal gait also requires 40° of hip flexion and 10° of internal rotation and external rotation.

Patient Evaluation

History

The evaluation of a patient with hip pain requires careful attention to the history, physical examination, and radiographic studies. The character, nature, and duration of the patient's pain should be documented. Acute or recent onset pain will more commonly be associated with trauma or infection. Chronic and gradually progressive pain is associated with arthritic conditions. Intra-articular pain is usually described as a deep, aching pain. Pain from the hip joint will commonly be noted anteriorly in the groin or posterior to the greater trochanter. Hip pain can radiate down the inner and anterior thigh to the knee with little or no pain in the area of the hip. Only rarely will hip pain radiate distal to the knee. In adolescent patients, it is not uncommon for hip pathology to present as knee pain. Therefore a thorough physical and radiographic evaluation of the hips is necessary to identify the pathology in these patients. Posterior pain and buttock pain is more commonly associated with lumbar spine pathology. Spine pain also will more commonly radiate down the posterior thigh and below the knee. The insidious onset of a deep boring pain, and pain that awakens the patient at night, suggests either infection or neoplastic disease.

Hip pain is commonly aggravated by activity and relieved by rest. Patients will report difficulty donning and doffing their shoes and socks and difficulty with toenail care on the involved extremity. As the pain progresses, patients will begin to have pain with prolonged sitting and at night as they try to sleep. Patients with hip arthritis will report that if they sit for a prolonged period of time and then get up to walk, the hip feels out of place or painful for the first few steps. This feeling usually will resolve quickly after a few minutes of walking.

The use of a cane, walking stick, or crutch should be documented. The patient may also have begun to take over-the-counter anti-inflammatory medication or pain relievers. The medication and the amount the patient is taking, as well as the level of relief that is provided, need to be recorded. The patient's walking tolerance can be measured in terms of blocks the patient can walk, or in terms of how many minutes the patient can be ambulatory doing activities such as grocery shopping or walking in a mall. Documentation of the above data will give a detailed picture of the degree of pain and the patient's functional limitations.

Patients should also be questioned about past problems with the hip such as hip dislocation at birth, delays in ambulation as an infant, and any bracing as a child. If previous surgery or trauma to the hips has occurred, this should be explored in detail. The past medical history and any medications the patient is taking should be noted. This information can have implications for the patient's hip problems and may have an impact upon what treatment may be instituted.

Physical Examination

The most important aspect of the physical exam in patients with hip disease is to evaluate their gait pattern. This will reveal important information about the patient's ambulatory status and their pain. Patients with significant hip pain will manifest a coxalgic gait. This gait pattern is represented by a reduced stance phase on the painful leg and the shoulders lurch laterally over the affected hip. Patients with mild pain or weakness in the abductor muscles may have a stance phase equal to the opposite leg, but the shoulders will continue to lurch over the affected leg. This lurch results in moving the center of gravity closer to the center of rotation of the hip, which in turn reduces the force necessary to stabilize the pelvis in stance phase. This gait is referred to as a Trendelenburg gait (equal stance phase and the shoulders lurching over the affected hip).

The hip should be inspected for previous scars, swelling, bruises, or abrasions. The region then should be palpated to identify areas of focal tenderness such as over the greater trochanter, sciatic nerve, or anterior hip capsule. The range of motion of the hip should then be determined. Normal range of motion of the hip is flexion to 130°, extension to 20°, adduction to 30°, abduction to 40°, internal rotation to 30°, and external rotation to 70°. When assessing the range of motion of the hip, it is important to stabilize the lumbar spine. Motion in the lumbar spine may be attributed to the hip if the examiner is not careful. The Thomas test will stabilize the lumbar spine to measure for a flexion contracture of the hip (Fig. 11.6). Movement of the pelvis with abduction and adduction can be accurately assessed by placing a

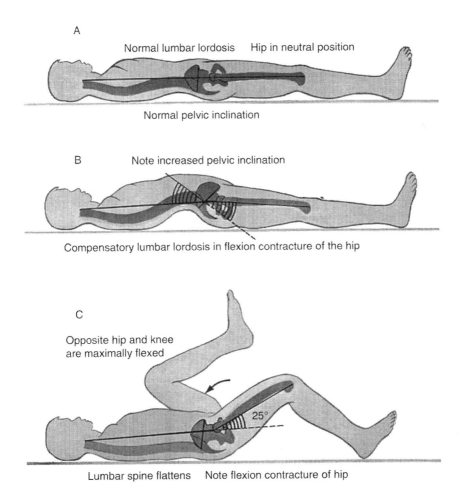

Fig. 11.6 Diagrammatic representation of the Thomas test to assess hip flexion contracture (Adapted from von Lanz T, Wachsmith W. *Praktische Anatomic*. Berlin, Julius Springer; 1938: 157) (From Tachdijian MO. *Pediatric Orthopaedics*. 2nd ed. Philadelphia, PA, WB Saunders; 1990:28. Reprinted with permission)

hand on the opposite anterior superior iliac spine and recording the patient's motion as the amount of motion prior to pelvic abduction.

To assess the function of the hip abductor muscles, the patient should be standing and the involved leg lifted off the floor. The patient should stand on the uninvolved leg and the pelvis should remain level. The patient then stands on the involved leg and lifts the uninvolved leg off the floor. If the pelvis is level, the patient has normal strength of the abductor muscles. If the pelvis is noted to be lower on the elevated leg, the abductor muscles are weak or the hip which is weight-bearing is painful. This is referred to as the Trendelenburg sign.

A careful neurologic exam and lumbar spine exam are essential to assessing the possibility of spine pathology producing pain radiating to the hip. Patients with significant arthritic disease in the hip will also commonly have spine pathology as well. Hip arthritis and restriction in hip range of motion can exacerbate spine pathology. The limited range of motion of the hip will result in increased motion at the lumbo-sacral junction. This can aggravate degenerative facet arthropathy and lumbar stenosis. Replacement of the hip and improvement in the range of motion in the hip, however, can relieve stress from the lumbo-sacral junction and subsequently relieve the patient's pain.

In addition, the pulses should be palpated in the foot and ankle. Significant reduction may indicate vascular insufficiency and may require further evaluation. Vascular compromise may impair wound healing or may lead to acute vascular crisis in the early post-operative period if this is not recognized and treated prior to any elective hip procedure. In addition, if any significant vascular reconstruction has been done in the area of the involved hip, care needs to be taken at the time of surgery to avoid damage to the previous reconstruction.

Radiographic Evaluation

Routine radiography of the pelvis and hips is the most useful study in evaluating hip pathology. Standard anteroposterior (AP) radiography of the pelvis will reveal the lower lumbar spine, sacro-iliac joints, innominate bone, pubic symphysis, hip joint, and proximal femurs. Frequently, in unilateral disease, the normal side can be used for comparison (Fig. 11.7). Lateral views of the proximal femurs can also be helpful in defining pathology and in determining the size and location of a pathologic lesion. Four pelvic oblique views can be obtained to further evaluate the pelvis and acetabulum, particularly in cases of trauma; these are the inlet, outlet, and Judet views. Judet views are 45° pelvic oblique views. They are useful for examination of the acetabulum, including the anterior and posterior columns (Figs. 11.8, 11.9, 11.10, and 11.11). The inlet and outlet views are useful for patients with pelvic trauma in order to evaluate for any superior or inferior translation of the hemipelvis.

Computerized tomography (CT) of the pelvis is most helpful in evaluating trauma. In some centers, this modality has replaced and certainly augments the use of oblique pelvic radiography. CT imaging is particularly helpful in demonstrating

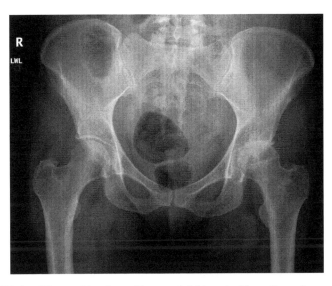

Fig. 11.7 This is a 75-year-old patient with severe left hip pain. The radiograph reveals a normal right hip and advanced arthritic changes in the left hip. The left hip demonstrates a lateral femoral neck osteophyte, subchondral sclerosis of the subchondral bone, and a subchondral cyst in the femoral head

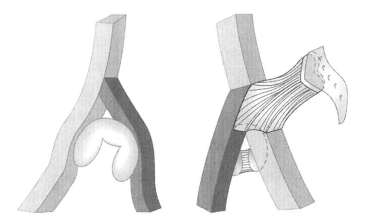

Fig. 11.8 Graphic depiction of the anterior and posterior columns of the acetabulum. *Left*, diagram of left acetabulum viewed from outside. Note that the anterior column (*light*) is larger than the posterior column (*dark*) and that both columns support the horseshoe-shaped articular surface. *Right*, view of the left acetabulum viewed from inside the pelvis. The sciatic buttress (stippled) connects both columns to the axial skeleton through the sacro-iliac joint (From Brandser E. Fractures. *Diagnosis and Treatment*. In: David Moehring H, Greenspan A, eds. ©2000 Current Medicine Group LLC)

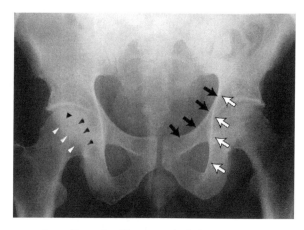

Fig. 11.9 Anteroposterior radiograph with arrows depicting the anterior and posterior wall of the right hip (black and white arrows, respectively). The left hip demonstrates the iliopectineal line of the anterior column (*black arrows*) and the ilio-ischial line of the posterior column (*white arrows*) (Brandser E. *Fractures: Diagnosis and Treatment*. In: David Moehring H, Greenspan A, eds. ©2000 Current Medicine Group LLC)

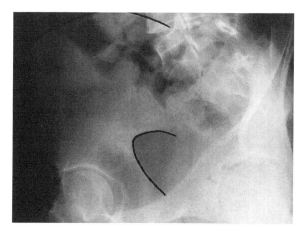

Fig. 11.10 Right posterior oblique view with right acetabulum highlighted. This view is also called the iliac oblique view and shows the posterior part of the acetabulum and greater sciatic notch, facilitating evaluation of fractures that extend into this region. The edge of the anterior wall can be seen on this view. The iliac wing is seen en face and it is therefore the best view for detecting fractures that extend proximally into the iliac wing. The obturator ring is poorly seen in this view (From Brandser E. *Fractures: Diagnosis and Treatment*. In: David Moehring H, Greenspan A, eds. ©2000 Current Medicine Group LLC)

fractures in the posterior pelvis and sacrum, which may be poorly visualized in routine radiography. Fractures to the acetabulum are well visualized on CT scan images (Figs. 11.12 and 11.13). CT images can clearly delineate the extent of the fracture as well as demonstrate any intra-articular fragments, which may be present. The

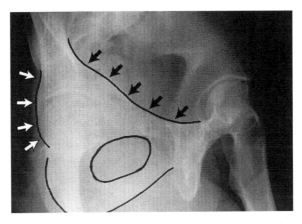

Fig. 11.11 Left posterior oblique, also called the obturator oblique for the right acetabulum. Note that the obturator ring is well seen; the anterior portion of the iliopectineal line (*black arrows*) and the posterior wall (*white arrows*) are seen well. In the presence of a both column fracture, this is the best view to demonstrate the spur sign. Obturator ring fractures can occur in several places, usually the inferior portion of the ring at the ischiopubic junction or the anterior and superior portions of the ring, at the puboacetabular junction (From Brandser E. *Fractures: Diagnosis and Treatment.* In: David Moehring H, Greenspan A, eds. ©2000 Current Medicine Group LLC)

Fig. 11.12 CT image of an acetabular fracture showing a small posterior lip fragment and a larger anterior wall fragment (From Greenspan A. *Fractures: Diagnosis and Treatment.* In: H. David Moehring H, Adam Greenspan eds. ©2000 Current Medicine Group LLC)

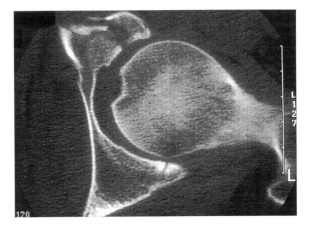

CT can also be converted into a three-dimensional image to more clearly demonstrate the fracture pattern. CT imaging can also be utilized to demonstrate other non-traumatic pathology. For example, anterior osteoarthritis, which may be subtle on the plain radiographs, can readily be appreciated on CT images.

Magnetic resonance imaging (MRI) of the hips is indicated in patients where a peri-articular lesion is suspected, labral pathology is suspected, or to evaluate for the

Fig. 11.13 CT image of an
acetabular fracture involving
the dome of the acetabulum
(From Greenspan A.
*Fractures: Diagnosis and
Treatment.* In: David
Moehring H, Greenspan A.
©2000 Current Medicine
Group LLC)

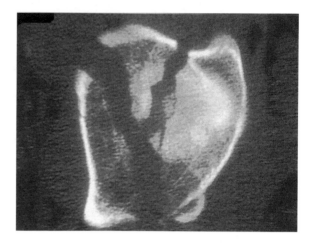

Fig. 11.14 Coronal section
of magnetic resonance
imaging (MRI) of a patient
with steroid-induced
osteonecrosis of the right
femoral head. Note the loss of
signal within the superior
region of the head (From
Mabrey J. *Current
Orthopedic Diagnosis and
Treatment.* In: Heckman JD,
Schenck RC, Agarwal A.
©2002 Current Medicine
Group LLC)

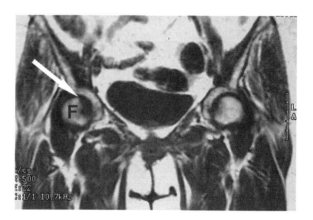

presence of avascular necrosis (AVN) of the femoral heads (Fig. 11.14). MRI is a
very sensitive and specific tool for the evaluation of AVN. It can readily demonstrate
the avascular segment prior to changes on the plain radiographs. MRI can also be
helpful in demonstrating a tear in the acetabular labrum. This is best demonstrated
by the use of MR arthrography. MR contrast material is injected intra-articularly and
an MR of the hip is obtained. The contrast will outline the labrum and any defect in
labrum can be identified.

The Tc99-MDP bone scan can be used as a sensitive indicator of osseous pathology in the pelvis. Metastatic disease, occult fractures, infection, or osteomyelitis can
be identified. The bone scan is most helpful as a general skeletal screening tool for
metastatic disease. The bone scan is very sensitive, but is not specific. Therefore,
other studies such as MRI or CT may be necessary to fully evaluate the nature and
extent of any identified the pathology.

Hip aspiration and arthrography can be helpful in the evaluation of pathology. Aspiration can be helpful in evaluating hip sepsis in both a native hip and after hip arthroplasty. Aspiration is best performed under fluoroscopic guidance to ensure proper entry into the small joint space of the hip. An arthrogram can then be utilized to confirm the intra-articular position of the needle. Arthrography is also utilized to assess for loosening of a hip prosthesis. The contrast material can be seen flowing around the loosened implant, demonstrating the separation of the implant, cement, and bone. Not infrequently patients will present with a history of both hip and spine pathology. Injection of local anesthetic, with or without a corticosteroid medication, into the hip under fluoroscopic guidance can be helpful in differentiating the pain coming from the hip with that coming from the spine. If the intra-articular local anesthetic results in significant relief of pain, the pain is most likely intra-articular in origin. If the local anesthetic agent does not alter the pain, extra-articular pathology or spine disease should be investigated.

The patient's history and physical examination direct the use of these radiographic techniques. The appropriate use of these diagnostic tests can result in cost-effective and accurate diagnosis and properly directed treatment.

Hip Pathology

A variety of soft tissue conditions can affect the hip. These are not uniformly associated with trauma or injury; however, an injury can be the inciting event. Trochanteric bursitis is a common condition of the hip. The pain results from inflammation within the trochanteric bursa. This is located over the lateral aspect of the greater trochanter under the fascia lata. It is associated with pain over the lateral aspect of the hip in the region of the greater trochanter. The pain is a deep ache centered over the greater trochanter with radiation both proximally to the pelvic brim and distally, occasionally all the way to the knee. Patients often complain of pain while seated, or upon arising from a chair, as well as pain that awakens them from sleep when lying on the involved side. The pain is exacerbated by adduction of the hip with the knee extended. No pathologic changes are noted on either plain radiographs or MRI. The treatment consists of stretching the fascia lata and the iliotibial band, and non-steroidal anti-inflammatory medications. If these conservative measures are unsuccessful, the patient may benefit from physical therapy with the use of local modalities such as ultrasound and iontophoresis. These modalities can be augmented with a corticosteroid injection into the bursa. If these non-operative modalities fail to relieve the pain, the bursa can be surgically excised. However, this option is rarely required and is not routinely successful.

The iliotibial band and the trochanteric bursa can also be involved in the snapping hip. The iliotibial band snapping over the trochanteric bursa and the greater trochanter causes this condition. This is not always painful. The treatment is similar to that for trochanteric bursitis. Snapping in the hip can also occur anteriorly. The iliopsosas tendon can snap over the anterior aspect of the hip where the tendon exits the pelvis over the anterior pelvic brim. This results in an anterior snap with flexion and extension. The amount of pain associated with the snap is variable. The treatment is directed toward alleviation of the pain. Non-steroidal anti-inflammatory medications can be helpful at alleviating the pain. Stretching of the iliopsosas with hip extension can also help to reduce the symptoms.

Another cause of a snapping hip is a tear in the acetabular labrum. The acetabular labrum is a dense, fibro-cartilaginous structure that is attached to the acetabular rim. This structure can be injured similar to a meniscal injury in the knee. The labrum is more prone to injury in patients with acetabular dysplasia. In this condition, the acetabulum is shallow and the labrum hypertrophies and is weight-bearing. A tear in the acetabular labrum presents clinically with pain in the hip anteriorly, particularly with internal rotation. This is also commonly associated with a click noted when the hip is flexed and extended. The diagnosis can be confirmed with an MRI obtained after the injection of intra-articular contrast dye. The accuracy of this assessment is approximately 85%; without the intra-articular contrast, the accuracy is only 50–60%. When a tear is identified, no treatment is necessary if the pain is mild. If, however, the patient has pain or if the click is activity limiting, then the tear should be excised or repaired. This is normally done by hip arthroscopy.

Intra-articular loose bodies can occur either as a result of trauma or as a result of synovial chondromatosis. In synovial chondromatosis, the synovium will develop osteochondral loose bodies that will be free in the articular space. In the knee, these loose bodies cause a great deal of mechanical symptoms such as locking. In the hip, there is not enough free space for the loose body to cause locking. However, these loose bodies can restrict motion and cause pain. Synovial chondromatosis can be difficult to diagnose. The plain radiographs are usually normal or will demonstrate the very subtle stippled calcifications of the osteochondral fragments. An MRI or CT scan can be helpful in demonstrating the loose bodies and the expansion of the synovial space and effusion. The treatment is surgical. An open arthrotomy is performed and the fragments removed. Synovectomy can be performed although care should be taken to preserve the vascularity of the femoral head.

Avascular necrosis is a condition that most commonly affects the femoral head. However, this condition can also affect the proximal humerus, knee, and talus. The specific mechanism causing AVN is unclear. Several factors have been associated with increased risk of developing this condition. The most common factors are trauma to the femoral head or neck, systemic corticosteroid administration, and excessive alcohol intake. In addition to these factors, there is a long list of other less common factors such as hemoglobinopathies, metabolic conditions, and inflammatory conditions, which can cause AVN. However, in as many as one-third of patients with non-traumatic AVN, no specific etiology can be identified, and thus these cases are identified as idiopathic AVN.

In all cases of AVN there is compromise of the blood supply of the femoral head. This most commonly occurs in the anterior, superior portion of the femoral head, leading to necrosis of a portion of the subchondral bone. If the avascular segment is large and in a weight-bearing area, the stability of the subchondral bone will be compromised as the necrotic trabeculae weaken. This process occurs over

6–24 months. While an MRI or Tc99-MDP bone scan can demonstrate the lesion early (see Fig. 11.14), the plain radiographs are frequently normal after the segment becomes avascular. Over time the round femoral head will weaken and then develop an area of collapse. At this point, the joint is no longer round and congruent and, without intervention, frequently will progress to degenerative arthritis.

The lesion of AVN has a very typical pathologic and radiographic pattern. The lesion is most commonly in the anterior and superior subchondral bone of the femoral head. There are several distinct zones to the lesion. The outer zone is an area of increased vascularity and inflammation that is in response to the necrotic segment. The next layer is a dense area of sclerotic bone, which is laid down around the necrotic segment in an attempt to heal the lesion. However, this simply serves to wall off the lesion and prevents vascular invasion and healing of the lesion. Inside the sclerotic bone is the necrotic bone with the trabecular structure that is relatively intact. Histologically, the necrosis of the bone is demonstrated by trabecular bone with empty lacunae. Closer to the subchondral bone is the area of collapse of the trabecular bone. The outer layer is composed of the subchondral bone and articular cartilage. Radiographically, a subchondral radiolucent line that is referred to as a crescent sign demonstrates this region. Frequently, after collapse of the subchondral region, there will be a defect through the cartilage and the subchondral bone that will allow articular fluid to enter the necrotic area. This will further impair healing of the lesion.

In early cases prior to collapse of the femoral head, attempts can be made to save the femoral head and restore viability to the necrotic bone. There are several surgical variations; all involve drilling a core tract into the avascular portion of the femoral head in an attempt to restore vascularity to the necrotic bone and possibly heal the lesion. Several techniques have been described to augment this procedure. These include the use of autologous cancellous bone grafting, bone graft substitutes, allograft cortical or cancellous bone, or one of the patient's fibulae on a vascular pedicle to place vascularized bone into the lesion.

Of patients who have documented AVN that is untreated, 70% will require a total hip replacement within 5 years. Patients who have had a core decompression type procedure will require a total hip replacement in 30–35% of cases by 5 years. The results are improved compared to the natural history; however, the success rate is less than optimal. Vascularized fibular grafting has demonstrated an improvement in the survivorship of the involved hip in a few centers. However, this requires highly specialized surgical technique and can lead to significant weakness in foot and ankle function on the involved side after harvesting the fibula.

For patients with small lesions that have already undergone subchondral collapse, an osteotomy may be done to rotate the necrotic collapsed segment out from under the weight-bearing area of the hip. However, commonly the lesion is extensive and not enough viable bone remains to allow the necrotic segment to be rotated out of the weight-bearing area of the hip. As the AVN progresses and the hip becomes severely degenerated, a hip replacement offers the most reliable means of restoring function and relieving pain. Many of these patients are relatively young to receive a total hip replacement. The average age of patients with AVN is approximately

35–45 years. The results of arthroplasty in this population have not been as successful as in patients with osteoarthritis. Newer, more durable bearing surfaces hold promise for this younger, more active patient population.

Hip Arthritis

A wide variety of arthritic conditions can affect the hip joint. While the medical therapy can vary based upon the specific diagnosis, the operative treatments fall into several broad categories and will be discussed as such. Arthritis is defined as any condition that results in articular cartilage damage with resulting pain and limitation of the motion of a joint. Hip arthritis can be divided into several broad categories (Table 11.1).

Table 11.1 Classification of hip arthritis

Category	Examples	Etiology
Osteoarthritis	Primary osteoarthritis	Idiopathic
	Secondary osteoarthritis	Congenital
		Developmental
		Avascular necrosis
		Post-traumatic
Inflammatory arthritis	Rheumatoid arthritis	Immunogenic
	Ankylosing spondylitis	
	Psoriatic arthritis	
	Systemic lupus	
Infectious	Pyogenic	*Staphylococcus aureus, S. epidermidis*, gonococcal
	Lyme disease	*Borrelia*
	Non-pyogenic	*Mycobacterium*
Other	Crystals	Gout, pseudogout
	Hemophilia	Hemosiderin deposition

The clinical presentation of hip arthritis is a gradual increase in pain and limitation of motion. Frequently patients will complain of a reduction in their ability to walk for distances. Patients will also notice a marked stiffness in the joint when they have been sitting for a period of time and go to stand. The joint will feel out of place or stiff. This symptom will resolve usually after a few steps. As the arthritis progresses and the joint begins to lose motion, patients will also notice a reduction in their ability to care for their own toenails and have difficulty with activities such as putting on socks or stockings and tying their shoes. A limp will also commonly occur in patients with hip arthritis, particularly after long walks or at the end of the day.

Radiographic and etiologic criteria can assist in dividing the patients into two broad categories, osteoarthritis and inflammatory arthritis, based upon the history and the radiographic appearance of the hip joints. Osteoarthritis has four classic features on plain radiography: localized joint space narrowing, subchondral sclerosis, osteophyte formation, and subchondral cysts (see Fig. 11.7). In rheumatoid arthritis, a classic example of an inflammatory arthritis, the radiographic features are peri-articular osteopenia and erosions, diffuse or global joint space narrowing, and occasionally subchondral cysts. In inflammatory arthritis of the hip, protrusio deformity of the femoral head beyond the ilio-ischial line can be noted as well. In most cases of arthritic disease in the hip, no additional studies other than plain radiography are necessary for the evaluation.

The non-operative treatment will vary based upon the specific diagnosis. Osteoarthritis, whether primary or secondary, is treated in a similar fashion. The treatment for the majority of patient's with osteoarthritis is non-operative. There are five primary interventions in the non-operative management of the patient with osteoarthritis (Table 11.2). These five interventions can be used in isolation or in combination based upon the specific clinical situation in which the patient presents. Non-steroidal anti-inflammatory drugs (NSAIDs) can be very effective in reducing the pain and improving function. However, there is a large individual variation in the efficacy and side effects with each of these agents. Therefore, patients should be tried on several NSAIDs from different chemical classes prior to abandoning this limb of therapy. The principal side effect of NSAID is gastrointestinal (GI) intolerance with the possibility of ulcer formation. NSAIDs can also affect renal and hepatic function; and in the long-term use of these agents, renal and hepatic function test should be followed. In addition, these medications can affect platelet function and may have an adverse effect on bleeding times. These medicines should not be used in patients requiring anticoagulation therapy or within 5–7 days prior to any surgical intervention.

Table 11.2 Primary interventions in the non-operative management of osteoarthritis

Non-steroidal anti-inflammatory medications
Physical therapy
Intra-articular injection of corticosteroids
Assistive devices
Modification of activities

The cyclo-oxygenase-2 (COX-2) inhibitors were thought to offer lower side effects compared to the non-specific cyclo-oxygenase inhibitors which represent the majority of NSAIDs on the market. However, their safety was brought into question in several large clinical trials which suggested an increased rate of cardiac and vascular events after long-term use at high doses. The COX-2 inhibitors do have the advantage of a lesser effect on platelet function and have been shown to be safe for patients on anticoagulation therapy, which allows them to be safely used in the peri-operative setting.

Intra-articular corticosteroid injections are helpful for the treatment of an acute exacerbation in pain. Intra-articular injections are more beneficial in the treatment of shoulder and knee and knee pathology compared to the hip. They have not been as widely utilized for arthritis of the hip, in part due to the difficulty ensuring the injection is in fact intra-articular. Fluoroscopy is helpful in confirming proper placement of the needle. Injection of the hip with local anesthetic can be helpful in differentiating referred back pain from intra-articular hip pathology. Also, there are patients who will have a strong referred pain from the hip to the knee. In these patients, an intra-articular hip injection will relieve the knee pain and confirm the site of origin of the knee pain. However, injections are limited in their ability to provide long-term relief of symptoms. Corticosteroid injection for arthritis should not be done more than three times per year. If the patient requires more frequent injections for pain control, other therapeutic measures or surgery should be considered. Repeated injection of the joint is not indicated. This will result in acceleration of the articular cartilage degeneration and increases the risks of complications, such as infection.

Physical therapy can be beneficial in reducing pain and improving range of motion for osteoarthritis (OA) involving the knee or shoulder; however, limited benefit has been found for the treatment of OA involving the hip. If this modality is to be utilized, it should be done early in the course of OA. As the arthritis progresses, therapy will only serve to exacerbate an already painful joint. However, all patients should be encouraged to maintain aerobic fitness to maintain their joint function as well as their general health. Activities such as swimming and cycling have minimal repetitive impact and are excellent for aerobic fitness. Activities such as running and racquet sports can further damage an arthritic joint and should be discouraged in a patient with hip arthritis. As the arthritis progresses, the patient will be able to do less and less and become more sedentary. As this occurs, the symptoms will also increase in severity.

Assistive devices, including crutches, cane, and a walker, can be quite effective in the relief of stress across the joint surface during ambulation in patients with OA involving the lower extremities. A cane used in the contralateral hand of a patient with isolated hip arthritis can reduce the joint reaction force by as much as 30%. However, the use of these devices is associated with a significant change in a patient's perception of themselves and their global health status. So while this modality can be helpful in relieving symptoms and maintaining mobility, it will commonly meet resistance from the patient.

Modification of activities is one of the most significant aspects in the non-operative management of arthritis. This includes modification in a patient's activities of daily living and self-care. Modification of the patient's parking, as well as obtaining devices to assist in putting on shoes and socks, can be very helpful for patients with limitations due to hip arthritis. The reduction in certain activities such as running or racquet sports can improve the joint symptoms. However, this will result in a gradual progressive decrease in the patient's quality of life. The level of social interaction and activities in which the patient can comfortably participate can become markedly reduced. Modification of activities should also address patients who are overweight. Reduction in weight can significantly improve a patient's symptoms, increase mobility, and improve global health status. In addition, reduction in weight will reduce the stress placed upon the joint replacement if they require surgery.

The non-operative management of a patient with OA involves all of the above therapies. However, as the arthritis progresses, pain and limitation of activities will continue to increase. When the patient fails to achieve acceptable symptomatic relief with the non-operative regimen, joint replacement should be discussed. No significant change in the complexity of the surgery or outcome will be noted in patients with hip arthritis who delay operative intervention with non-operative treatment. Therefore, the timing of the surgical intervention is based entirely upon the patient, the patient's pain, and limitations of daily activities.

Surgical Management

Most hip pathology can be managed with one of several options; these include arthroscopy, osteotomy, arthrodesis, and arthroplasty (hemiarthroplasty or total hip arthroplasty). Each option has specific indications and contraindications, which will be discussed in the next few sections.

Arthroscopy

Hip arthroscopy is in its infancy compared to this technique in the knee. The indications for hip arthroscopy are growing and now include the removal of loose bodies from the hip joint, addressing acetabular labral pathology, bone resection procedures for femoral-acetabular impingement, synovial disease, snapping hip syndrome from the iliopsoas tendon or iliotibial band, and identification of articular cartilage defects. The technique requires the use of special equipment due to the more extensive soft tissue envelope around the hip compared to the knee. The soft tissue envelope also limits the mobility of the arthroscope within the hip. In addition, the hip capsule is quite thick and the articular space quite small. Traction is required to gain visualization of the hip joint. The portals must be opened with care to avoid injury to the neuro-vascular structures surrounding the hip. These issues have presented challenges to the widespread use of this technique, but its application is rapidly expanding.

Arthrotomy

Arthrotomy involves surgical opening of the hip joint. Many of the indications for hip arthroscopy are also indications for hip arthrotomy, such as removing loose bodies or to address acetabular labral lesions. However, hip arthrotomy can also address the drainage of hip sepsis and hip synovectomy. The hip joint can be exposed and opened either from the anterior aspect or the posterior aspect. Anterior approaches are more commonly utilized as this approach is less likely to injure the blood supply to the femoral head which arises from the medial femoral circumflex vessels along the posterior intertrochanteric line.

The hip joint is normally entered from the acetabular edge, with care taken to preserve the acetabular labrum. If the labrum is torn, it can either be excised or repaired, depending upon the condition and nature of the tear. It may be necessary to apply traction to the leg to allow inspection of the hip joint. Any loose bodies or fragments can be removed. If the indication for arthrotomy is synovectomy, it may be necessary to open the hip both from the posterior and from the anterior aspect. This does increase the risk of post-operative avascular necrosis; however, the synovium of the hip cannot be removed from a single approach.

Osteotomy

Osteotomy involves redirecting the articular surface to move damaged cartilage from the weight-bearing areas of the joint and place a less damaged area of the articular surface in the weight-bearing area of the hip joint. Osteotomy can also reduce joint forces by realigning the bone of the pelvis or proximal femur to yield a larger area of contact to distribute the force of weight-bearing. During osteotomy, the bone of the pelvis or femur is transected, redirected, and then fixed rigidly (Fig. 11.15). If the arthritis is localized to only one region of a joint, performing an osteotomy can move the damaged cartilage away from the weight-bearing area and transfer undamaged articular surfaces into the high-stress area. This will result in reduced pain and prolong the functional life of the patient's native joint. Prerequisites for an osteotomy are that the patient has an adequate range of motion of the joint, that the joint is stable, and that the articular damage involves only a limited area of the joint. If extensive arthritis or an inflammatory arthritis is present, an osteotomy will not be successful.

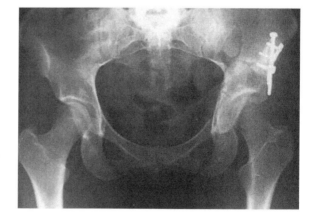

Fig. 11.15 Anteroposterior radiograph of a 26-year-old female 6 months after a left pelvic osteotomy was performed to deepen her acetabulum and improve coverage of the femoral head. Her primary diagnosis was developmental dysplasia of the hip, which left her with a shallow left acetabulum

In properly selected patients, hip osteotomies can have a success of greater than 80% at 8–10 years follow-up. For young patients with focal articular damage, osteotomy can provide an acceptable result and allow them to retain their own hip joint. This can delay or possibly eliminate the need for replacement with artificial materials that can wear or become loose. Acetabular osteotomy for developmental dysplasia of the hip can make subsequent total hip arthroplasty easier by redirecting the acetabular bone stock and providing better coverage for an acetabular component. However, osteotomy of the proximal femur can make a future hip replacement more difficult by altering the anatomy of the proximal femur. This may require an additional osteotomy to reconstruct the femur at the time of total hip replacement.

Arthrodesis

Arthrodesis involves the fusion of the proximal femur to the pelvis. This can provide a strong, stable, painless lower extremity. The patient can return to even heavy labor without the risk of loosening or damaging the arthrodesis. Arthrodesis is indicated in patients who are young with unilateral hip disease with no symptoms or disease involving the lumbar spine, contralateral hip, or the ipsilateral knee. Patients with an inflammatory arthritis or non-traumatic AVN are relatively contraindicated for arthrodesis, as these diseases are frequently bilateral. Several studies looking at the long-term results of arthrodesis have found good results lasting greater than 20 years. However, the hip is no longer mobile, and over 15–20 years, the arthrodesis can result in low back pain and pain in the ipsilateral knee. Several reports have noted that between 50 and 60% of patients complain of pain in the back or knee at 25–50 years follow-up. This technique has become less common due to the better options that are now available in total joint bearing surfaces that seem to provide a more durable and functional solution.

Hip Replacement Surgery

Total hip replacement (THR) is a common operation today. Approximately 300,000 replacements are performed each year. The primary goal of hip replacement is to relieve pain and improve mobility. This can routinely be accomplished in over 95% of patients. Long-term studies have demonstrated excellent results, with survivorship ranging from 65 to 90% at 30 years of follow-up.

In total hip replacement, both the socket (acetabulum) and the ball (femoral head) are replaced with metal and plastic parts. The socket is commonly replaced with a metal shell impacted into the prepared acetabular space with a modular plastic, metal, or ceramic liner (Figs. 11.16 and 11.17). The ball is replaced by a metal ball attached to a stem that goes inside the proximal canal of the femur. Two principle types of implants are used: those inserted with bone cement and those inserted without cement which are designed to allow bone to grow onto or into a porous metal

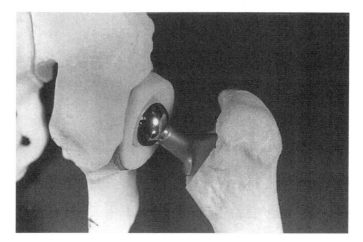

Fig. 11.16 Total hip arthroplasty with the acetabular component press-fit onto the pelvis and the femoral component inserted into the femoral canal, with the femoral head articulating with the polyethylene liner)

Fig. 11.17 Anteroposterior radiograph of an uncemented total hip arthroplasty

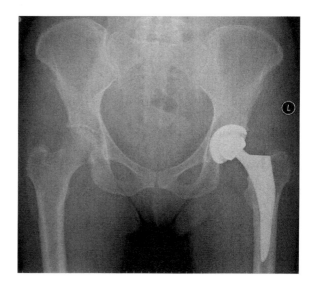

surface. Both techniques have excellent long-term follow-up data supporting their effectiveness. The cemented technique has seen a dramatic decrease in use over recent years due to the successful results of the uncemented designs that are thought to be easier to insert and remove the need for an additional possible mode of failure, the cement interface.

Most uncemented stems have a press-fit design which allows for rigid, stable fixation at the time of implantation, since the prosthesis is slightly larger than the bony space which is prepared by broaches, creating a tight wedging effect. Proximal tapered designs have a wedge-shaped taper in the stem, which provides an enhanced level of bony contact in the proximal femur, providing more physiologic loading of the femur with weight-bearing. Longer porous-coated stems have a cylindrical design of the stem which provides a large area of bony contact in the diaphysis of the femur. This moves the load transfer distally and can stress shield the proximal femur, leading to gradual resorption of the unloaded bone over time. These designs are commonly used in revision cases where the proximal femur is deficient. The key aspect of successful implantation of an uncemented stem is solid fixation at the time of surgery. Initial instability can occur if the stem is undersized relative to the femoral canal or due to improper technique. This leads to micro-motion at the bone–prosthesis interface, causing the creation of a fibrous union. This can produce thigh pain that may or may not resolve with time. Initially, this is treated with limited weight-bearing and NSAIDs. If the pain persists, revising the stem becomes necessary.

Total hip arthroplasty is performed from either an anterior, posterior, transtrochanteric, or minimally invasive (MIS) approach. The transtrochanteric approach, which can be used in revision or complex procedures, utilizes an osteotomy of the greater trochanter to mobilize the abductors to gain access to the hip joint. This has the advantage providing excellent exposure by lifting the abductors superiorly, allowing visualization of both the anterior and posterior columns of the acetabulum. In addition, advancing the trochanter distally to tighten the abductors and reduce the risk of post-operative dislocation can increase the stability of the total hip. However, historically there has been a trochanteric osteotomy non-union rate of 5–15%. Trochanteric non-union will result in a persistent limp and an increased rate of hip dislocation post-operatively.

The posterior approaches are commonly used for total hip replacement. The dissection is carried posterior to the trochanter. The short external rotators are divided and a posterior capsule is opened. This creates a defect in the posterior capsule. The hip is dislocated posteriorly by flexion, adduction, and internal rotation. The posterior approach provides an excellent extensile exposure to the pelvis, hip, and femur. In addition, the gluteus medius and minimus are preserved, optimizing the function of the hip abductors post-operatively. However, post-operatively patients are at risk for a posterior dislocation with flexion, adduction, and internal rotation. The dislocation rate after a posterior approach is 1–3% in primary total hip replacement.

Anterior approaches to the hip are also commonly employed for total hip replacement. These approaches enter the hip from in front of the greater trochanter by detaching a portion of the gluteus medius and minimus. The anterior capsule is then opened, and the hip is extended, adducted, and externally rotated to dislocate the femoral head and the arthroplasty completed. This approach can yield extensile exposure proximally and distally. This leaves the posterior capsule intact, protecting the patient from a posterior dislocation. The rate of instability is 1–2% in most series. However, by detaching a portion of the gluteus medius from the trochanter, the muscle is weakened. This can lead to a greater incidence of limp and pain in the post-operative period. Furthermore, if the repair of the detached gluteus medius pulls off of the trochanter, the patient may be left with a persistent Trendelenburg limp.

Currently there is a great deal of interest in minimally invasive approaches for hip replacement, which include anterior and posterior approaches. The purpose is to reduce peri-operative pain and to speed recovery. These techniques, when combined with aggressive pain management protocols, have shown promise in improving the early recovery of the patient. While this is a significant benefit, it must be emphasized that proper surgical placement and technique is required for long-term success. Any short-term benefit from MIS surgery must not come at the expense of long-term results.

The patient is mobilized early after a total hip replacement, often beginning physical therapy on the day of surgery. The best exercise in the post-operative period is walking. Hip abduction exercises may be done with a posterior approach. However, if an anterior approach was utilized, active abduction exercises should be delayed to allow the gluteus medius repair to heal.

If the posterior approach is used, patients need to be careful not to flex the hip beyond 90° and to keep their legs abducted and neutrally rotated for the first 6 weeks to prevent the femoral head from dislocating out of the acetabular component. The rate of instability and the position of greatest instability vary with the approach used for the arthroplasty as outlined above. With anterior approaches, the greatest instability is with extension and external rotation. The patients usually report a dislocation occurring while they are standing and pivoting or while they are supine in bed with the legs adducted and the feet externally rotated. In contrast, posterior instability occurs when the hip is in a flexed, adducted, and internally rotated position. Patients are at risk of instability when they are getting out of a chair, getting off the toilet seat, or getting out of an automobile. The rate of dislocation is greatest in the first 6 weeks post-operatively while the soft tissues are healing. If a dislocation does occur within the first 6 weeks, the rate of recurrent instability is approximately 30%, with the majority having a single event. However, if the first dislocation occurs after the first 6 months, the rate of recurrent instability increases to 60%, with the majority of patients having recurrent instability, often requiring revision surgery to address the problem.

The treatment of a dislocated hip is to first reduce the hip, usually with conscious sedation. If this is unsuccessful, general anesthesia may be required. The patient is often placed into a brace or a knee immobilizer for a period of 6 weeks and can weight-bear as tolerated. If the patient does have recurrent instability, revision may be necessary. Prior to revision, it is helpful to determine the precise position of the components. Plain radiography can accurately determine the vertical inclination of the component; however, it is the degree of anterior rotation of the component that is a greater factor in instability after total hip replacement. Accurate assessment of the anterior rotation of the component can be best assessed by the use of CT imaging. If CT scan imaging cuts are also taken through the femoral condyles, the rotation of both the femoral and acetabular components can be determined. This information is important to aid in identifying the cause of the recurrent instability and to plan appropriate reconstructive surgery to correct the problem.

Aseptic loosening of the implant from bone occurs at a low rate with modern techniques. Many studies have shown that, at 10 years, approximately 90–95% of patients retain their original implant. This drops to 80–85% at 20 years, and approximately 65% at 30 years. The rate of loosening of the femoral component is usually less than that of the acetabular component. Acetabular loosening tends to increase over time due to osteolysis or stress shielding of the bone behind the more rigid metallic cups.

The survival of implants in patients less than 50 years of age is less than that noted in older patients. This is related to the higher demands and higher activity level in this younger group of patients. In an attempt to reduce the rate of aseptic loosening after THR in this younger patient population, surgeons have tried to achieve implant fixation directly to bone with increased use of uncemented stems. This can be achieved through the use of porous surfaces made of small beads or wires sintered onto the base stem. If this surface is closely approximated to bone, and no significant motion occurs at the interface, bone trabeculae will interdigitate and grow into the porous surface and secure the implant. The wedge-shaped designs of current stems help to achieve early stability while bone ingrowth occurs over time. It is also important to have minimal motion between the polyethylene liner and the metal shell. Motion and wear can occur at this interface, as well as on the articulating interface. This leads to the development of wear debris which loosens the metal shell, or it can cause a mechanical failure of the polyethylene liner and require revision surgery (Fig. 11.18). In addition, it is important to have high-quality locking mechanisms and thick polyethylene liners for acetabular components. The current recommendations are for a polyethylene thickness of at least 6 mm.

Most designs limit the amount of screw holes in the metal shell which are used for ancillary fixation with screws to fix the shell to bone prior to bone ingrowth. The holes in the shell can provide a direct conduit for wear debris to the implant bone interface. This debris can lead to an osteolytic reaction and subsequent loosening of the acetabular shell. Most surgeons attempt to avoid the need for holes by press fitting the metal shell on the bone by under-reaming the acetabular bed and then inserting a slightly larger metal shell into the acetabular bed. This can provide excellent initial stability and eliminate the need for screws and screw holes. In cases of abnormal anatomy and osteopenic bone, or in revision cases, screws are routinely indicated to supplement early stability.

Loosening appears to be primarily related to the generation of polyethylene wear debris from the articulation. Several new technologies have been developed to reduce wear from the articulation in a total hip replacement. The first new concept was to improve the polyethylene. This was accomplished by cross-linking the polymer strands within the material by means of free radical production using radiation. Think of a polymer as a bowl of cold spaghetti. If a strand of spaghetti is pulled, the whole strand can be teased from the bowl. If some of the strands are cut, and then these shorter strands are linked to other strands, it will be more difficult to pull out a strand and also more difficult to pull out a long strand. This logic applies to cross-linked polyethylene. The wear rate is reduced by 10-fold and the debris produced is of much smaller particles.

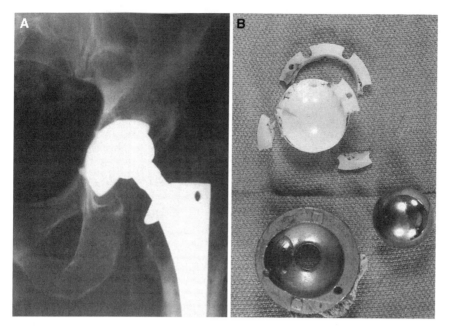

Fig. 11.18 (**a**) Anteroposterior radiograph of the left hip of a 52-year-old male 5 years after a non-cemented total hip arthroplasty demonstrates a markedly eccentric position of the femoral head within the acetabular component. (**b**) Photograph of retrieved acetabular component and femoral head of this patient. The polyethylene is fragmented and was found displaced within the shell, allowing the femoral head to articulate with the metal acetabular shell

However, even with cross-linking, the plastic is the weak link and debris is produced from wear of the polyethylene. Two other alternatives are now available. These are referred to as hard on hard interfaces. Metal on metal and ceramic on ceramic are both available. By using much harder materials for the articulation, the wear rate and debris production can be reduced by up to a 1000-fold. With less debris and less wear, a much longer functional life is hoped for these articulations. These new articulations, however, also have some limitations. Metal on metal involves the use of a cobalt–chromium femoral head on a cobalt–chromium acetabular liner. This articulation has been in clinical use for approximately 30 years. Early designs failed early due to design problems. The early heads were made of equal dimension to the acetabular opening, which would result in binding of the head within the acetabulum and the component would loosen. Current designs have reduced the size of the head relative to the acetabulum by a very small amount. This allows for lubrication of the interface and less friction known as triboliogy, eliminating the problem of acetabular loosening. However, metal debris is produced in the form of small metal ions which are detectable in the blood, lymphatics, and urine of patients with metal on metal hip articulations. The long-term effects of this are unknown, but there is a concern since the ions continue to be produced over the entire life of the joint replacement. The metal on metal bearing surface also has the advantage of using very large femoral head designs which can improve stability and range of motion by increasing the head to neck ratio and maximizing the jump distance necessary for the head to dislocate. Many surgeons allow patients to participate in higher impact activities with hard on hard bearing surface implants. However, recent problems have begun to appear with patients developing painful hips and no evidence of gross loosening. It is thought that some patients develop a hypersensitivity to the metal debris particles, leading to pain and, in some cases, significant synovitis. Early investigation suggests that a vertical placement of the acetabular component can lead to edge loading and subsequent increase of wear debris. Further studies are needed to help clarify the situation.

Ceramic on ceramic is the other hard on hard interface and results in the least amount of wear debris of all the currently used articulations for total hip arthroplasty. However, it is limited by the strength of the ceramic material. Ceramic implants can be prone to fracture and when a ceramic implant fails, it results in a catastrophic failure. The ceramic fragments are very hard and abrasive, resulting in rapid extensive wear of the metallic implants that are attached to the bones. Frequently, the metal components attached to the bones and the ceramic articulation all need to be removed after a fracture. The remaining particles in the soft tissue surrounding the joint lessen the success rates of revision surgery after ceramic fracture. Recently, a phenomenon of "squeaking hips" has been reported in which patients develop audible squeaking when actively moving their hip replacement. It is thought that improper placement of the components leads to this problem and can require revision surgery.

Currently wear and loosening are the most worrisome complications, which are being addressed by improvements in materials and designs. However, the current devices have such high success rates that determining if new technologies are truly an improvement will need at least 10 years of clinical follow-up. All of the new devices need to be evaluated not only for their benefits but also for the real and potential limitations.

Complications

The most frequent complication after THR is thromboembolic disease (TED). This includes deep venous thrombosis (DVT) and pulmonary embolism. Early in the history of THR, the rate of fatal pulmonary embolism was 1–2%. However, at that time patients were kept on bed rest for as long as 2–3 weeks and kept up to 6 weeks in the hospital. Early mobilization of patients has undoubtedly contributed to the significant reduction in the rate of fatal pulmonary embolism. However, significant reduction has also occurred through the use of anticoagulant prophylaxis, regional anesthesia, shorter operating times, and lower blood loss. In the United States, THR is considered a significant risk factor for TED and therefore the routine use of medical and/or mechanical prophylaxis has been recommended. At present, the rate of TED ranges between 5 and 20%. The rate of fatal pulmonary embolism is low, approximately 0.01%. The principal methods of prophylaxis are low-dose Coumadin (warfarin), aspirin, low molecular weight heparin, and pneumatic compression stockings. Coumadin is started the evening prior to surgery or on the day of surgery. It is recommended that the therapy be continued for 3–6 weeks post-operatively. The medication needs to be monitored closely to keep the level within a safe range. The international normalized ratio (INR) is targeted at approximately 2.0. It has been shown in many studies to be a safe and effective method of prophylaxis. However, the monitoring of Coumadin is of particular concern. Occasionally patients will have a dramatic elevation of their prothrombin time (PT) and INR with the first dose. This will lead to a risk of post-operative bleeding and hematoma at the operative site. As the length of stay in the hospital has decreased to 3–4 days or less, this has made the use of Coumadin increasingly difficult. It frequently will take 5–7 days to get a patient equilibrated on a steady dose of Coumadin. This is more difficult to accomplish in the outpatient setting. Currently this is managed with the use of home nursing services and frequent monitoring.

Low molecular weight heparin (LMWH) formulations were developed in part to provide safe, effective prophylaxis against thromboembolic disease. Subcutaneous unfractionated heparin has been used historically in the general surgical population. It has not been found to be effective in the orthopedic population. Intravenous unfractionated heparin is effective prophylaxis and treatment of thromboembolic disease. However, it requires even greater monitoring when used intravenously as it fully anticoagulates the patient immediately. If this occurs within the first 3 days post-operatively, the incidence of wound hematoma is greater than 50%; thus this is infrequently used in the post-operative orthopedic patient. Low molecular weight heparin is more selective in the interruption of the coagulation cascade creating a more controlled effect, and patients do not require monitoring. The current protocols are for 10 days to 4 weeks of therapy. Most studies demonstrate efficacy comparable with or better than Coumadin for total hip replacement. The disadvantage of LMWH is the significant risk of bleeding and wound complication, which occurs at a rate of approximately 4%.

Aspirin has been used for DVT prophylaxis historically. Aspirin irreversibly inhibits platelet function and theoretically will reduce the rate of formation of DVT. Little data directly supports the routine use of aspirin in THR; however, several studies demonstrate acceptable prophylaxis with the use of aspirin and hypotensive epidural anesthesia (HEA). HEA is an excellent anesthesia technique for THR; however, it requires careful patient monitoring and a dedicated anesthesia team. This form of anesthesia results in reduced blood loss while maintaining blood flow in the lower extremities. This reduces the need for transfusion post-operatively, which has been shown to increase the risk of DVT. In addition, the reduction in blood loss results in less activation of the coagulation cascade, again minimizing the risk of DVT. While this technique has been shown to be very effective, it has not been widely applied due to concerns about the reduction of mean arterial pressure in elderly patients, which may result in stroke, renal failure, or myocardial infarction.

Dislocation of the prosthetic femoral head from the acetabular component occurs in 1–3% of patients after THR. Post-operatively patients are instructed to not bend their replaced hip beyond 90°, to keep their legs abducted and in neutral rotation. These restrictions should be followed closely for the first 6 weeks following surgery. After this time, the patient should have formed a sufficient pseudocapsule to protect against dislocation. However, a replaced hip is always at greater risk for dislocation compared to a native hip joint. The majority of patients who dislocate their hip in the early post-operative period can be reduced without additional surgery and protected with a hip abduction brace or knee immobilizer for 6 weeks to allow healing of the pseudocapsule. In addition to patient compliance, the other etiologies for dislocation are component malposition, excessive soft tissue laxity, and impingement of the prosthetic or osseous structures resulting in levering of the femoral head out of the acetabulum. If a patient recurrently dislocates, revision surgery may be indicated.

The most devastating complication after THR is deep sepsis. Early post-operative infection occurs in approximately 0.3–0.5% of cases after primary THR. Late infection resulting from hematogenous spread can occur in 1–2% of patients. If detected within the first 2 weeks post-operatively, aggressive open debridement and synovectomy combined with intravenous antibiotics may be successful. However, if the infection recurs after debridement or is detected beyond 2 weeks of symptoms, treatment consists of a two-stage explantation procedure. This involves the stage one removal of the prosthetic components and all cement. The prosthesis is left out for at least 6 weeks. An antibiotic impregnated spacer is placed at the time of debridement, which provides a local depot of antibiotics at the site of the infection, and improves mobility and maintains soft tissue tension during the treatment period. Appropriate intravenous antibiotics are administered for 6–8 weeks and the patient is monitored for clinical signs of infection. If lab values normalize (white blood cell [WBC], erythrocyte sedimentation rate [ESR], C-reactive protein), the joint can be aspirated after antibiotics have been stopped for at least 2 weeks. If this is negative, the second-stage reimplantation can be done. The success rate for this technique is often greater than 90%. If the pathologic organisms are highly virulent and resistant to antibiotic therapy, reimplantation can be delayed for more than 12 months.

Heterotopic ossification (HO) can form around a THR in 5–25% of cases. Heterotopic bone is histologically bone tissue. It forms within the muscle around the hip after arthroplasty. There is a metaplasia that occurs, forming a bone matrix that becomes calcified over the first 6–12 months after the surgery. Most commonly the presence of HO will not compromise the clinical result. Associated risk factors are patients with hypertrophic osteoarthritis, males, over the age of 65, HO formation after previous surgery, and ankylosing spondylitis.

Heterotopic ossification is graded according to Brooker. Grade one consists of isolated islands of bone within the soft tissue between the femur and pelvis. Grade two is bone protruding from the proximal femur or pelvis with greater than 1 cm of separation. Grade three consists of bone protruding from the femur and/or pelvis with less than 1 cm between the bones. Grade four is radiographic ankylosis, with no visible space between the bone protruding from the femur and pelvis. Grades one and two are rarely symptomatic. Grade three patients usually have stiffness and mild pain. Patients with grade four usually have marked stiffness and can be very symptomatic.

Patients who are at high risk for this complication can receive prophylaxis using indomethacin or low-dose radiation therapy. Once HO forms, the patients should be encouraged to maintain range of motion and activity, but passive stretching and passive range of motion should be avoided. Surgical intervention, in which the HO is excised, is indicated in patients with significant restriction of motion and pain. This occurs most commonly in patients with grade three and four HO. Surgery should be delayed until the HO is mature. This usually takes 12–24 months and is indicated by mature appearance on plain radiography, uptake similar to the uninvolved bone of the pelvis on a Tc-99MDP bone scan and normal serum alkaline phosphatase level. Attempts to remove the bone prior to maturity have an increased rate of recurrence. After the bone is excised, the patient should receive prophylaxis to prevent recurrence. The prophylaxis is as above with either indomethacin or radiation therapy. Radiation therapy is preferred in most patients as it is usually a one-dose regimen of 700–800 cGy and can be administered either immediately pre-operatively or within the first 2 or 3 days post-operatively. In this way the entire treatment regimen is delivered in a controlled setting compared to indomethacin, which is administered for as long as 6 weeks. The rate of recurrence after excision and prophylaxis is approximately 5–20%.

The limitations to the long-term fixation of a total hip arthroplasty are loosening and wear. As the implant, particularly the polyethylene liner, wears, the debris that is produced is released into the local tissues. The body has no mechanism to digest or eliminate the polyethylene debris. However, the local macrophages in the area recognize the material as a foreign substance and try to eliminate the debris. The macrophages ingest the material and try to digest it with catabolic enzymes and super-oxides, which fails to alter the material. As the debris accumulates within the cell, it breaks down, releasing the polyethylene, enzymes, and oxides into the local environment. This results in a local bone lysis that creates cysts in the bone and dissects along the fixation of the implant or cement and bone. If allowed to continue, the lysis leads to loosening.

Loosening can also result from mechanical failure of the implant bone interface. The cement mantle can fragment or fracture, leaving the implant loose. In non-cemented fixation, the implant can also loosen. This can occur due to the implant never actually bonding to the bone with bone ingrowth; a fibrous tissue forms instead. This fibrous tissue may not be sufficient to maintain stable fixation of the implant. The implant will then migrate slowly, best appreciated on serial radiographs. This will require revision to provide a stable implant.

Similar to the indications for primary arthroplasty, these are elective surgeries. However in the revision setting, it is important to follow the patient closely with plain radiographs. If an accelerated pattern of bone loss is noted, revision surgery should be performed prior to the loss of an extensive amount of bone. The greater the loss of bone at the time of revision, the greater the difficulty in obtaining stable fixation for the revision components. This may also lead to a higher rate of repeated revision for aseptic loosening.

Summary

As noted initially, disorders involving the hip and femur are manifested by alteration in a patient's ability to ambulate. These can be diagnosed and treated by obtaining a careful history, thorough physical examination, and the appropriate use of radiographic studies. When proper diagnosis is made for most non-traumatic disorders, it is usually best to begin with a non-operative approach. If the non-operative treatment alternatives are not successful, then operative intervention is indicated and will result in an excellent outcome in the majority of patients.

Suggested Reading

1. Bauer TW, Parvizi J, Kobayashi N, Krebs V. Diagnosis of periprosthetic infection. *J Bone Joint Surg Am.* 2006;88:869–882.
2. Brooker AF, Bowerman JW, Robinson RA, Riley LH Jr. Ectopic ossification following total hip replacement. Incidence and a method of classification. *J Bone Joint Surg Am.* 1973;55(8):1629–1632.
3. Byrd JW. Hip arthroscopy. *J Am Acad Orthop Surg.* 2006;14(7):433–444.
4. Callaghan JJ, Templeton JE, Liu SS, et al. Results of Charnley total hip arthroplasty at a minimum of 30 years. A concise follow-up of a previous report. *J Bone Joint Surg Am.* 2004;86-A(4):690–695.
5. Collier JP, Sutula LC, Currier BH, et al. Overview of polyethylene as a bearing material: comparison of sterilization methods. *Clin Orthop Relat Res.* 1996;333:76–86.
6. Evans BG. Late complications and their management. In: Callaghan JJ, Rosenberg AG, Rubash HE, eds. *The Adult Hip.* New York, NY: Lippincott-Raven; 1998:1149–1161.
7. Garvin KL, Evans BG, Salvati EA, Brause BD. Palacos gentamicin for the treatment of deep periprosthetic hip infections. *Clin Orthop Relat Res.* 1994;298:97–105.
8. Healy WL, Lo TC, DeSimone AA, Rask B, Pfeifer BA. Single-dose irradiation for the prevention of heterotopic ossification after total hip arthroplasty. A comparison of doses of five hundred and fifty and seven hundred centigray. *J Bone Joint Surg Am.* 1995;77(4):590–595.
9. Hoaglund FT, Steinbach LS. Primary osteoarthritis of the hip: etiology and epidemiology. *J Am Acad Orthop Surg.* 2001;9(5):320–327.
10. Jazrawi LM, Kummer FJ, DiCesare PE. Alternative bearing surfaces for total joint arthroplasty. *J Am Acad Orthop Surg.* 1998;6(4):198–203.
11. Meehan J, Jamali AA, Nguygen H. Prophylactic antibiotics in hip and knee arthroplasty. *J Bone Joint Surg Am.* 2009;91(10):2480–2490.
12. Steinberg ME. Early diagnosis, evaluation, and staging of osteonecrosis. *Instr Course Lect.* 1994;43:513–518.
13. Trousdale RT, Ekkernkamp A, Ganz R, Wallrichs SL. Periacetabular and intertrochanteric osteotomy for the treatment of osteoarthrosis in dysplastic hips. *J Bone Joint Surg Am.* 1995;77(1):73–85.
14. Wiklund I, Romanus B. A comparison of quality of life before and after arthroplasty in patients who had arthrosis of the hip joint. *J Bone Joint Surg Am.* 1991;73(5):765–769.

15. Willert HG, Bertram H, Buchhorn GH. Osteolysis in alloarthroplasty of the hip. The role of ultra-high molecular weight polyethylene wear particles. *Clin Orthop Relat Res.* 1990;258:95–107
16. Woo RYG, Morrey BF. Dislocations after total hip arthroplasty. *J Bone Joint Surg Am.* 1982;64(9):1295–1306.

Chapter 12
The Knee

Brian G. Evans and Mark W. Zawadsky

This chapter will discuss the anatomy, biomechanics, and pathology of the knee. The function of the knee is provided primarily by the soft tissue. Therefore, injury to these soft tissue structures will have significant impact upon the stability of the knee.

Anatomy

The osseous anatomy of the knee consists of the proximal tibia, the distal femur, and the patella (Fig. 12.1). The distal femur consists of the medial and lateral condyles, the medical and lateral epicondyles, femoral trochlear groove, and the intercondylar notch. The medial condyle is larger and extends slightly distal compared to the lateral condyle. Both condyles are covered with articular cartilage. The trochlear groove lies on the anterior aspect of the distal femur between the medial and lateral femoral condyles. This surface is also covered by the articular cartilage and serves as the site of articulation of the patella. The lateral rim of the trochlear groove is frequently more prominent than the medial side to allow for proper patellar tracking along the femur.

The epicondyles serve as the site of insertion of several important structures. The deep and superficial medial collateral ligaments (MCL) attach to the medial epicondyle. The proximal margin of the medial epicondyle is enlarged and serves as the site of insertion of the adductor magnus (the adductor tubercle). The lateral or fibular collateral ligament (LCL) attaches to the lateral epicondyle. Inferior to the attachment of the LCL is the insertion of the popliteus muscle at the junction

B.G. Evans (✉)
Department of Orthopedic Surgery, Georgetown University Medical Center, Washington, DC 20007, USA
e-mail: evansb1@gunet.georgetown.edu

S.W. Wiesel, J.N. Delahay (eds.), *Essentials of Orthopedic Surgery*,
DOI 10.1007/978-1-4419-1389-0_12, © Springer Science+Business Media, LLC 2010

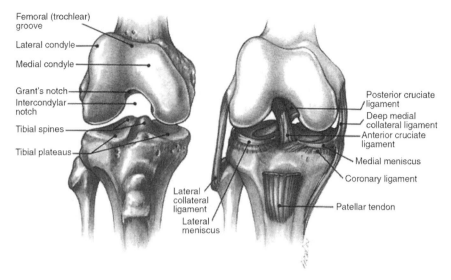

Fig. 12.1 Bony anatomy and major ligamentous structures of the flexed knee joint (*anterior view*)

of the lateral condyle and epicondyle. The medial and lateral heads of the gastrocnemius muscle originate from the medial and lateral posterior femoral condyles. The intercondylar notch is the site of the femoral attachment of the cruciate ligaments. The anterior cruciate ligament (ACL) attaches in the posterior lateral aspect of the notch and the posterior cruciate ligament (PCL) attaches in the anterior medial aspect of the notch.

The proximal tibial surface is composed of the medial and lateral plateaus and the intercondylar eminence. The medial plateau is larger and extends further posterior compared to the lateral plateau. The surface of the medial plateau is slightly concave. The lateral tibial plateau is in fact slightly convex. Both of the tibial plateaus are covered with articular cartilage. The intercondylar eminence is the site of attachment menisci and the cruciate ligaments.

The patella is a sesamoid bone within the tendon of the quadriceps mechanism. There are two major facets on the patella, the medial and lateral facets. There is significant variability in the size and orientation of these facets. However, normally the lateral facet is broader and the medial facet is more acutely oriented to the femoral trochlea.

The osseous anatomy of the knee provides little to the stability of the knee. Stability and function are therefore provided by the complex soft tissue envelope around and in the knee (Figs. 12.2 and 12.3). The soft tissue components of the knee can be divided into several components: static restraints (ligaments), dynamic restraints (muscles and tendons), and the menisci. The static restraints are represented by the medial collateral ligament (MCL), lateral collateral ligament (LCL), anterior cruciate ligament (ACL), and posterior cruciate ligament (PCL). These

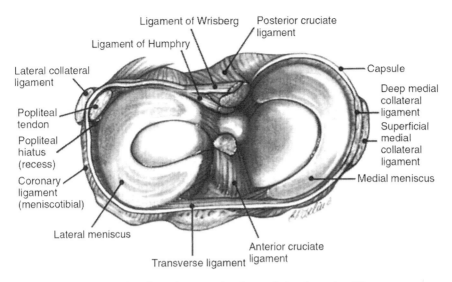

Fig. 12.2 Cross section of the knee demonstrating the menisci and associated ligaments

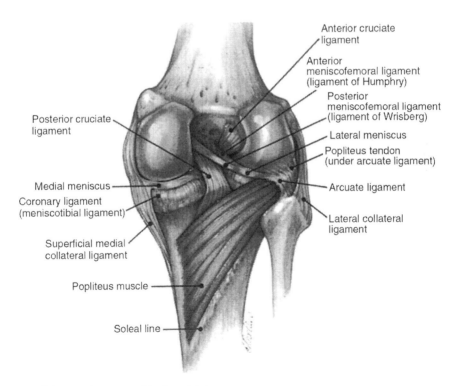

Fig. 12.3 Posterior aspect of the knee joint

structures resist valgus and varus stress as well as anterior and posterior translation of the tibial relative to the femur. The MCL consists of two layers. The deep MCL spans from the medial epicondyle of the femur to the proximal tibial border, just below the medial tibial plateau. The superficial MCL has the same femoral origin; however, the ligament has a broad tibial insertion extending 6–10 cm below the tibial plateau along the posterior medial border of the tibia. The LCL is a more discrete band along the lateral aspect of the knee. It spans from its origin on the lateral femoral epicondyle and inserting not on the proximal tibia but instead on the fibular head.

The ACL resists the anterior translation of the tibia relative to the femur. The ligament runs from the anterior aspect of the tibial eminence to the posterior lateral aspect of the femoral notch. The PCL resists posterior translation of the tibia relative to the femur and resists hyperextension of the knee. The ligament extends from the posterior aspect of the intercondylar eminence and proximal tibia in the midline to the anterior medial aspect of the femoral intercondylar notch.

The dynamic restraints in the knee are the muscles and tendons which cross the knee joint. These are broadly divided into muscles which act to extend and those which act to flex the knee. The extensor muscles are the quadraceps femoris and the tensor facia lata. The quadriceps is a group of four muscles all inserting onto the patella and patellar tendon, which in turn inserts upon the anterior tibial tubercle. The muscles that make up the quadriceps are the rectus femoris, vastus lateralis, vastus medialis, and vastus intermedius. These are all supplied by the femoral nerve. The tensor fascia lata originates upon the pelvic brim and inserts at Gerdy's tubercle on the proximal anterior lateral tibia. The tensor fascia lata is innervated by the superior gluteal nerve.

The primary flexors of the knee are the hamstring muscles—semimembranosis, semitendonosis, and the biceps femoris—and the sartorius and gracillis. The hamstring muscles originate on the ischium and insert on the posterior medial and lateral proximal tibia. They receive their innervation from the sciatic nerve; all are innervated by the tibial division of the sciatic nerve except the short head of the biceps which is innervated by the peroneal division of the sciatic nerve. The sartorius originates from the anterior superior iliac spine and the gracillis originates from the pubis. Both of these muscles with the semitendonosis insert into the proximal medial tibia in the pes anserine (goose's foot, relating to the appearance of the three tendons inserting together). The sartorius is innervated by the femoral nerve and the gracillis by the obturator nerve.

The other muscles that serve to flex the knee are the gastrocnemius and popliteus which extend from the posterior aspect of the femoral condyles to the calcaneous and proximal tibia, respectively.

The menisci are two crescent-shaped cartilaginous structures attached to the proximal tibial surface. These structures serve two purposes in the knee. They increase the surface area for weight bearing, therefore, reducing the peak stress in the articular cartilage. They also provide a small degree of stability to the knee by changing the relatively flat tibial articular surface to a cupped surface. The menisci are composed of dense organized cartilage tissue.

Biomechanics of the Knee

The mechanical axis of the lower extremity extends from the center of rotation of the hip to the center of the ankle joint. This normally crosses the knee joint in the lateral third of the medial tibial plateau. The normal anatomic alignment of the knee is 5–7° of valgus. When the knee is loaded, the medial compartment receives 60% of the weight-bearing stress and the lateral compartment receives 40% of the weight-bearing stress. This difference in the applied load in the normal knee is why the medial tibial plateau and medial femoral condyle are larger than the lateral side. Patients with significant angular deformity of the knee will have altered weight bearing, resulting in increased stress in the medial (with varus or bow-legged deformity) or lateral (with valgus or knock-knee deformity) compartment. The increased stress will frequently result in early arthritis in the overused compartment of the knee.

The highest joint forces, however, are found in the patello-femoral articulation. Forces as high as three to five times the body weight across the patello-femoral articulation can be noted for activities such as stair climbing and jumping. The function of the patella is to provide a mechanical advantage to the quadriceps tendon. The patella moves the line of pull of the quadriceps further away from the center of rotation, therefore, acting as a lever and reducing the force required to extend the knee. Patients who have had the patella removed because of arthritis or trauma are noted to have approximately 30% reduction in the force in the quadriceps compared to patients with a patella.

Evaluation of the Painful Knee

History

The history should begin with the chief complaint and how long the patient has noticed the problem: the specific location of pain, any radiation, the nature of the pain (ache, burning, stabbing, etc.), and any exacerbating or ameliorating factors. The relationship of the pain with activity and rest is important to note in particular. Pain in the musculoskeletal system will commonly be relieved with rest. Severe pain that is present at rest suggests a septic process or neoplasm, which may be primary or metastatic.

Frequently knee problems begin with an injury. Detailed history describing the injury can be very helpful in determining the structures that are injured. The nature of any external force contacting the knee and the position of the knee at the time of injury should be elicited. Did an audible or palpable pop occur at the time of the injury? Shifting or abnormal movement of the knee may also have been noted at the time of injury. The degree and nature of any swelling around the knee are important to record. In addition to the description of injury, it is helpful to inquire about the patient's ability to use the knee after the injury: was the patient able to weight bear, was the onset of pain or swelling immediate or delayed, could the patient flex or extend the knee after injury are important questions to ask the patient after knee injury.

In addition to pain, patients with knee problems will complain of mechanical problems in the knee. Patients may note an inability to fully bend or straighten the knee. This is referred to as locking of the knee. Locking can be a result of a loose body in the knee becoming lodged between the femoral condyle and tibial plateau, similar to a wedge "door stop." The patients who note intermittent locking of the knee will usually be able to relieve the locked knee by gently moving the knee without weight bearing. This maneuver allows the loose fragment to be released from between the femur and tibia and motion will be restored. However, inability to fully flex and extend the knee can also be noted in patients with large effusions and in patients with ligament injuries.

Instability is another frequent complaint of patients with knee injuries. Patients will observe that their knee will shift or buckle with particular activities. Instability can result from two general etiologies. The first is ligamentous injuries. As noted previously, the stability of the knee is a result of the ligaments which cross from the tibia to the femur. Disruption of the ligaments will result in alteration of knee function; the knee may shift or sublux with activity. The second common cause of a knee buckling or giving way is problems in the patello-femoral joint. Instability of the patella in the trochlear groove will result in a giving way sensation as the patella subluxes. Damage to the articular surfaces of the patella or the trochlear groove will result in pain as the patella tracks over the trochlea. This can occasionally lead to a sharp acute pain which will lead to the quadriceps releasing its contraction while the patient is weight bearing on the leg as a result of a primitive reflex arc. The patient will note a giving way or buckling sensation in the knee and a few patients may actually fall as a result.

The majority of knee complaints are aggravated by activities. The specific problems the patient has encountered are important to note. Patients will commonly have difficulty ascending and descending stairs. Frequently descending stairs will be the most symptomatic as this places high stress across the patello-femoral joint. Bicycling can also aggravate the patello-femoral joint. Activities that involve quadriceps contraction with the knee in flexion may result in subluxation in patients with patellar instability. Patients with meniscal tears will have difficulty squatting and may notice snapping or pain when rising from a chair or ascending stairs. Activities that involve stopping and turning or cutting will result in the knee shifting or giving way if there is insufficiency in the collateral or cruciate ligaments.

Physical Examination

Physical examination of the patient with a knee complaint begins inspection. Observation of the alignment of the lower extremity should demonstrate a normal 5–7° valgus (knock-knee) angle at the knee when a patient is standing. Deformity of the leg in varus or valgus beyond the normal 5–7° can be associated with either a ligamentous or osseous deficiency. Any swelling, bruising, or ecchymosis should be recorded.

Next, the evaluation should focus on the patient's gait. Normal gait requires the range of motion from 0 to 65° of flexion. The gait should have a smooth cadence with the length of each step being equal on the left and right sides. The knee should not demonstrate any sudden shift to either the lateral or medial side. If abnormal lateral motion is noted this is recorded as a medial or lateral thrust, respectively.

The knee should then be examined with the patient sitting with their legs over the edge of the examining table. The position of the patella should be anterior and symmetric. The patellar tracking can then be followed by asking the patient to flex and extend the knee with the examiner palpating the patella. There should be little lateral movement. Crepitus may also be noted as a grinding sensation between the patella and the femoral trochlear groove.

The knee should then be examined with the patient supine. For all aspects of the examination the contralateral knee can be used as a normal control. Effusion or fluid within the knee can be assessed by placing both hands on the knee with one below the patella and one above the patella. Any fluid in the knee can then be displaced and palpated proximally and distally. The knee can be palpated to determine the specific site of maximum tenderness. The range of motion of the knee is measured with the knee in straight extension as 0° of flexion; normal full flexion is approximately 135°.

The collateral ligaments are then assessed by stabilizing the thigh with one hand and placing a varus or valgus stress on the knee with the other hand. A normal knee will have a small amount of medial and lateral laxity in the collateral ligaments. However, any laxity which is excessive or if pain is elicited should be noted. The cruciate ligaments can also be assessed. The anterior cruciate ligament is best assessed using the Lachman test. The examiner should stand by the patient's feet. The femur is stabilized with one hand holding the distal medial thigh. The tibia is then held with a thumb at the lateral joint line. The examiner then attempts to displace the tibia forward in relation to the femur. Translation less than 5 mm should be noted and the anterior cruciate ligament should be felt to "snap taut" in the normal knee. Injury to the posterior cruciate ligament can be demonstrated by noting the degree of recurvatum (back-knee) which can be obtained passively compared to the contralateral knee. Also, with both knees flexed 60–90° and the patient supine, the tibia on the deficient side will be noted to sag posteriorly compared to the uninjured leg when viewed from the side. Comparison to the contralateral knee is very important for examination of the collateral and cruciate ligaments.

The menisci are examined by palpation of their outer margin along the joint line at the proximal tibial articular surface. In addition, meniscal tears can be detected by the McMurray maneuver. This is done by flexing the knee internally and externally rotating the tibia and then extending the knee with a valgus force applied. If a reproducible snap is palpated or pain elicited at the joint line, this is suggestive of a tear. Patients with meniscal tears will also report pain when asked to squat down with the knees flexed.

Imaging

All of the available imaging techniques have been utilized in the evaluation of patients with knee problems. Plain radiographs are the most commonly obtained studies (Fig. 12.4). Plain radiographs are helpful in the evaluation of fractures and subluxation of the joint; also the condition of the articular surfaces can be investigated. The standard series of routine X-rays of the knee should include a standing anteroposterior (AP) radiograph of both knees, a lateral view and a merchant or "sunrise view." The sunrise view is a view taken with the knee in 45° of flexion with the beam directed inferiorly and parallel to the patellar articular surface. There should be a space of 5–10 mm between the ends of the femoral condyles and the tibial surface and beneath the patellar surface and the femoral trochlea. This "clear space" is in fact occupied by the articular cartilage.

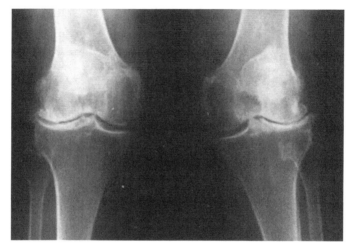

Fig. 12.4 Standing AP radiograph of both knees in a 70-year-old female with osteoarthritis of both knees with a valgus (knock-knee deformity) of both knees. Note the asymmetric space between the medial and lateral femoral condyles and the tibial surface

Routine radiography is an excellent tool for the evaluation of the knee for trauma, arthritis, and alignment. Plain radiographs, however, only demonstrate the osseous structures. As mentioned earlier, the soft tissues provide stability and allow the knee to function. Arthrography has been used in the past to evaluate the knee for meniscal pathology. However, this technique was inaccurate and invasive. The development of arthroscopy allows the direct visualization of the structures within the knee in a minor surgical procedure. However, this technique is also invasive and while arthroscopy is accurate, the procedure is relatively expensive compared to an imaging modality alone. Nuclear medicine studies are of limited use in the knee. These studies are sensitive; however, the specificity of these studies is limited. Magnetic

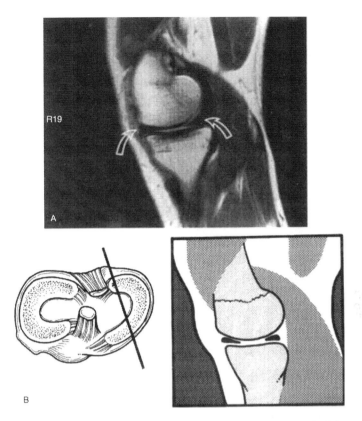

Fig. 12.5 (**a**) Normal T_1-weighted magnetic resonance imaging (MRI) sagittal image of the medial meniscus. (**b**) Schematic illustration showing the section cut of (**a**)

resonance imaging (MRI) has provided a dramatic step forward in the ability to diagnose soft tissue injury to the knee. MRI provides accurate and non-invasive evaluation of all of the soft tissue structures within the knee (Fig. 12.5). MRI is currently the study of choice for the evaluation of intra-articular pathology within the knee.

Knee Pathology

Soft tissue injury is common in the knee. A knee with a bloody effusion after an injury has an incidence as high as 80% of significant soft tissue injury. The differential diagnosis of a post-traumatic bloody effusion in the absence of an intra-articular fracture is a meniscal tear, an ACL tear, or a patellar dislocation.

Meniscal Tears

Tears of the meniscus can occur in two settings. One is the result of a specific injury. This usually involves a twisting injury with the knee in some flexion. Swelling and pain are noted immediately after the injury. There is increased pain with attempts at movement and there is a limitation in the range of motion. Pain with squatting down or arising from a chair is commonly reported. The torn meniscus can block the motion. Occasionally the knee can be gently manipulated to reduce the torn meniscal fragment and motion will be restored. However, the fragment will frequently redisplace and intermittent locking may occur. This form of tear is usually in younger patients with stout meniscal tissue.

In older individuals, the meniscal tissues soften and the edge becomes frayed. As this occurs, the frayed edges can become entrapped between the edges of the bone initiating a tear which can extend into the meniscal substance. This tear can occur with little or no trauma with minimal swelling and pain initially. The diagnosis is made by joint line pain, effusion, and rarely locking. Patients with locking will frequently require arthroscopic surgery to debride the torn portion of the meniscus. In older patients with meniscal tears, if the tear does not cause locking it frequently can be treated with nonsteroidal anti-inflammatory (NSAI) medications and an intra-articular corticosteroid injection. These treatments will reduce the effusion and pain. With continued activity, the soft meniscal tissue can be worn down and a stable edge reestablished.

Ligament Injuries

Injury to the ligamentous structures manifest by instability in the knee. In addition to pain and swelling, patients will report a sense of the knee shifting or giving way. This may be with only specific activities, such as descending stairs or when turning on the loaded extremity. The initial management of these injuries is rest, ice, and elevation. A splint or knee immobilizer can also be helpful to protect the knee. As the initial pain subsides, it is important to begin to work on restoring the range of motion using a brace to protect the injured ligament. As the pain further decreases, strengthening is begun. If the knee remains unstable after the strengthening program is completed, the patient may be a candidate for surgical reconstruction.

Patello-Femoral Pathology

The patello-femoral joint is one of the most common areas of pain in the knee. Common complaints are anterior knee pain which is aggravated by activities involving high loads on a flexed knee, such as stair climbing or bicycling. This pain can be the result of degenerative changes in the patello-femoral articulation or a result of maltracking of the patella within the trochlear groove. A grinding or snapping sensation may also be noted. Pain is usually relieved by rest, however, if the patient is sitting for a prolonged period of time with the knee flexed, such as in a theater, on a plane, or during a long car ride, anterior knee pain will result. Frequently patients will try to change the position of the knee to relieve their discomfort. This symptom is referred to as movie sign and is indicative of degenerative changes in the patello-femoral joint. Softening of the articular surface is referred to as chondromalacia patella. This can be a primary problem or it may be secondary to excessive trauma to the joint due to maltracking of the patella within the trochlear groove.

The treatment of these conditions is primarily non-operative. Improving the patellar tracking can be done through a series of exercises to retrain the quadra-ceps and through patellar mobilization exercises. The exercise program needs to be maintained for a minimum of 6–8 weeks to demonstrate benefit. The symptoms can frequently be recurrent. If the symptoms are recurrent and do not respond to the non-operative regimen and patellar maltracking is evident, operative intervention may be indicated. Operative intervention is directed at correcting the patellar tracking and to maximize the quadraceps function with postoperative physical therapy.

Arthritis

The management of arthritic symptoms within the knee is similar to the management of arthritis elsewhere. The non-operative management of arthritis within the knee consists of a five-modality approach. The first line of therapy is the use of NSAI agents. These medications will reduce the pain and swelling associated with the knee. Although all of the NSAI drugs (NSAIDs) function in a similar fashion, there is a wide variation in individual patient response. Therefore, minimally two or three different NSAIDs should be tried. The most common side effect of this course of treatment is gastritis and gastrointestinal (GI) intolerance.

The second line of treatment of arthritis is the selected use of intra-articular corticosteroid medication. This can be effective in patients who have an acute exac-erbation of the arthritic pain. The injection can quiet their pain and restore them to a baseline level of discomfort. The injection should not be utilized for the control of baseline pain. If the injection is required at a frequency of greater than once every 6–8 weeks, some other course of treatment should be initiated, such as surgery. If the knee is injected more frequently than —two to three times per year, the corticosteroid may have a detrimental effect on the articular cartilage.

Physical therapy can be very helpful in the treatment of arthritis of the knee. As the soft tissue sleeve is very important to the function of the knee, optimizing func-tions of the soft tissues can reduce the symptoms of arthritis. The physical therapy should be directed at maintaining the range of motion of the knee and optimizing the strength of the quadriceps and the hamstring muscles. In the late stages of degener-ative arthritis, physical therapy may worsen the patient's symptoms and should be limited to a program within the patient's tolerance.

Assistive devices such as a cane or crutch may aid in the management of arthritis of the knee. This can limit the stress across the painful knee and improve the patient's walking tolerance. The final approach to the management of arthritis of the knee is modification of activities. This includes alterations of the patient's activities such as sports, work environment, and possibly even assisting in arranging special parking for the patient. Frequently patients with significant knee arthritis are also overweight. Weight loss in these patients can significantly reduce symptoms and the need for other treatment modalities. As the force across the knee joint may be —three to five times the patient's body weight, weight loss can have a significant impact on a patient's knee symptoms.

Surgical Reconstruction for Arthritis

When all non-operative measures have failed to relieve the symptoms of knee arthritis, surgical intervention should be contemplated. The surgical correction of knee arthritis can be separated into treatments which retain the patient's articular surfaces and knee replacement. Non-replacement options include the use of arthroscopy to "clean out" the knee; this procedure can remove the small cartilage fragments that accumulate in arthritic joints and debride any loose articular fragments and degenerative meniscal tears. The pain relief from this procedure, however, is short-lived, lasting only 3–6 months. Patients should be informed preoperatively that if extensive arthritis is noted during arthroscopy, there is a possibility that the pain may be worse after surgery. In that setting, the patient is a candidate for knee replacement.

Patients with osteoarthritis of the knee will frequently develop angular deformities. The most common deformity is varus angulation of the knee. This results from erosion of the medial compartment of the knee. As the deformity progresses, a greater portion of the weight-bearing stress is concentrated in the medial compartment of the knee. Osteotomy is a procedure to realign the articulation. The proximal tibia is transected and a wedge of bone is removed from the lateral aspect or a wedge can be inserted on the medial side. This will result in a correction of the alignment and the varus deformity. It also redistributes some of the weight-bearing stress to the lateral compartment and can result in improved symptoms in the knee. The result is generally successful for 5–10 years. Osteotomy is contraindicated in knees which are stiff or unstable. When the symptoms return, knee replacement surgery is indicated.

Arthrodesis or fusion of the knee is an option for the management of young active patients, particularly physical laborers. This will result in a stiff straight knee that will allow the patient to ambulate and stand for long periods of time without difficulty. However, significant limitations also exist. The gait pattern is significantly abnormal. In addition, patients will have difficulty sitting, particularly in confined spaces such as public transportation and theaters. Resection arthroplasty is a procedure where the articular surfaces are resected and a fibrous pseudoarthrosis forms within the joint space. Pain may be decreased; however, the knee is significantly unstable, requiring a brace for ambulation. Arthrodesis and resection arthroplasty are not commonly performed. Currently these procedures are reserved for the management of a failed total knee replacement.

Total knee replacement (TKR) is commonly utilized to relieve the symptoms of knee arthritis and restore function (Fig. 12.6). Approximately 250,000 arthroplasties

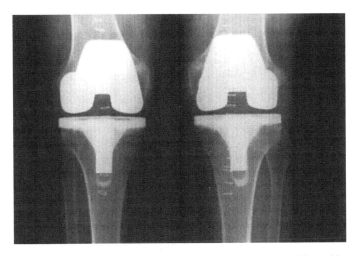

Fig. 12.6 Standing AP radiograph of both knees 2 weeks after one stage bilateral knee replacements in the 70-year-old female whose preoperative radiograph is shown in Fig. 12.4

are performed annually in the United States; the average age of patients receiving a TKR is 65–70 years. Successful results can be obtained in over 95% of patients with survivorship at 10–15 years of 90%. All components are currently fixed with polymethylmethacrylate (PMMA) bone cement. Non-cemented components, those used with porous ingrowth surfaces for bone ingrowth, have been associated with a higher incidence of loosening and pain. However, advances in non-cemented fixation may yield improved results in the future.

The proximal tibia is cut perpendicular to the long axis of the shaft and the femoral articular surface is cut using specific guides to remove the femoral trochlea, distal and posterior femoral condyles. The anterior cruciate ligament is removed; however, the posterior cruciate ligament can be resected or retained depending on the design of implant chosen. For proper function of the arthroplasty the MCL, LCL, and, if retained, PCL must be carefully balanced. The components are then fixed to the surfaces of the tibia and femur with bone cement. The patella is normally resurfaced as well after resecting the articular surface parallel to the anterior surface.

The patient is mobilized into a chair on the first postoperative day and full weight bearing may be allowed immediately. However, a knee immobilizer should be utilized to protect the knee from acute flexion while walking. This is continued until the quadraceps function returns. The critical element of the postoperative therapy is the restoration of motion. If motion is not restored within the first 3–6 weeks, maturation of scar tissue will prevent major gains in motion after that point. Many patients can be safely discharged at 3–4 days after surgery.

Frequently, however, these patients will require physical therapy after discharge from the hospital to continue to work on the range of motion and ambulation in the first few weeks after surgery. While the total rehabilitation period after total knee replacement is between 3 and 6 months, patients are functionally mobile after 2–3 weeks. Knee replacement can be performed bilaterally in one stage in medically healthy patients (Fig. 12.6). The initial increase in debilitation postoperatively is offset by a reduction in the overall period of rehabilitation after sequential unilateral TKR.

Aseptic loosening of the implants after TKR occurs at a low rate. Several studies have documented a 15-year survivorship of greater than 90% and less than 0.5% per year rate of aseptic loosening after cemented TKR. If a TKR is noted to be loose prior to 5 years, it should be evaluated for deep infection. Deep sepsis is associated with early loosening after total knee replacement. Young age, marked obesity, and high demand will also negatively impact the long-term survival of the replacement. To date, the best data for non-cemented TKR is equal to the cemented replacement. Several studies suggest poorer results when cement is not used, particularly for fixation of the tibial component. Increased tibial loosening and pain have been noted with these devices. At present, due to the generally increased cost for non-cemented porous-coated implants and poorer clinical results, the use of these devices is difficult to justify.

The majority of complaints after cemented TKR are from the patello-femoral joint, which can be the result of poor soft tissue alignment at the time of arthroplasty. This may lead to painful subluxation or dislocation of the patellar component. If inadequate bone is resected from the patella at the time of resurfacing, a marked increase in the patello-femoral stress can be noted which may become painful. Some surgeons have advocated not resurfacing the patella; however, several studies now demonstrate a higher rate of patello-femoral complaints after TKR without patellar resurfacing. If significant patello-femoral arthritis exists at the time of arthroplasty, patients with weights greater than 60 kg and heights greater than 160 cm will have more pain postoperatively if the patella is not resurfaced.

The most common complication after TKR is thromboembolic disease (TED). The rate of deep venous thrombosis ranges from 25 to 50% of cases in patients evaluated with venography or duplex Doppler analysis. Similar to patients receiving total hip replacement (THR), it is currently recommended that all patients receive some form of prophylaxis against TED. Mechanical methods, such as the pneumatic compression stockings, appear to have a greater benefit after THR compared to TKR. Low-dose Coumadin (warfarin), aspirin, and low molecular weight heparin are currently the most commonly utilized medications. New oral anticoagulants are currently under investigation and may have a significant role in the future.

Deep infection occurs at a rate of approximately 1% after TKR for osteoarthritis over the life of the implant. The most common organisms are skin flora primarily *Staphylococcus aureus* and *S. epidermidis*. In particular to knee replacement, the relatively thin soft tissue envelope at the inferior aspect of the skin incision can lead to wound dehiscence and allow entry of the flora into the joint. Any area of skin breakdown after TKR should be treated aggressively to prevent deep infection. This is particularly true in patients with prior incisions and in those with diabetes or significant vascular disease.

If a deep infection is established, the only way to eradicate the infection is to remove the implants and all of the bone cement and thoroughly debride the joint. An antibiotic impregnated cement spacer is then placed into the joint space and the patient should receive 6 weeks of intravenous (IV) antibiotics. The serum bactericidal titers of the IV antibiotics should exceed 1:8. After 6 weeks, the knee can be reimplanted if adequate soft tissue and bone remain. However, due to the inevitable scarring, the clinical result is compromised.

Occasionally after TKR, the range of motion of the knee does not progress well after surgery. If the patient is less than 2–6 weeks after surgery, a gentle manipulation of the knee in the operating room under anesthesia may be beneficial. If the motion cannot be restored, particularly if the patient is beyond 6 weeks after replacement, additional surgery may be necessary to restore functional range of motion.

Summary and Conclusions

The knee is a complex joint with function provided by the combination of osseous and soft tissue structures. The soft tissue envelope plays a significant role in the pathology of the knee and in the management of these conditions. With careful history, physical examination, and appropriate use of the available diagnostic modalities, knee pathology can be accurately determined and successful treatment instituted. Successful management of knee pathology includes treatment of the specific etiology but optimal management of the soft tissue envelope with directed physical therapy is essential to an optimal outcome.

Suggested Reading

1. Heck DA, Murray DG. Biomechanics in the knee. In: Evarts CM, ed. *Surgery of the Musculoskeletal System.* 2nd ed. New York, NY: Churchill Livingston; 1990:3243–3254.
2. Rand JA, Ilstrup DM. Survivorship analysis of total knee arthroplasty. Cumulative rates of survival of 9200 total knee arthroplasties. *J Bone Joint Surg Am.* 1991; 73(3):397–409.
3. Stern SH, Insall JN. Posterior stabilized prosthesis. Results after follow-up of nine to twelve years. *J Bone Joint Surg Am.* 1992; 74(7):980–986.
4. Windsor RE, Bono JV. Infected total knee replacements: *J Am Acad Orthop Surg.* 1994; 2:44–53.

Chapter 13
The Foot and Ankle

Paul S. Cooper

Introduction

An overview of orthopedics would not be complete without an understanding of
the foot and ankle. This area of the body is often forgotten in the scheme of things
and yet is one of the most common sources of complaints in any physician's office.
Painful feet are seen in emergency rooms and family practitioner's offices. Ankle
discomfort is seen in medical clinics and on the sidelines of recreational sporting
activities. This chapter is meant to familiarize the student of medicine, be it an actual
medical student, resident, or practitioner, with the anatomy, diagnostic tools, and
some common conditions that affect the foot and ankle.

Bones and Joints

The bony anatomy of the foot and ankle consists of the distal tibia and fibula in the
leg and the 26 major bones that compose the foot. The tibia distally terminates into
the metaphyseal plafond with its medial malleolus. The lateral surface of the distal
tibia has a sulcus to accommodate the adjacent fibula, forming the distal tibiofibular joint. The distal fibula which lies laterally and slightly posterior to the tibia is
held there by the inferior tibiofibular ligaments. The fibula forms the lateral malleolus of the ankle joint. The relationship of the fibula to the tibia is not static. With
ankle dorsiflexion, the fibula laterally translates, proximally migrates, and externally
rotates.

The ankle is a diarthrodial joint (Figs. 13.1 and 13.2). It consists of an articulation between the talus and the mortise of the tibia and fibula. Dorsiflexion of
the ankle joint is coupled with eversion of the foot and plantar flexion is combined
with inversion. The distal fibula provides a static buttress over the talus laterally and

P.S. Cooper (✉)
Department of Orthopedic Surgery, Georgetown University Medical Center, Washington,
DC 20007, USA
e-mail: cooperpa@gunet.georgetown.edu; pcoope@mac.com

S.W. Wiesel, J.N. Delahay (eds.), *Essentials of Orthopedic Surgery*,
DOI 10.1007/978-1-4419-1389-0_13, © Springer Science+Business Media, LLC 2010

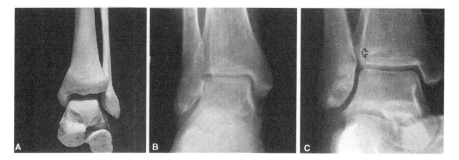

Fig. 13.1 (**a, b**) Photographic diagrammatic, and radiologic anatomy of the normal ankle in anterioposterior views. (**c**) Note equal width of cartilage spaces and alignment of lateral talus with posterior cortex (*arrow*) on mortise view. (From Weissman BNW, Sledge CB. *Orthopedic Radiology*. Philadelphia, PA: Saunders; 1986. Reprinted with permission)

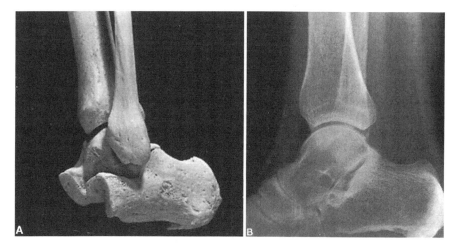

Fig. 13.2 Photographic (**a**) and radiologic (**b**) anatomy of the normal ankle in lateral projection. (From Weissman BNW, Sledge CB. *Orthopedic Radiology*. Philadelphia, PA: Saunders; 1986. Reprinted with permission)

also bears 1/6 of the transmitted weight during the stance phase of gait. The foot is composed of seven tarsals, five metatarsals, and 14 phalanges. Three anatomic groupings are defined for descriptive purposes: the hindfoot, the midfoot, and the forefoot (Fig. 13.3). The hindfoot consists of the talus and calcaneus bones. The talus consists of a body, neck, and head. Two-thirds of the talus is covered by articular cartilage. There are no muscle or tendon attachments on this bone. The talar dome is the superior portion of the body which articulates with the mortise of the tibia and fibula. The dome is wider anteriorly, which allows for stability in the mortise during dorsiflexion. Posteriorly, a sulcus is formed between the posterolateral

Fig. 13.3 Anatomic regions of the foot. (From Weissman BNW, Sledge CB. *Orthopedic Radiology*. Philadelphia, PA: Saunders; 1986. Reprinted with permission)

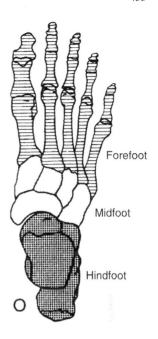

Forefoot

Midfoot

Hindfoot

and posteromedial tubercles to accommodate the flexor hallucis longus (FHL) tendon. The inferior surface of the talus articulates with the corresponding facet of the calcaneus to create a subtalar joint. The calcaneus is the largest bone in the foot, with its longitudinal axis directed dorsally and laterally. Its superior surface articulates with the talus and three facets—anterior, medial, and posterior—to form the subtalar joint (Fig. 13.4). The large posterior facet articulates with the corresponding articular facet on the inferior surface of the talus. The middle facet overlies the sustentaculum tali (a dense, medial projection of the calcaneus that contains a groove to accommodate the FHL tendon sheath) and is often merged with the anterior facet. The middle facets and anterior facets articulate with the undersurface of the talar head.

The midfoot consists of the navicular, cuboid, and three cuneiform bones. The tarsonavicular bone articulates with the talar head and lies medially to the cuboid bone. It functions as a keystone for the medial longitudinal arch of the foot. The distal surface is composed of three facets that articulate with the medial, middle, and lateral cuneiform bones, respectively. This is also the insertion site for the posterior tibial tendon. In 10% of people, an unfused accessory navicular bone may be present. The cuboid bone forms an articulation with the calcaneus proximally and the fourth and fifth metatarsals distally. Laterally, a groove accommodates the peroneus longus tendon as it courses plantarly. Three cuneiform bones have distal articulations with the first, second, and third metatarsals and contribute to the

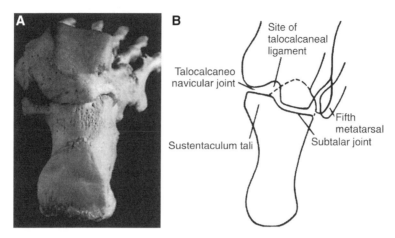

Fig. 13.4 Photographic (**a**) and diagrammatic (**b**) anatomy of the normal ankle in tangential calcaneal (Harris) projection. (From Weissman BNW, Sledge CB. *Orthopedic Radiology*. Philadelphia, PA: Saunders; 1986. Reprinted with permission)

formation of part of the tarsometatarsal, or Lisfranc's joint (Fig. 13.5). The middle cuneiform bone is shorter axially, adding to greater stability in the second tarsometatarsal joint. This is also known as the keystone.

The forefoot consists of the metatarsal and phalangeal bones. Five metatarsals terminate distally with articulations to the proximal phalanges creating metatarsal phalangeal (MTP) joints. The fifth metatarsal is a prominent styloid process proximally to which the peroneus brevis attaches. Each of the lesser toes, two through five, has three phalanges—a proximal, middle, and distal phalanx—and the hallux has only two phalanges, proximal and distal. Each distal phalanx terminates in a tuft of bone and serves as an anchor for the toe pad. Underlying the first MTP joint are the two sesamoid bones. Tibial (medial) and fibular (lateral) sesamoid bones are encased by the flexor hallucis brevis tendon (FHB) which inserts at the base of the proximal phalanx.

Ligaments

The ligamentous structures of the ankle joint (Fig. 13.6) include the medial deltoid ligament complex and the lateral ankle ligament complex. The deltoid joint ligament medially has both superficial and deep components and is the primary contributor to medial stability of the ankle joint. The lateral ligament complex consists of three major ligaments including the anterior talofibular ligament (ATFL), the calcaneofibular ligament (CFL), and the posterior talofibular ligament (PTFL). These contribute to lateral stability of the ankle joint.

Ligaments of the ankle syndesmosis include the anterior tibiofibular, posterior tibiofibular, and interosseous ligaments. Injuries to these ligaments may occur with

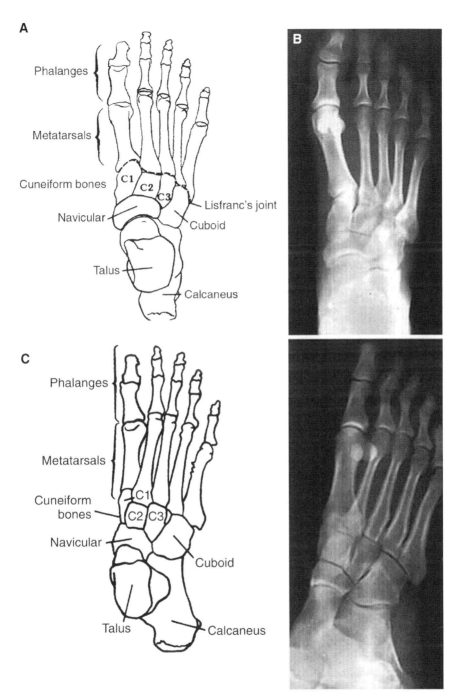

Fig. 13.5 Photographic, diagrammatic, and radiologic anatomy of the normal foot in posteroanterior (**a, b**) and internal oblique (**c, d**) projections. (From Weissman BNW, Sledge CB. *Orthopedic Radiology*. Philadelphia, PA: Saunders; 1986. Reprinted with permission)

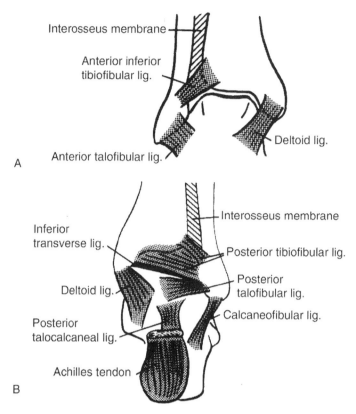

Fig. 13.6 The tibiofibular syndesmosis. The syndesmosis consists of the interosseous membrane, the anterior and the posterior inferior tibiofibular ligaments, and the inferior transverse ligament. (**a**) Anterior view; (**b**) posterior view. (From Weissman BNW, Sledge CB. *Orthopedic Radiology*. Philadelphia, PA: Saunders; 1986. Reprinted with permission)

hyperdorsiflexion and external rotation, creating a "high-ankle sprain" which is seen especially in athletes. Ligamentous support of the subtalar joint is contributed by the CFL, the ligaments of the anterior capsule, the posterior subtalar joint capsule, the interosseous talocalcaneal ligaments, and the ligaments of the tarsal canal. The midfoot joints are stabilized by multiple ligaments as well as the intrinsic bony architecture of the wedge-shaped cuneiform bones. Little motion occurs through the midfoot. Stabilizing ligaments include the bifurcate ligament, a V-shaped structure composed of the lateral calcaneonavicular and medial calcaneocuboid ligaments. They insert on the anterior process of the calcaneus, navicular, and cuboid bones, respectively. Superficial and deep plantar ligaments span from the calcaneus to the cuboid bone and metatarsals. These serve as static stabilizers of the longitudinal arch. Another important structure is the plantar aponeurosis (or plantar fascia). This thick fibrous structure runs from the plantar surface of the calcaneus to distally insert into the metatarsals. It stabilizes the arch during gait (Fig. 13.7). There is

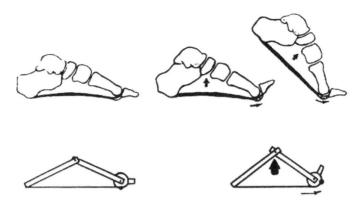

Fig. 13.7 Plantar aponeurosis and windlass mechanism provide stability to the longitudinal arch of the foot when the first metatarsophalangeal joint is forced into dorsiflexion and it secondarily plantar flexes the first metatarsal. (From Mann RA. The great toe. *Orthop Clin North Am.* 1989;20(4):520. Reprinted with permission)

no true transverse interosseous ligament between the first and second metatarsal bases. Instead, there is an oblique plantar ligament that connects the first cuneiform bone to the second metatarsal. It is known as Lisfranc's ligament. Stabilizing the MTP joints is a deep transverse metatarsal ligament as well as medial and lateral collateral ligaments.

Muscles

The muscles of the leg are encased in four leg compartments: the superficial and deep posterior compartments, the lateral compartment, and the anterior compartment. The superficial posterior compartment includes the gastrocnemius, the plantaris, and the soleus muscles. This compartment houses the main plantarflexors of the ankle (Fig. 13.8) that are innervated by the tibial nerve. The tendon fibers of the soleus merge with the gastrocnemius tendon fibers to firm the tendo calcaneus or Achilles tendon. The Achilles tendon rotates 90° to insert on the posterior-superior tuberosity of the calcaneus. The deep posterior compartment contains three muscles which invert the foot and serve as secondary plantar flexors. These muscles are the tibialis posterior muscle, the flexor digitorum longus (FDL) muscle, and the flexor hallucis longus muscle. The lateral compartment, innervated by the superficial peroneal nerve, contains the peroneus longus and peroneus brevis muscles, the main evertors of the foot. The deep peroneus longus muscle courses distally underneath the cuboid to insert on the base of the first metatarsal and medial cuneiform bone. The peroneus brevis inserts on the base of the fifth metatarsal. The anterior leg compartment contains the tibialis anterior, the extensor hallucis longus (EHL), and the

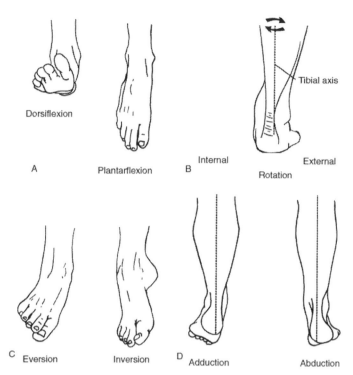

Fig. 13.8 Motions of the foot and ankle. (**a**) *Plantar flexion* and *dorsiflexion* refer to movement of the foot downward or upward. *Supination* and *pronation* refer to rotation of the foot internally or externally around the longitudinal axis of the foot. (**b**) *Internal rotation* and *external rotation* of the foot refer to motion around the vertical axis of the tibia. (**c**) *Eversion* directs the sole laterally, whereas *inversion* refers to rotation of the foot until the sole is directed medially. (**d**) *Adduction* and *abduction* describe motion of the forefoot toward or away from the midline. (From Weissman BNW, Sledge CB. *Orthopedic Radiology*. Philadelphia, PA: Saunders; 1986. Reprinted with permission)

extensor digitorum longus (EDL) muscles. These muscles serve as the primary dorsiflexors of the ankle and foot. These muscles are innervated by the deep peroneal nerve.

The intrinsic muscles of the foot are arranged in four plantar layers and there is a single dorsal muscle, the extensor digitorum brevis (EDB). The EDB is innervated by the deep peroneal nerve. The first superficial layer of the intrinsic plantar muscles includes the flexor digitorum brevis (FDB), the abductor hallucis, and the abductor digiti minimi (ADM) muscles. The second layer contains the muscles for toe motion and includes the quadratus plantae and lumbrical muscles as well as the tendons of the FHL and FDL. The third layer includes the flexor hallucis brevis, abductor hallucis, and the adductor hallucis (ADH) tendon. These muscles assist in first and fifth toe function. The fourth and deepest layer of intrinsic muscles contains the seven interosseous muscles and the insertions of the peroneus longus and anterior and posterior tibial tendons. The interossei are divided into two groups with four dorsal interossei and three plantar interossei. The dorsal interossei are involved in toe adduction and the plantar interossei are involved in toe abduction.

Nerves and Vessels

The neurovascular structures of the foot and ankle include five major nerve branches and three arteries. The tibial and common peroneal nerves are terminal branches of the sciatic nerve which arises from the lumbosacral plexus. The common peroneal nerve from L5 branches into the superficial peroneal nerve and deep peroneal nerve. The superficial peroneal nerve courses through the lateral compartment and exits the lateral compartment approximately 10–15 cm above the lateral malleolus through a fascial defect and continues subcutaneously to provide sensory innervation of the dorsal aspect of the foot and toes. The deep peroneal nerve courses through the anterior compartment with the anterior tibial artery, continues into the foot with the dorsalis pedis artery to provide innervation to the intrinsic foot muscles including the EDB and EHB muscles, and terminates as a cutaneous nerve in the first web space. The tibial nerve, a branch of S1, travels through the popliteal fossa into the deep posterior compartment. It courses medial to the Achilles tendon, enters the tarsal tunnel just posterior to the medial malleolus, and divides into the median and lateral plantar nerves. The medial and lateral plantar nerves supply motor and sensory function to the plantar aspect of the foot. The sural nerve is a sensory branch of the tibial nerve and provides sensation to the posterolateral hindfoot and lateral border of the foot. The saphenous nerve courses along the anteromedial aspect of the lower limb posterior to the greater saphenous vein and provides sensation to the medial side of the ankle.

Vascular supply to the foot and ankle is derived from the anterior and posterior tibial arteries and peroneal arteries. The anterior tibial artery becomes the dorsalis pedis in the foot. The posterior tibial artery divides into the medial plantar artery and lateral plantar artery to supply the plantar structures in the foot. The peroneal artery branches from the posterior tibial artery and travels posterior to the interosseous membrane, deep to the FHL muscle, terminating at the distal tibiofibular joint.

The major structures of the venous system of the leg include the greater saphenous vein and the lesser saphenous vein. The greater saphenous vein courses anteromedial to end in the femoral vein. It drains the dorsum of the foot. The lesser saphenous vein runs posterior to the fibula and drains the lateral foot and arch.

Gait Cycle

The gait cycle consists of one heel strike to the next heel strike of the same foot. It is traditionally divided into a *stance phase* that makes 62% of the cycle and the *swing phase* that makes the remaining 38% of the cycle. At initial heel strike, the lower extremity is in internal rotation. The ankle joint is plantar flexed and the subtalar joint is everted. The transverse tarsal joint is unlocked to allow shock absorption. Anterior compartment muscles are active in helping decelerate the limb. At foot flat, the lower extremity externally rotates, the ankle joint dorsiflexes, and the subtalar joint begins to invert. This increases stability throughout the midfoot in anticipation of push-off. Anterior compartment muscles become inactive. Intrinsic muscles of the foot become active and the posterior compartment calf muscles are contracting. At pre-swing, the ankle joint is in plantar flexion.

Clinical Evaluation of the Foot and the Ankle

History and Physical Examination

A complete medical and surgical history, the mechanism of injury, and the duration of the symptoms should be elicited. The location and quality of pain should be documented. Existing systemic disorders should be ruled out with an emphasis on diabetes and gout. Musculoskeletal history involving the spine and lower extremities is helpful. A physical examination should be done with both stockings and shoes removed. Gait patterns should be determined, with the patient walking both toward and away from the examiner. The stance phase or station should be examined with emphasis placed on the relationship of the hindfoot with the forefoot and longitudinal arch. Once inspection has been completed, examination of the bony and soft tissue structures follows. The area should be examined for the presence of edema, effusion, skin temperature changes, and previous sites of surgery or trauma. Systemic examination can be divided into the ankle, hindfoot, midfoot, and forefoot subgroups. When examining the ankle, note any effusion. Range of motion of the ankle is normally 20° of dorsiflexion and 40–50° of plantar flexion. Loss of ankle dorsiflexion may be associated with a tight Achilles tendon, posterior capsular contracture, or bony impingement. Limitation of dorsiflexion with the knee in full extension that improves passively with the knee flexed to 90° indicates a contracture of the gastrocnemius muscle. Ligamentous laxity should be evaluated in comparison with the contralateral ankle joint and palpation of the tendons should be performed to note evidence of subluxation or dislocation. Midfoot examination involves selective palpation of the bony anatomy to isolate specific joint or joint involvement. Forefoot examination should include MTP joint motion with any documentation of subluxation and pain.

Pulses and sensation are vital to the evaluation. Both the dorsalis pedis and posterior tibial artery should be documented for strength and quality. Sensation evaluation should document intact levels in all nerve distributions around the foot, for pin, light touch, and vibratory. In addition, the Semmes-Wienstin monofilament test is applied in the diabetic patient to quantitate protective sensation. A failed test at the 5.07 level indicates a loss of sensation and signifies a risk for skin ulceration.

Radiology of the Foot and Ankle

Radiographic studies of the foot and ankle require weight bearing X-rays when possible. Important views involve the anteroposterior (AP), lateral, and oblique views of the foot and AP, lateral, and mortise views of the ankle. The AP view of the foot can be used to assess forefoot and midfoot pathology. The lateral view of the foot shows the relationship of the talus and calcaneus to that of the midfoot, forefoot, and ankle joint. The medial oblique view is used to evaluate the lateral tarsometatarsal joints. Other studies are available to assess the sesamoids, the calcaneus, or the subtalar joint. The sesamoid view involves the X-ray beam directed tangential to the plantar surface of the sesamoid region while the patient's toes are in hyperextension. Harris axial heel view is used to assess the calcaneal tuberosity and is important in calcaneus fractures or tarsal coalitions. Ancillary radiographic studies include computed tomography (CT) (Fig. 13.9), magnetic resonance imaging (MRI), and radionuclide studies. MRI can be used to assess soft tissue structures such as soft tissue tumors, osteomyelitis, avascular necrosis, bone tumors, chondral lesions, and tendon abnormalities. CT is best to assess bone abnormalities including sequestrum and nonunions.

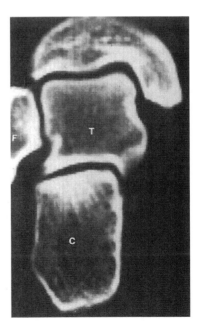

Fig. 13.9 Normal anatomy seen on computerized tomography: coronal section through the ankle and subtalar joint. *C*, calcaneus; *F*, figula; *T*, talus. (From Weissman BNW, Sledge CB. *Orthopedic Radiology*. Philadelphia, PA: Saunders; 1986. Reprinted with permission)

Diseases of the Foot and Ankle

This overview of the pathologic states that affect the foot and the ankle is discussed by diagnostic category. This is not meant to be an exhaustive catalog of every affliction, but rather a representative sampling of the more common disease states that mandate medical care.

Trauma

Ankle

Injuries of the ankle mortise include pilon fractures, ankle fractures, and syndesmotic injuries.

Pilon Fractures

Pilon fractures involve the intraarticular fractures of the tibial metaphysis which extend to the weight bearing portion of the tibia. There is often extensive comminution. Nondisplaced pilon fractures may be treated nonoperatively with immobilization in a cast; however, since these are often displaced injuries, treatment consists of some type of operative fixation. Initially and temporarily, an ankle-spanning external fixator may be applied to maintain length and ankle joint reduction until soft tissue swelling subsides within 1–2 weeks. At that point, open reduction and internal fixation using screws and a plate can be done. In high-energy injuries with soft tissue compromise, external fixation may be the definitive treatment.

Ankle Fractures

Ankle fractures are discussed in Chapter 2.

Syndesmosis Injuries

With disruption of the syndesmotic ligaments, a diastasis, or separation, of the distal tibia and fibula can occur. This injury is often associated with higher grades of ankle fractures when medial stability is compromised by a medial malleolar fracture or a deltoid tear. Definitive diagnosis of a syndesmotic injury can be made with stress X-rays which show a diastasis at the distal tibial and fibular joint. If this exists, reduction and stabilization of the syndesmosis are achieved with screw placement across the tibial and fibular joint or tibial and fibular syndesmosis. The trans-syndesmotic screw should remain in place for a minimum of 12–16 weeks and is then removed.

Fractures to the Hindfoot

Fractures of the hindfoot involve the calcaneus, talus, and navicular bones.

Talus Fractures

The talus articulates with the ankle, calcaneus, and navicular bones and is covered by articular cartilage on 60% of its surface (Fig. 13.10). Since the majority of the talus is covered by articular cartilage and there are no muscle or tendinous attachments, there is limited space for blood vessels to enter this bone, making the blood supply tenuous. The blood supply enters the talus at the neck and travels retrograde into the body and the dome (Fig. 13.11). Fractures of the talus, depending

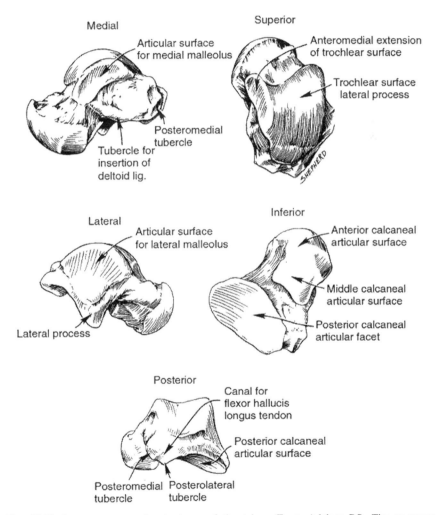

Fig. 13.10 Important anatomic structures of the talus. (From Adelaar RS. The treatment of complex fractures of the talus. *Orthop Clin North Am.* 1989;20(4):692. Reprinted with permission)

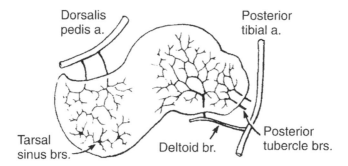

Fig. 13.11 Extraosseous and intraosseous circulation of the talus. (From Adelaar RS. The treatment of complex fractures of the talus. *Orthop Clin North Am*. 1989;20(4):693. Reprinted with permission)

upon the severity, can often disrupt this blood supply. Fractures of the talus typically occur through the neck and result from an acute dorsiflexion injury. Standard radiographs with CT scans are usually adequate to demonstrate the nature of the fracture. Treatment is tailored to restore normal talar anatomy. If nondisplaced, conservative nonsurgical treatment with cast immobilization can be used. If displaced, often anatomic reduction and rigid fixation is the best approach. This is done in an effort to prevent avascular necrosis which can result as a disruption of the tenuous blood supply. Hawkins' classification of talar neck fractures categorizes these fractures into three patterns (Fig. 13.12): Type I is a nondisplaced fracture of the neck, Type II is a displacement of the neck fracture with subluxation or dislocation of the talar body from the subtalar joint, and Type III is a neck displacement fracture with

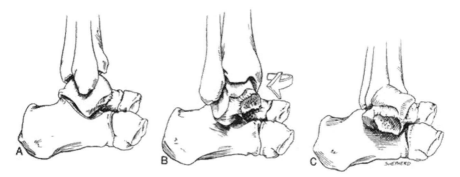

Fig. 13.12 Classification of talus neck fractures: (**a**) Class I; (**b**) class II; (**c**) class III. (Modified from Hawkins LG. Fractures of the neck of the talus. *J Bone Joint Surg*. 1970;52A:991–1002; and from Adelaar RS. The treatment of complex fractures of the talus. *Orthop Clin North Am*. 1989;20(4):696. Reprinted with permission)

subluxation or dislocation of the body from both the ankle and the subtalar joints. A fourth pattern, which has been described, involves a displaced neck fracture which includes dislocation of the talonavicular joint. The incidence of avascular necrosis increases significantly with each increase in type. Radiographic signs of intact vascularity of the talus are demonstrated by the crescent or "Hawkins" sign at 8–10 weeks out from injury.

Calcaneus Fractures

The calcaneus is the most commonly fractured tarsal bone. Fractures are classified as intraarticular or extra-articular. Calcaneus fractures are often seen when an axial load is applied to the foot, resulting from falls or motor vehicle accidents. Patients typically present with severe pain and swelling. Radiographs including the axial heel view in addition to CT scanning can fully define the injury. Closed treatment of these fractures is reserved for nondisplaced fractures or poor surgical candidates with severe soft tissue compromise or complicated medical conditions. Open reduction and internal fixation is indicated for displaced intraarticular fractures and significantly displaced extra-articular fractures. Surgical intervention should not proceed until the soft tissues and excessive swelling have stabilized. Assessment of this can be done by observation of wrinkling of the lateral hindfoot soft tissues. If soft tissues are not amenable to open reduction and internal fixation, other techniques including percutaneous fixation and external fixation may be utilized. Despite anatomic reduction and adequate treatment, these patients often develop subtalar stiffness and symptomatic osteoarthritis. Salvage would consist of a subtalar fusion without bone loss, or an intercalary tricortical graft to restore axial height.

Injury to the Midfoot

The midfoot injuries include those of the tarsonavicular, cuboid, cuneiform, and tarsometatarsal joints. Injuries to the Lisfranc (tarsometatarsal) joints include subtle sprains to frank fracture dislocations. Bony architecture is similar to that of a Roman arch and designed for stability. The keystone of the arch is the second metatarsal, which has a wedge-shaped base that is recessed between the medial and lateral cuneiform bones. Strong plantar interosseous ligaments provide the main support for the tarsometatarsal joints. There is an absence of an intermetatarsal ligament between the first and second metatarsal joint which makes this area susceptible to injury. The "Lisfranc ligament" spans the plantar lateral aspect of the medial cuneiform bone and the medial base of the second metatarsal and resists lateral translation of the lesser metatarsals. Mechanisms of Lisfranc injury include a direct crush injury to the midfoot and an indirect twisting-type injury when an axial load is applied to the heel with the foot in fixed equinus, as in motor vehicle accidents or sporting activities. Up to 20% of these injuries are missed on initial evaluation because of their potential subtle nature. It is important to obtain standard three-view radiographs of the injured foot and look for the appropriate signs of injury.

Treatment involves anatomic reduction of the involved joints with rigid fixation via percutaneous method or open reduction internal fixation. Over 80% of patients develop posttraumatic arthrosis and stiffness, necessitating a fusion of the involved joints in the most refractory cases.

Ankle Sprains

Ligamentous disruptions, partial and complete, are common about the ankle. The most common ligament to be injured is the anterior talofibular ligament (Fig. 13.13). Inversion stress testing can elicit pain and demonstrate instability on radiographs (Fig. 13.14). Partial injuries can be treated with either a cast or fracture boot or a brace. A complete ligament disruption (grade III) particularly if the deltoid ligaments are similarly involved may require surgical repair. Repairs are divided into anatomic and non-anatomic. Anatomic repairs involve repairing the ligaments primarily and reinforcing the injured tissues with a second layer utilizing the inferior extensor retinaculum (modified brostrum). Non-anatomic repairs require reconstructing the ligaments with a "cable" using either local tissue (spitting the peroneus brevis) or allograft.

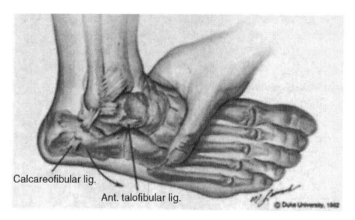

Fig. 13.13 Inversion stress testing, or the talar tilt. (From Lasseter TE Jr, Malone TR, Garrett WE Jr. Injury to the lateral ligaments of the ankle. *Orthop Clin North Am.* 1989;20(4):631. Reprinted with permission)

Injuries of the Forefoot

Fractures of the sesamoid bones occur relative to direct trauma or use or both injuries associated with hyperdorsiflexion of the first metatarsal phalangeal joint. Bipartite sesamoid bones (congenital separation of the two poles of the sesamoid) occur in approximately 25% of individuals, the majority involving the tibial sesamoid bone.

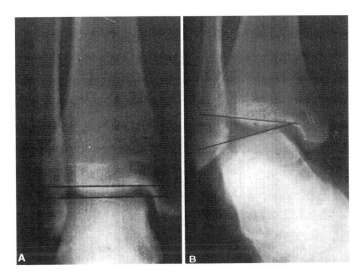

Fig. 13.14 (**a**) Anteroposterior view of the ankle prestress. (**b**) Anteroposterior view of the ankle with inversion stress reveals marked lateral ligament injury. (From Lasseter TE Jr, Malone TR, Garrett WE Jr. Injury to the lateral ligaments of the ankle. *Orthop Clin North Am.* 1989;20(4):632. Reprinted with permission)

If the sum of the parts is greater than the adjacent sesamoid, then a congenital condition is more likely. Management is mostly conservative. Phalangeal fractures may be either displaced or nondisplaced and angulated. Closed manipulation is often needed under local anesthetic; then taping the affected toe to the adjacent toe as a splint mechanism or "buddy taping" is done with wearing of a stiff-soled shoe or sandal.

Acquired Deformities of the Foot and Ankle

Deformities of the Forefoot

Hallux Valgus

This is a condition of medial prominence of the first MTP joint with lateral drifting of the big toe (Fig. 13.15). It is almost exclusively related to shoe wear. Radiographically, it is defined as an MTP joint angle of more than 15° and an angle between the first and second metatarsals that is more than 9°. Symptoms include pain, swelling, and inflammation over the medial first MTP joint related to shoe wear. Range of motion of the first MTP joint should be assessed and AP and lateral radiographs are taken to determine the degree of hallux valgus deformity, the associated metatarsus primus varus, joint congruity, and degenerative changes, as well as position of the sesamoids. Treatment of hallux valgus deformity in the early stages is conservative and includes shoe modification to a high, wide toe box and a soft

Fig. 13.15 Classic
abnormalities in a bunion: 1,
hallux valgus; 2, the
exostosis; and 3, metatarsus
primus varus. (From Mann
RA. The great toe. *Orthop
Clin North Am.*
1989;20(4):524. Reprinted
with permission)

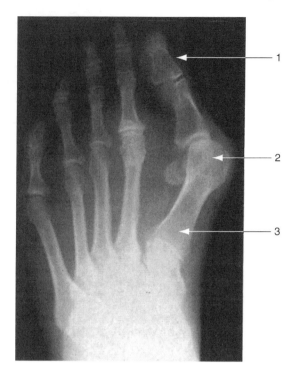

leather upper portion of the shoe. Orthotic devices can be helpful. When conservative measures are not successful, surgical procedures are recommended. These include a simple exostectomy, soft tissue repair, proximal metatarsal osteotomy, distal metatarsal osteotomy, resection arthroplasty, proximal phalangeal osteotomy, and arthrodesis. In cases of mild to moderate hallux valgus angles (<30°) where the joint is congruous, a distal type of procedure like the chevron osteotomy is indicated. In more severe angled bunions with incongruous joints, a proximal osteotomy in conjunction with a distal soft tissue release is best suited. Contraindications to surgery include generalized spasticity, severe pes planovalgus deformity, ligamentous laxity as seen in Marfan's and Ehlers-Danlos' syndromes and vascular or soft tissue insufficiency.

Hallux Varus

This is a medial deviation of the great toe at the MTP joint. Causes include complications from overcorrection of hallux valgus surgery or rupture of the conjoined tendon as seen in rheumatic conditions. Treatment in early or flexible cases consists of an abductor hallucis release with transfer of the extensor hallucis brevis. In more advanced cases, salvage with fusion of the metatarsophalangeal joint will leave satisfactory results.

Hallux Rigidus

Hallux rigidus is painful loss of motion at the first MTP joint (Fig. 13.16). Patients present with an enlarged, warm, and swollen first MTP joint, with a decreased range of motion, predominantly in dorsiflexion. Shoes with elevated heels tend to increase pain. Initial treatment is conservative with orthotic devices and shoe modifications to reduce the stress across the first MTP joint. Surgical intervention includes resection arthroplasty, cheilectomy, metatarsal or phalangeal osteotomy, or arthrodesis. The approach is the same for all procedures—the extensor hallucis longus tendon is lateralized through a dorsal incision. If a cheilectomy is performed, the dorsal 25% of the metatarsophalangeal joint is resected. In advanced cases, the joint surfaces are denuded, and the joint is positioned in a rectus position with the ground, typically at 15° dorsiflexion and valgus. A metal plate or screws provide definitive fixation.

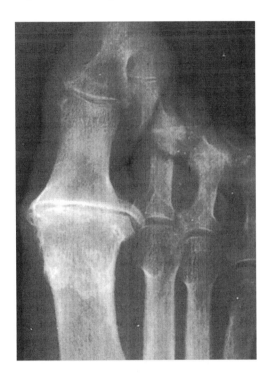

Fig. 13.16 Hallux rigidus. The posteroanterior view of the great toe metatarsophalangeal joint shows the marked cartilage loss, flattening of articular surfaces, and hypertrophic lipping that resulted in severe loss of motion. (From Weissman BNW, Sledge CB. *Orthopedic Radiology.* Philadelphia, PA: Saunders; 1986. Reprinted with permission)

Injuries of the Tendons of the Foot and Ankle

Tendinitis is a nonspecific term for a variety of pathological conditions of tendons. Tendinitis is the inflammatory process of the structures of the connective tissue structure surrounding a tendon. Tendinosis is intratendinous degeneration.

Management is often conservative with rest and immobilization with anti-inflammatory medications. Common disorders of tendons are those involving the peroneal tendon complex, the anterior tibial tendon, the Achilles tendon, the posterior tibial tendon, and the FHL tendon.

Peroneal Tendon Pathology

Peroneal tendon disorders include injury and degeneration of the peroneus brevis or longus and instability of the peroneal tendon complex. Peroneus brevis tendon injuries may manifest as tenosynovitis, a longitudinal split in the tendon, and sub-luxation or frank dislocation of the tendon. The patient may have a history of an inversion supination sprain. Radiographic studies are often normal. Indications for operative treatment are persistent pain and failure of conservative treatment with cast immobilization for 2–3 weeks and physical therapy. Goals of surgery are to reconstruct the superior peroneal retinaculum, perform a tenosynovectomy when applicable, and repair any longitudinal splits in the tendon.

Anterior Tibial Tendon Pathology

Injuries of the anterior tibial tendon are rare. Tenosynovitis may result from irritation by shoe wear, but is often attributed to an underlying rheumatic condition. Full rupture is due to wear associated from the superior border of the extensor retinaculum. Often when the tendon ruptures, proximal retraction results in a mass above the ankle joint, so called pseudotumor. Surgery is indicated for a young, active individual with an acute rupture. Neglect will result in a profound foot drop requiring an ankle–foot orthosis (AFO) long term.

Achilles Tendon Disorders

Disorders of the Achilles tendon include peritendinitis, tendinosis, partial and complete rupture, and insertional tendinitis with retrocalcaneal bursitis. Achilles tendinitis is painful inflammation and degeneration of either the surrounding peritenon (peritendinitis) or tendon (tendinosis) or both that occurs proximal to the insertion site of the Achilles in the calcaneus. This is often seen in runners with tight Achilles tendons and poor flexibility. Treatment is often conservative with a period of immobilization to allow inflammation to subside and followed by physical therapy and stretching of the Achilles tendons daily, except in advanced cases of tendinopathy. When conservative measures fail, debridement of the Achilles tendon can be done surgically where the tendon is approached medially, split longitudinally to debride, and repaired side to side. When tendinitis occurs at the Achilles tendon insertion onto the posterior aspect of the calcaneus, it is called "insertional Achilles tendinitis." Often, there is an enlarged posterior-superior calcaneal process called a

Haglund's deformity. This tendinitis is also associated with a retrocalcaneal bursitis which is inflammation of the bursa directly anterior to the Achilles tendon at its insertion. Conservative treatment includes a period of immobilization, heel lifts to shorten the Achilles tendon and take the pressure off the insertion, stretching exercises through physical therapy, and modification of shoe wear. When conservative measures fail, surgery consists of debridement of the insertion Achilles tendonopathy, and resection of the calcaneal posterior-superior tuberosity, in addition to reattachment of the Achilles tendon.

Ruptures of the Achilles tendon can be acute or chronic. They commonly occur in middle-aged men at the hypovascular zone of the Achilles tendon approximately 3–5 cm above the insertion site due to the "watershed" of proximal and distal blood supply. Ruptures occur because of forceful eccentric contraction of the elongating tendon. They rarely result from direct trauma. Symptoms include severe pain at the back of the calf. Patients often describe being hit in the back of the leg and an audible "pop." Palpating a defect above the Achilles insertion with the patient in a prone position confirms the diagnosis. Two findings are consistent with complete rupture of the tendon. The first is loss of passive resting tension in comparison to the opposite extremity which causes the foot to be at right angle to the remainder of the lower extremity. Normal tone with the tendon intact is approximately 25° of plantarflexion passive. The second finding is performing the Thompson test, which is done with the patient's foot hanging over the edge of the examination table in a prone position. The midcalf is squeezed. If the tendon is intact, the ankle passively plantar flexes. If the tendon is ruptured, no plantar flexion occurs. In difficult cases, MRI or ultrasound can confirm the diagnosis.

Treatment of an acute rupture of the Achilles tendon can be conservative or surgical. Nonoperative management includes immobilization in a plantar flexed position, non-weight bearing, for approximately 3 months. This should be reserved for elderly, less active patients with a medical history that makes surgery dangerous. Disadvantages of conservative management include a higher re-rupture rate and weaker push-off than that of surgical repair. Surgical repair includes direct repair of the ends of the Achilles tendon. Potential complications involve wound complications, infection, and sural nerve injury. Treatment of chronic neglected ruptures includes bracing with an ankle–foot orthosis or complex surgical reconstruction including flexor hallucis longus tendon transfer to fill the defect.

Posterior Tibial Tendon

Overuse of the posterior tibial tendon causes conditions that range from mild tendinitis to complete rupture and asymmetrical flatfoot deformity. Posterior tibial tendon dysfunction etiologies include trauma, inflammatory arthropathies, or nutritional degenerative conditions. Predisposing factors include hypertension, obesity, diabetes, steroid exposure, and prior surgery or trauma. Early stages include pain, swelling, and fullness localized to the posterior and medial hindfoot. As the tendon continues to deteriorate and becomes dysfunctional, a progressive asymmetrical flatfoot deformity develops with lateral hindfoot impingement and peroneal tendonitis. Clinical exam may show tenderness and swelling over the posterior medial hindfoot, a secondary Achilles tendon contracture, and weakness with resistive plantar flexion and inversion. Patients are unable to perform a single stance heel rise and often show a "too-many-toes sign" when visualizing the foot from behind in a standing position. Too-many-toes sign refers to an advanced collapse of the arch with the heel in significant valgus. The toes are abducted more on the affected foot than the unaffected foot and show more prominently on exam. Weight bearing X-rays may show uncovering or "sag" of the talar head by the navicular on both AP and lateral views; the normal angle is close to zero. The forefoot and midfoot are abducted in relation to the hindfoot. MRI can confirm tenosynovitis versus tendinosis. Treatment options are determined by the stage of dysfunction and presentation. Stage I, which is very mild tendon weakness without flatfoot deformity, can be addressed with orthotics, anti-inflammatory medicines, and physical therapy. A period of cast immobilization is needed to allow a decrease in inflammation. Stage II, which involves posterior tibial tendon disruption and the presence of a flexible flatfoot deformity, can be treated conservatively with orthotics or surgically, which involves repair of the posterior tibial tendon. In advanced cases, reconstruction is accomplished by using the adjacent flexor digitorum longus tendon as a transfer. Alone, tendon repair or reconstruction will yield a 50% failure within 2 years post-reconstruction unless a bone procedure is added. Options include either medial displacement calcaneal osteotomy or lateral column lengthening at the anterior one-third calcaneus. Stage III, which involves a rigid foot or with advanced arthritis, can be treated conservatively with orthotics or surgically with the appropriate joint fusions. Typically, a triple arthrodesis involving fusions of the subtalar, talonavicular, and calcaneo-cuboid joints is recommended.

Heel Pain

Plantar heel pain is one of the most common and most disabling conditions of the foot. There are many causes including tumors, infection, stress fractures, inflammatory arthropathies, and neuropathies. The most common cause of plantar heel pain is associated with chronic injury of the plantar fascial origin. This heel pain syndrome is also known as heel spur syndrome and plantar fasciitis. Typical pain occurs at the plantar medial aspect of the heel. Onset is insidious and often patients recall no trauma. Classic pain and stiffness occurs when arising from bed and taking the first step on the floor in the morning. Symptoms often decrease after prolonged walking. High-heeled shoes typically alleviate symptoms, whereas barefoot walking and wearing flat shoes may increase symptoms. Physical examination shows point tenderness on the plantar medial heel. Often, there is a tight Achilles tendon complex with limited ankle dorsiflexion. Occasionally, fat pad or heel pad atrophy is present. Radiographs include a lateral X-ray which may show a plantar heel spur

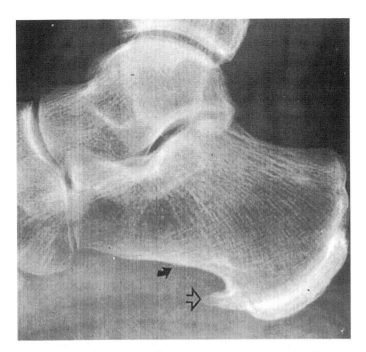

Fig. 13.17 Calcaneal spurs. The normal plantar spur (*open arrow*) has smooth margins, no sclerosis or erosion, and no adjacent soft tissue swelling. Very small spurs are present at the insertions of the long plantar ligament (*arrow*) and the Achilles tendon. (From Weissman BNW, Sledge CB. *Orthopedic Radiology*. Philadelphia, PA: Saunders; 1986. Reprinted with permission)

(Fig. 13.17). This is often associated with a flexor digitorum brevis origin and can signify a chronic condition. It is important to rule out a calcaneal stress fracture and tumor via X-rays. Treatment is almost always conservative consisting of rest, anti-inflammatory medication, orthotic devices, and aggressive stretching. Isolated stretching of the gastroc-soleus complex and plantar fascia is important. Surgery is typically reserved for chronic conditions that have lasted over 6 months to a year and involves partial release of the plantar fascial origin in addition to tarsal tunnel decompression.

Arthritic Conditions of the Foot and Ankle

Causes of ankle joint degeneration include primary osteoarthritis, posttraumatic arthritis, avascular necrosis, osteochondritis dissecans, synovial chondromatosis, and rheumatologic conditions. Conservative management includes anti-inflammatory medications, bracing, and intraarticular cortisone injections. Surgical management is dependent on the extent and location of the arthrosis. Options are split between reconstruction and salvage. For early to intermediate stage or focal involvement, options include joint debridement either arthroscopically or open, low tibial osteotomy, osteochondral auto or allograft replacement, and distraction arthroplasty. Salvage procedures include ankle arthrodesis (fusion) or a total ankle replacement. While the main advantage with fusion is permanency, the downside is that stress transference into adjacent joints leading to osteoarthritis can occur. Ankle replacement avoids this problem by maintaining ankle motion; however, longevity of the implant may require revision surgery over a lifetime.

Rheumatoid Arthritis

Rheumatoid arthritis is a systemic disease that commonly involves the foot as there are many joints lined with synovium (Fig. 13.18). It affects both the synovial lining of the joint and the surrounding tendons. Physical examination shows an antalgic gait, generalized swelling, and decreased motion in the joints of the foot. Weight bearing radiographs of the foot and ankle are essential for showing deformity and often show a valgus angulation of either the ankle or subtalar joint.

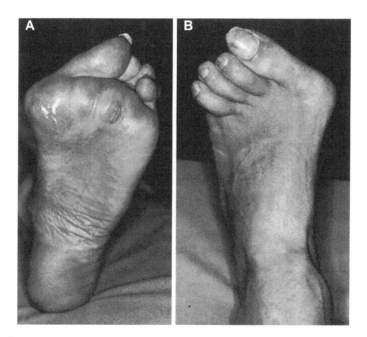

Fig. 13.18 Plantar (**a**) and dorsal (**b**) views of the foot of a patient with rheumatoid arthritis with characteristic dislocation of all toes, which tend to drift off into marked hallux valgus with dorsal displacement of the phalanges onto the metacarpals. The metacarpal heads become very prominent in the sole of the foot, and large, painful callosities are common. (From Bogumill GP. *Orthopaedic Pathology: A Synopsis with Clinical and Radiographic Correlation*. Philadelphia, PA: Saunders; 1984. Reprinted with permission)

Treatment options include conservative management such as patient education, activity modification, intermittent steroid injections, optimizing medical management, shoe modifications, and the use of an ankle–foot orthosis. Surgical options include simple synovectomy, arthrodesis, and total ankle arthroplasty.

Infections

Both the bones and joints of the foot can be involved in musculoskeletal septic processes such as osteomyelitis and septic arthritis.

Puncture Wounds

Puncture wounds in the foot can be caused by many objects including glass, nail, and plant and animal parts. Typically, the puncture occurs through the sole of the sneaker and enters the foot (Fig. 13.19). Since the insole of a sneaker can be colonized with the *Pseudomonas* organism, care should be taken to treat the patient with an infection from a puncture wound for this organism. Patients frequently present late with a swollen cellulitic foot. A complete blood count (CBC) and sedimentation rate can occasionally be abnormal. Standard radiographs and a bone scan can

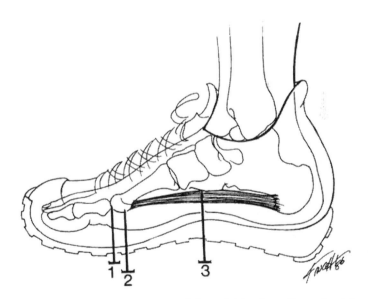

Fig. 13.19 Puncture injury sites: 1, metatarsophalangeal joint; 2, cartilage of metatarsal head; 3, plantar fascia. (From Clinton JE. Puncture wounds by inanimate objects. In: Gustilo RB, Gruninger RP, Tsukayama DT, eds. *Orthopaedic Infection: Diagnosis and Treatment*. Philadelphia, PA: Saunders; 1989. Reprinted with permission)

confirm the diagnosis. When bone or joint involvement is extensive, aggressive surgical debridement is mandatory for satisfactory resolution. Appropriate antibiotic coverage is required until the infection has resolved.

Paronychia

A paronychia is an infection of the medial or lateral nail fold, often seen in the great toe (Fig. 13.20). Paronychiae are often seen in an abnormally growing nail, which penetrates the skin of the lateral nail fold, introducing bacteria.

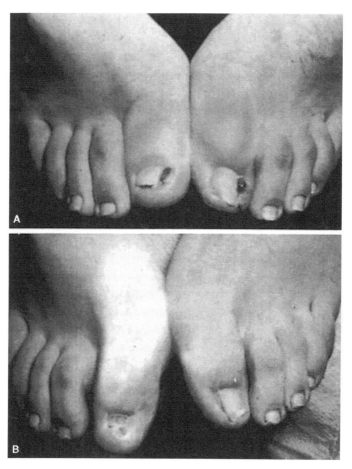

Fig. 13.20 (**a**) Bilateral infected ingrowing of both edges of the big toenails. The toenail of the right big toe was practically completely separated from its bed and was avulsed. The operation, which was performed under a local anesthetic, consisted of bilateral resection of all onychogenic tissue in the longitudinal grooves. (**b**) Sixteen months after surgery. (From Lapidus PW. The toenails. In: Jahss M, ed. *Disorders of the Foot*, Vol I. Philadelphia, PA: Saunders; 1982. Reprinted with permission)

A soft tissue abscess forms and a paronychia develops. Decompression of the abscess is done under local anesthesia and removing the lateral portion of the nail often allows temporary relief. With more chronic paronychial infections, more aggressive nail procedures including either partial or total nail ablation may be required.

Diabetic Foot Infections

People with diabetes can develop a sensory neuropathy which prevents them from protective sensation. Because of abnormal pressures unremitting for 20 min or more, ulcerations which allow bacterial inoculation and infection to develop may result. Typical scenarios in which this can happen is after a pedicure or from the abrasions of a poorly fitting shoe (Figs. 13.21 and 13.22). With abscesses and ulcers, both acute and chronic septic arthritis and osteomyelitis are frequently the end result. Charcot arthropathy, a noninfectious degradation of joints, may coincide, making diagnosis difficult with that of osteomyelitis. Aggressive treatment of any infection in the diabetic foot is mandatory for salvage. Medical management of the diabetes is crucial and the patient must be under strict diabetic control. Intravenous antibiotics are almost always necessary in the acute scenario. Antibiotics are often broad spectrum due to the polymicrobial nature of these infections.

Tumors

A complete discussion of soft tissue and bone tumors is beyond the scope of this chapter; however, a few specific lesions are mentioned here.

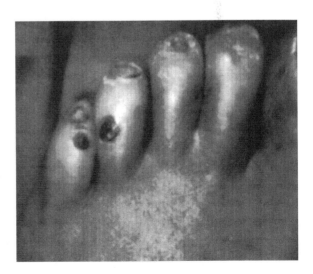

Fig. 13.21 This diabetic patient had recently obtained new shoes. The two small, dorsal ulcers were exquisitely painful. Note the blanching of the toes distal to the ulcers. (From Harrelson JM. Management of the diabetic foot. *Orthop Clin North Am.* 1989;20(4):606. Reprinted with permission)

Fig. 13.22 One day of new shoe wear produced the ulcers seen over the fifth metatarsal head and lateral sides of the fourth and fifth toes. (From Harrelson JM. Management of the diabetic foot. *Orthop Clin North Am.* 1989;20(4):606. Reprinted with permission)

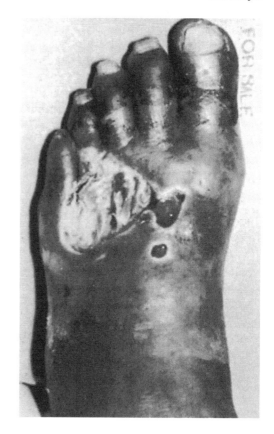

Soft Tissue Lesions

The anterolateral ankle is the common site for the development of a ganglion cyst as well as soft tissue lipomas. These are both benign lesions and excision can be performed if symptoms warrant. Thickening of the plantar fascia on the plantar surface of the foot can be palpated on some patients. Sometimes these thickenings are large, firm nodules known as plantar fibromas. They are benign and should be treated conservatively at all costs.

Bone Tumors

Common bone tumors include enchondroma, a benign cartilage tumor that can occur in the short tubular bones such as the phalanges. The chondromyxoid fibroma (Fig. 13.23) is another benign cartilage tumor that can affect the bones of the foot. It is usually managed by curettage of the lesion. Occasionally, a bone cyst can form in the calcaneus. Pathologic fracture through this can occur and may, in fact, be the chief complaint at a patient's presentation. Treatment usually requires curettage and

Fig. 13.23 Chondromyxoid fibroma. This lesion has a tendency for localization in small bones of the hands and feet. A sharply circumscribed defect in the proximal phalanx of the great toe is shown here. (From Bogumill GP. *Orthopaedic Pathology: A Synopsis with Clinical and Radiographic Correlation.* Philadelphia, PA: Saunders; 1984. Reprinted with permission)

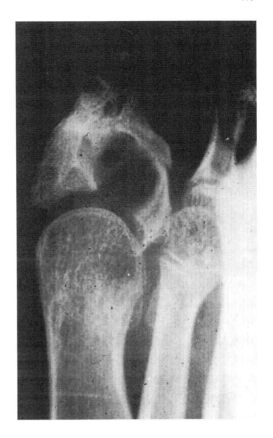

bone grafting. It is uncommon to have metastatic disease to the small bones of the foot. When seen, one should suspect the lung as the primary site of the patient's disease.

Complex Regional Pain Syndrome

This disabling disorder of unknown pathophysiology has a variable symptom complex with many hypothesized causes and mechanisms. Renamed from the limited descriptive term reflex sympathetic dystrophy, complex regional pain syndrome (CRPS) is more common in women than men, and more common in adults than children. It can occur after a minor injury with no nerve involvement, or after a significant injury with nerve involvement. Patients present with disproportionate extremity pain, swelling, autonomic symptoms (i.e., changes in sweating, skin discoloration), and motor symptoms (i.e., weakness). Diagnosis of any obvious, treatable causes of pain should be done prior to definitively selecting CRPS as the diagnosis. Treatment involves extensive therapy and pain relief with desensitization through medication or nerve blockade.

Summary and Conclusions

Numerous conditions affect the foot and ankle, and foot pain remains a very common presenting complaint. A knowledge of anatomy and common foot and ankle problems can provide the diagnostician adequate tools to treat patients. The last figures in this chapter provide algorithms that can assist in the diagnosis and treatment of foot and ankle pain. Figure 13.24 can assist in the diagnosis and treatment of patients with foot and ankle complaints resulting from an acute injury. Figure 13.25 provides steps to evaluate and treat patients that have foot and ankle pain without a history of an acute injury, but with radiographic evidence of deformity or pathology. Figure 13.26 should provide some structure to the diagnosis and treatment of

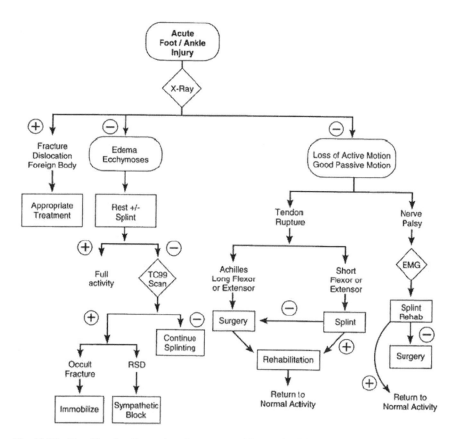

Fig. 13.24 Algorithm for diagnosis and treatment of foot and ankle pain with acute injury

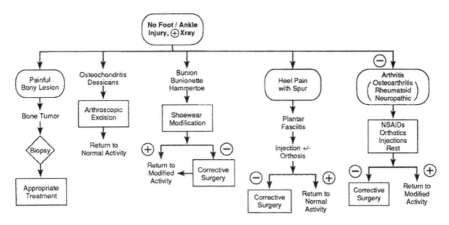

Fig. 13.25 Algorithm for diagnosis and treatment of foot and ankle pain with no injury and positive radiograph

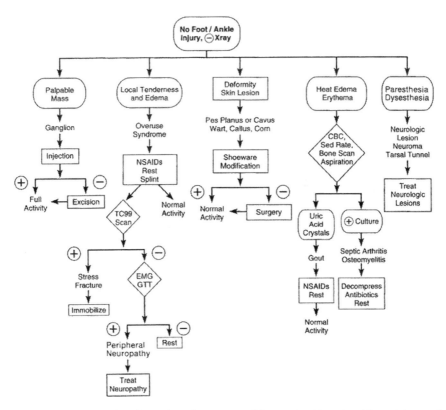

Fig. 13.26 Algorithm for diagnosis and treatment of foot and ankle pain with no injury and negative radiograph

patients with foot and ankle complaints without injury and no radiographic evidence of deformity or pathology. These are not comprehensive algorithms, but should provide some guidance when encountering patients with foot and ankle complaints.

Suggested Reading

1. Cooper PS. The foot and ankle. In: Wiesel SW, Delahay JN, eds. *Principles of Orthopaedic Medicine and Surgery.* Philadelphia, PA: WB Saunders; 2001:767–830.
2. Mann R, Coughlin M, eds. *Surgery of the Foot and Ankle.* 6th ed. Philadelphia, PA: Mosby; 1993.
3. Myerson M, ed. *Foot and Ankle Disorders.* Philadelphia, PA: WB Saunders; 2000.

Glossary

Abscess: a collection of purulent material which usually consists of bacteria, both alive and dead, and the by-products of local infection including viable and nonviable neutrophils, lymphocytes, and lysosomal enzymes. The presence of neutrophils within an abscess often results in a localized inflammatory reaction which can become systemic and life threatening if allowed to persist.

Acute osteomyelitis: bacterial colonization of bone or bone marrow with signs of acute inflammation and periostitis. Radiographic changes are usually present within the first 6 weeks.

Adjuvant therapy: therapy which is administered to assist in the treatment of a neoplasm. Adjuvant therapy can include radiation therapy or chemotherapy and usually is utilized to improve the results of a primary type of treatment (i.e., surgery).

Allograft: tissue for transplantation which is acquired from donated cadaveric sources. Musculoskeletal allografts are generally processed by either deep freezing or dehydration utilizing freeze-drying techniques. Sterilization is generally performed with either gamma radiation, aseptic acquisition in an operating room setting, or treatment with ethylene oxide.

Ankylosis: spontaneous bony fusion of a joint.

Antalgic gait: a type of limp characterized by shortening the stance phase of gait, in an attempt to relieve pain on weight-bearing.

Aponeurosis: a broad, flat tendon for common muscle insertion.

Apophysis: secondary ossification center which develops in response to tension and ultimately forms a process for muscular attachment.

Arthrodesis: fusion performed surgically between two articulating bones by removal of the joint cartilage, removal of cortical bone, bone grafting, and immobilization.

Arthrofibrosis: restricted joint motion due to formation of dense scar tissue around the articulation (contracture).

Arthroplasty: an operation to improve function and relieve pain caused by arthritis in a peripheral joint. Joint resection or replacement and interposition between joint surfaces are forms of arthroplasty.

S.W. Wiesel, J.N. Delahay (eds.), *Essentials of Orthopedic Surgery*,
DOI 10.1007/978-1-4419-1389-0, © Springer Science+Business Media, LLC 2010

Arthroscopy: a procedure to inspect, and operate on, the contents of a joint through a small portal utilizing a fiber-optic light source and specialized viewing and operative instruments.

Avascular necrosis: a pathologic condition in which the blood supply to the subchondral region of a joint is disrupted, leading to pain and possible collapse of the surface; commonly seen in the hip, knee, and shoulder.

Benign: a neoplasm which has local capability for growth, with well-differentiated cells that are not capable of vascular or lymphatic invasion. Benign neoplasms can be either latent, with limited local growth, or aggressive, with growth proceeding in a destructive manner.

Biopsy: the acquisition of material from a lesion, whether it be neoplastic or infectious, for diagnostic review. An adequate biopsy requires obtaining enough material for complete pathological review to arrive at a definitive diagnosis.

Bone cement: polymethylmethacrylate (PMMA), used as a filler to enhance the fixation of total joint components.

Bone graft: bone used to promote fracture healing, reconstruct a defect in bone, or enhance fusion by providing an organic matrix, osteoblasts, and hormonal factors that contribute to osteogenesis.

Bursa: a mesothelial-lined sac containing fluid located between tendon and bone to decrease friction.

Calcification: the deposition of calcium within a cartilaginous matrix. This occurs secondary to mineralization of an existing lobule of cartilage which may appear punctate, comma shaped, or popcorn-like on radiographs.

Callus: reparative tissue at the site of a fracture that evolves and matures, leading to fracture healing.

Cancellous bone: mature bone found in the epiphysis and metaphysis of long bones, and in flat bones, comprised of a three-dimensional lattice of trabecular bone that is less densely packed than cortical bone.

Chondrocyte: cartilage matrix-producing cells which rely on nutrition from synovial fluid and not blood vessels. These cells are often arranged in lacunae which are arranged in rather distinct layers.

Chondrolysis: disappearance of articular cartilage as a result of disintegration or dissolution of cartilage matrix and cells.

Chronic osteomyelitis: a chronic infection of bone, usually involving the presence of an involucrum or sequestrum, in addition to radiographic changes within the bone. Sclerosis surrounding chronic sites of radiolucency on radiographs and a sinus tract may be present. Chronic osteomyelitis generally requires at least 6 weeks in order to demonstrate radiographic changes.

Codman's triangle: a region at the periphery of a bone tumor which is formed secondary to the deposition of reactive bone underneath the periosteum. As the periosteum lays down new bone in response to stress, the bony trabecular patterns in this region are usually at a right angle to the underlying cortical bone. A Codman's triangle usually represents a rapidly growing tumor or osteomyelitis, with elevation of the periosteum off of the bone secondary to neoplastic tissue, bone edema, or purulent material.

Comminution: disruption of a fractured bone into more than two fragments.

Compartment syndrome: an increase in the resting pressure in a contained fibro-osseous compartment, such as the forearm or leg, resulting sequentially in decreased lymphatic drainage, decreased venous drainage, loss of arterial inflow, and finally death to the muscle contained in the affected compartment. Sequelae include contracture, pain, and severe functional disability.

Computerized axial tomography/computerized tomography (CAT/CT scan): an imaging modality which utilizes computer-generated analysis and imaging resulting from multi-planar exposure through either an extremity or the spine. These scans provide clinicians with excellent axial representation of body segments that were previously not available. Tissue density is graded based on Hounsfield units with dense structures being represented by a bright or white image.

Contracture: fixed loss of motion in one direction caused by hypertrophy and shortening of periarticular soft-tissue structures such as tendon, ligament, or capsule.

Cortical bone: mature, organized, densely packed bone, making up the periphery of flat bones and the diaphysis of long bones.

C reactive protein (CRP):   a plasma protein that rises in the blood with the inflammation from certain conditions. An acute phase reactant.

Crepitus: audible or palpable grinding, usually located in a peripheral joint, with motion.

Curettage: the mechanical removal of neoplastic or infectious tissue from a primary site. This generally involves entering a lesion and scraping its contents from within its lesional cavity and has the potential for leaving residual disease, at the microscopic level, in the periphery. This type of "intralesional resection" is generally utilized for benign neoplasms.

Cyst: a fluid-filled cavity which results from the production of fluid from a surrounding glandular membrane. The majority of cysts in orthopedic terminology, such as a simple bone cyst or aneurysmal bone cyst, are not true cysts, since the fluid does not directly result from the surrounding mesenchymal tissue present in the wall lining, but from the passive accumulation of fluid within the marrow cavity of bone.

Debridement: the removal of infected or devitalized bone, muscle, and skin. The purpose of debridement is to remove any material that can serve as a substrate which harbors bacteria and to enable antibiotics, via parental or local routes, to reach colonies of bacteria.

Delayed union: failure of a fracture to heal within the desired and expected time frame, with the potential still present for eventual union.

Developmental: pertaining to growth and differentiation.

Diarthrodial joint: a joint which consists of connections between two rigid parts of the musculoskeletal system which is lined by synovial tissue, lubricated by synovial fluid, and demonstrates appreciable ranges of motion. The ends of bones in diarthrodial joints are usually covered with hyaline cartilage.

Diaphysis: the tubular midportion of a long bone, consisting primarily of cortical bone.

Dislocation: loss of normal articular congruity of a joint, with no contact between opposing articular surfaces.

Dysostosis: an isolated disruption of normal bone growth with no identifiable etiology.

Dysplasia: intrinsic defect in normal bone growth, which may be localized or generalized.

Dystrophy: alteration in bone growth due to extrinsic defect, typically an endocrine abnormality.

Electromyography (EMG):   recording of the variations of electric potential or voltage from skeletal muscle. The EMG/nerve conduction velocity test is useful in determining the site of injury of a peripheral nerve or nerve root and in identifying peripheral neuropathy caused by metabolic abnormalities.

Enchondral ossification: bone formation following the template of a cartilaginous matrix.

Enchondroma: a benign tumor of bone, with a cartilaginous matrix, commonly occurring in the hand.

Epiphysis: a secondary ossification center, adjacent to the physis, which develops in response to compression and is covered by articular cartilage.

External fixation: the use of an extracorporeal device to stabilize a part of the skeleton, usually following an open fracture.

Fracture: a cortical disruption, ranging from incomplete and non-displaced to completely displaced.

Fracture healing: the process of biologic repair of a fracture in response to hormonal, biochemical, and mechanical factors. Fracture healing encompasses the phases of inflammation, soft callus, hard callus, and remodeling.

Free tissue transfer: one-stage transplantation of distant autogenous composite tissue from a donor site to a recipient site. Free tissue transfer can involve transplantation of muscle, fasciocutaneous tissue, or bone with or without attached soft tissue. This type of transfer requires immediate revascularization, utilizing microsurgical anastomosis of graft and recipient site arteries and veins.

Frozen section: the preparation of pathological sections from fresh tissue, used primarily in the operating room for rapid diagnosis which may impact on surgical decision making.

Ganglion: a soft, mucin-filled cyst arising from a tendon, tendon sheath, or joint capsule. Most common about the hand and wrist, and more common in women.

Gigantism (overgrowth):   hypertrophy of a single digit or entire limb, primarily involving soft tissues. Causes include neurofibromatosis, tumor, or vascular anomaly.

Haversian bone: cortical bone composed of vascular channels surrounded by mature (lamellar) bone.

Herniated nucleus pulposus (HNP):   Extrusion of gelatinous nucleus pulposus through the annulus fibrosus into the spinal canal or neural foramen. When an

HNP results in nerve root compression, radicular pain, numbness, or weakness may be seen. Herniated disc, ruptured disc.

Hydroxyapatite: the calcium mineral crystal component of bone.

Internal fixation: the use of an implant to stabilize the skeleton, usually after a fracture.

Involucrum: newly formed reactive bone, usually occurring at the interface between diseased bone and healthy tissue. An involucrum consists of viable bone which is the opposite of a sequestrum, which is composed of dead bone.

Joint reaction force: the force across a joint that results from a combination of weight-bearing and muscular contraction.

Kyphosis: forward bending of the spine, when viewed from the side, which is normal in the thoracic spine.

Laminectomy: removal of a lamina from its superior to its inferior margin, performed as surgical treatment for spinal stenosis or HNP. Laminotomy or hemilaminectomy refer to partial removal of the lamina.

Limbus: the hypertrophic fibrocartilagenous margin of the acetabular labrum seen in patients with developmental dysplasia of the hip.

Lordosis: backward bending, or "sway," of the spine when viewed from the side. Lordosis is normal in the neck and low back.

Low back strain: nonspecific term referring to acute onset of pain in the low back, occasionally radiating into the buttocks, with associated muscle spasm. Low back sprain, lumbago.

Magnetic resonance imaging (MRI): an imaging modality utilizing resonance phenomenon resulting in the absorption and/or emission of electromagnetic energy by nuclei or electrons in a static magnetic field. Magnetic resonance imaging requires unpaired electrons that are excited by exposure to a magnetic field with a particular signal being emitted once that field is removed. Differences in density of tissues are then represented on images as varying shades of gray, black, or white, depending on their concentration of hydrogen. The modality is extremely useful in the evaluation of musculoskeletal tumors, as well as disorders of the spine, knee, shoulder, and foot.

Malignancy: a neoplasm consisting of undifferentiated or dedifferentiated cells which have the active capability of vessel invasion, transport, and establishment of a secondary site of neoplastic growth in a distant organ.

Malunion: healing of a fracture in a nonanatomic position.

Membranous bone formation: bone formation occurring directly from a fibrous, mesenchymal, connective tissue template.

Metaphysis: the transition segment of a long bone from the enlarged end (epiphysis) to the tubular shaft (diaphysis). The funnel-shaped metaphysis is usually made up of abundant cancellous bone and, during growth, woven bone.

Metastasis: the deposition to secondary sites of neoplastic cells from a primary neoplasm.

Minimally invasive surgery: a technique used in total joint replacement and trauma surgery designed to minimize tissue dissection and disruption, with the goal of less pain and better short-term healing.

Myelopathy: noninflammatory dysfunction of the spinal cord resulting in long tract signs and symptoms, most commonly caused by mechanical compression in the cervical spine.

Neoadjuvant therapy: the application of adjuvant treatment, usually chemotherapy or radiation, prior to a primary procedure in an attempt to facilitate surgical removal of the primary tumor.

Neuroma: a nodule, frequently painful, developing in a nerve that has been partially or completely lacerated or traumatized.

Nonunion: failure of a fracture to heal within the upper range of time expected, with sequential radiographic documentation of a lack of any progression toward healing.

Nonsteroidal anti-inflammatory drugs (NSAIDs): these agents are in widespread use to treat arthritis as well as a variety of soft-tissue injuries and for pain relief. Gastrointestinal side effects are common.

Open fracture: a fracture which has come into contact with the outside, extracorporeal environment. Implications primarily relate to an increased risk of infection and impaired fracture healing secondary to soft-tissue injury.

Ossification: the deposition of mineral along osteoid matrix, produced by either normal (fracture healing) or malignant osteoblasts (osteosarcoma).

Osteoarthritis: noninflammatory degeneration of a diarthrodial joint characterized by loss of articular cartilage, effusion, crepitus, deformity, and pain. Radiographic changes include loss of joint space, subchondral sclerosis, cyst formation, and periarticular osteophytes.

Osteoblast: a type of differentiated mesenchymal cell that is essential for the process of osteogenesis or ossification. Osteoblasts alone can produce the organic intercellular substance or matrix which makes up bone tissue, called osteoid.

Osteoclasis: to manually fracture a bone, usually to correct malposition.

Osteoclast: bone resorbing cell.

Osteoconduction: a passive process by which bone grows on a surface. A physical, three-dimensional scaffold or matrix to facilitate bone repair.

Osteoinduction: an active process. A biologic response where chemical signals initiate bone formation.

Osteocyte: histologically and possibly biochemically inert osteoblast, usually present in bone which is not undergoing any active remodeling or repair.

Osteoid: organic component of bone.

Osteolysis: abnormal bone resorption seen on radiographs, often around a total joint prosthesis due to poly wear or infection.

Osteomalacia: metabolic disorder of bone characterized by inadequate mineralization of normal osteoid. Less common than osteoporosis, causes include Ca^{2+} deficiency and renal disease.

Osteomyelitis: infection involving bone (see acute and chronic osteomyelitis).

Osteoporosis: pathologic condition of bone characterized by a decrease in bone matrix with normal mineralization of the matrix that is present. Causes include postmenopausal estrogen deficiency, steroid usage, immobilization, and bed rest. Fractures of the spine, hip, wrist, and shoulder are common.

Osteotomy: surgical cutting and realignment of bone to change the mechanical environment of adjacent joints, posture, or appearance.

Pannus: hyperplastic, hypertrophic synovium seen in the inflammatory arthritides. Source of degradative enzymes.

Paresthesia: a "pins and needles" or "tingling" sensation in an extremity, typically along the distribution of a peripheral nerve or nerve root.

Pathologic fracture: a fracture occurring in bone that is of abnormal quality, from metabolic changes (e.g., osteoporosis), tumor, or infection.

Periosteum: thick fibrous tissue covering of a bone.

Physis (epiphyseal plate, growth plate): a highly specialized cartilaginous structure, at each end of long bones, through which longitudinal growth of the bone occurs. The physis regresses and closes at the end of active skeletal growth.

Polydactyly: the presence of an extra digit, either partial or complete. Most common in the hand, polydactyly may occur on either the ulnar or the radial side.

Press-fit technique: used to secure orthopedic implants, commonly total joint prostheses, where the bone is under-reamed compared to the implant, creating a tight initial fit of the component.

Prosthesis: a mechanical replacement for a removed portion of either bone or soft tissue. Prostheses include endoprostheses, which are internal replacements (joints, valves, etc.), and exoprostheses as would be used following an amputation.

Radial club hand: congenital absence of all or part of the radius, resulting in a near-normal hand attached to, but radially deviated on, the forearm.

Radicular pain: pain traveling down the extremity in a dermatomal distribution, often associated with paresthesia. Pain should typically extend distal to the elbow or knee to be considered radicular.

Radiculopathy: noninflammatory dysfunction of a spinal nerve with abnormal neurologic findings, most commonly secondary to a herniated nucleus pulposus or spinal stenosis.

Referred pain: sclerotomal pain in a region that shares a common embryologic origin with the diseased region, such as the trapezius and shoulders for cervical disc pathology or the buttocks and posterior thighs for the lumbar spine.

Remodeling: continuous process whereby older bone is removed and replaced with new bone, usually in response to mechanical stresses.

Rheumatoid arthritis: inflammatory arthritis characterized by morning stiffness, swelling of peripheral joints, subcutaneous nodules, pain, and deformity.

Rheumatoid factor: a blood marker that is usually, but not always, present in patients with rheumatoid arthritis. Some patients who do not have rheumatoid arthritis may have a positive rheumatoid factor.

Rotation tissue transfer: soft tissue, such as muscle, or bone which is transplanted for wound coverage from one local site to another without transecting the blood supply to the transplanted tissue.

Scintigraphy: a sensitive but nonspecific imaging modality for the diagnosis and staging of various orthopedic problems. The standard "bone scan" utilizes technetium 99m, a gamma-emitting radioisotope with a half-life of 6 h, coupled with methylene diphosphonate, a bone-seeking mineral material. Positive bone scans usually demonstrate increased uptake in areas of bony repair or destruction caused by neoplasm, fracture, infection, inflammation, or arthritis.

Sclerosis: a rim of host bone reaction around the periphery of a lesion, or in an area of degeneration, which appears white (radiopaque) on radiographs.

Scoliosis: coronal plane curvature, typically associated with rotation, leading to asymmetric rib or flank prominence. Common etiologies are idiopathic, neuromuscular, and congenital.

Segmental instability: abnormal motion pattern between adjacent vertebrae resulting in excessive motion under physiologic loads and causing, in some individuals, characteristic mechanical back or neck pain.

Septic arthritis: the presence of bacteria or their by-products within a diarthrodial joint.

Sequestrum: a microscopic or macroscopic island of necrotic bone found at the nidus of an infection within viable bone. Often, sequestered fragments are surrounded by purulent material and infected granulation tissue and occur secondary to devitalization of cortical bone.

Sourcil: from the French for "eyebrow"and refers to the thickened subchondral bone of the acetabulum.

Spinal fusion: arthrodesis of two or more adjacent vertebrae for painful or unstable conditions of the spine including spinal deformity, trauma, or degenerative segmental instability. Bone graft or bone-graft substitute is utilized and internal fixation may be used. Fusion may be performed anteriorly (interbody) or posterolaterally (intertransverse).

Spinal stenosis: narrowing of the spinal canal or neural foramen resulting in compression of the cord or nerve roots. Causes include congenital narrowing, degenerative changes, and spondylolisthesis.

Spondylolysis: defect of the pars interarticularis, most commonly a stress fracture that occurs during childhood; may be associated with back pain and lead to spondylolisthesis.

Spondylolisthesis: the forward slippage of a vertebrae on the one below it (most commonly L5 on S1). The most common types are isthmic (secondary to spondylolysis), degenerative (caused by degenerative instability of the disc and facet joints), or postsurgical.

Sprain: partial or complete injury to ligament resulting from excessive stretching.

Straight-leg raising (SLR) test: with the patient supine or seated, simultaneous hip flexion and knee extension places the sciatic nerve on stretch. Reproduction of ipsilateral sciatica (not back pain) constitutes a positive SLR sign.

Subluxation: partial dislocation of a joint, with some retained contact of the articular surfaces.

Syndactyly: webbing of the fingers, usually resulting from congenital failure of formation and commonly seen with other congenital abnormalities.

Synostosis: congenital fusion, either partial or complete, of adjacent bones. Synostosis is far more common in the upper than in the lower extremity and may involve the elbow, carpus, metacarpals, or phalanges.

Synovectomy: removal of the synovium (lining surface of a diarthrodial joint), for inflammatory conditions such as rheumatoid arthritis or infection.

Synovial membrane: a soft glandular tissue which lines diarthrodial joints and produces synovial fluid. The synovial membrane has a rich capillary network and serves both in phagocytosis of foreign debris and the production of synovial fluid.

Tension sign: a physical finding produced by placing the involved nerve root on stretch to assess for mechanical compression. A positive tension sign requires reproduction of pain, in a dermatomal distribution, down the extremity.

Trendelenburg gait: a type of limp, caused by ineffective hip abduction, marked by swaying the torso over the effected hip on weight-bearing.

Trendelenburg sign: an abnormal drooping of the pelvis, on single-leg stance, away from the effected side due to ineffective hip abduction secondary to neurologic or mechanical factors, or pain.

Two-stage explantation: a technique used to treat an infected total joint arthroplasty where the prosthesis is removed in stage one, an antibiotic-loaded spacer made of cement is placed in the joint, intra-venous antibiotics are administered until the infection is cured, followed by a second stage re-implantation of a new total joint

Ulnar club hand: congenital absence of all or part of the ulna, resulting in a near-normal hand attached to, but ulnarly deviated on, the forearm.

Valgus: malalignment of an extremity, in the coronal plane, with the apex of the deformity pointing to the midline ("knock-knees").

Varus: malalignment of an extremity, in the coronal plane, with the apex of the deformity pointing away from the midline ("bow-legs").

Volar: the palmar surface of the hand and forearm.

Wolff's Law: physiologic phenomenon whereby new bone forms in response to mechanical stress and resorbs in the absence of it ("form follows function").

Woven bone: immature bone found in the embryo and newborns, fracture callus, tumors, and osteogenesis imperfecta or Paget's disease.

Zone of transition: the boundary between what is perceived as normal bone and lesional tissue on radiographs. The zone of transition can be very sharply defined, indicative of a slow-growing process (benign tumor), or very poorly defined, indicative of an aggressive process (neoplasm or infection).

Index

Printed by Publishers' Graphics LLC

Printed by Publishers' Graphics LLC